Stroke and Atrial Fibrillation: An Integrated Study

Stroke and Atrial Fibrillation: An Integrated Study

Editor: Neta Allison

AMERICAN
MEDICAL PUBLISHERS
www.americanmedicalpublishers.com

AMERICAN
MEDICAL PUBLISHERS
www.americanmedicalpublishers.com

Cataloging-in-Publication Data

Stroke and atrial fibrillation : an integrated study / edited by Neta Allison.
p. cm.
Includes bibliographical references and index.
ISBN 978-1-63927-811-4
1. Cerebrovascular disease. 2. Atrial fibrillation. 3. Brain--Diseases.
4. Neglect (Neurology). I. Allison, Neta.
RC388.5 .S87 2023
616.81--dc23

American Medical Publishers,
41 Flatbush Avenue,
1st Floor, New York,
NY 11217, USA

ISBN 978-1-63927-811-4 (Hardback)

Contents

Preface

The world is advancing at a fast pace like never before. Therefore, the need is to keep up with the latest developments. This book was an idea that came to fruition when the specialists in the area realized the need to coordinate together and document essential themes in the subject. That's when I was requested to be the editor. Editing this book has been an honour as it brings together diverse authors researching on different streams of the field. The book collates essential materials contributed by veterans in the area which can be utilized by students and researchers alike.

Atrial fibrillation (A-fib) refers to a condition of an abnormal heart rhythm characterized by rapid and irregular beating of the atrial chambers of the heart. In this condition, heart's upper chamber shakes and quivers and does not squeeze and contract as it should. A-fib increases the risk of heart failure, stroke and other heart-related problems. Patients with A-fib are more likely to develop dementia and the occurrence of both conditions increases with age. A stroke is a life-threatening medical disorder, which occurs when the blood supply to a portion of the brain is cut off. It is a medical emergency that requires immediate treatment. In a situation, where a blood clot escapes from left atrial appendage and reaches the other part of the body, it can cut off the blood supply of the brain which causes a stroke. This book provides comprehensive insights into stroke, dementia and atrial fibrillation. It presents researches and studies performed by experts across the globe. This book is appropriate for students seeking detailed information in this area as well as for experts.

Each chapter is a sole-standing publication that reflects each author´s interpretation. Thus, the book displays a multi-facetted picture of our current understanding of application, resources and aspects of the field. I would like to thank the contributors of this book and my family for their endless support.

Editor

1

Impact of the Total Number of Carotid Plaques on the Outcome of Ischemic Stroke Patients with Atrial Fibrillation

Hyungjong Park [1,2], Minho Han [1], Young Dae Kim [1], Joonsang Yoo [2], Hye Sun Lee [3], Jin Kyo Choi [1], Ji Hoe Heo [1] and Hyo Suk Nam [1,*]

1 Department of Neurology, Yonsei University College of Medicine, Seoul 03722, Korea; hjpark209042@gmail.com (H.P.); UMSTHOL18@yuhs.ac (M.H.); neuro05@yuhs.ac (Y.D.K.); JKSNAIL85@yuhs.ac (J.K.C.); jhheo@yuhs.ac (J.H.H.)

2 Department of Neurology, Keimyung University School of Medicine, Daegu 42601, Korea; quarksea@gmail.com

3 Biostatistics Collaboration Unit, Yonsei University College of Medicine, university, Seoul 03722, Korea; HSLEE1@yuhs.ac

* Correspondence: hsnam@yuhs.ac

Abstract: Background: Atrial fibrillation (AF) shares several risk factors with atherosclerosis. We investigated the association between total carotid plaque number (TPN) and long-term prognosis in ischemic stroke patients with AF. Methods: A total of 392 ischemic stroke patients with AF who underwent carotid ultrasonography were enrolled. TPN was assessed using B-mode ultrasound. The patients were categorized into two groups according to best cutoff values for TPN (TPN ≤ 4 vs. TPN ≥ 5). The long-term risk of major adverse cardiovascular events (MACE) and mortality according to TPN was investigated using a Cox hazard model. Results: After a mean follow-up of 2.42 years, 113 patients (28.8%) had developed MACE and 88 patients (22.4%) had died. MACE occurred more frequently in the TPN ≥ 5 group than in the TPN ≤ 4 group (adjusted hazard ratio [HR], 1.50; 95% confidence interval [CI], 1.01–2.21; $p < 0.05$). Moreover, the TPN ≥ 5 group showed an increased risk of all-cause mortality (adjusted HR, 2.69; 95% CI, 1.40–5.17; $p < 0.05$). TPN along with maximal plaque thickness and intima media thickness showed improved prognostic utility when added to the variables of the $CHAD_2DS_2$-VASc score. Conclusion: TPN can predict the long-term outcome of ischemic stroke patients with AF. Adding TPN to the $CHAD_2DS_2$-VASc score increases the predictability of outcome after stroke.

Keywords: atrial fibrillation; cerebral infarction; carotid stenosis; ultrasonography; outcomes

1. Introduction

Atrial fibrillation (AF) is the most common cause of cardioembolic stroke and is associated with poor prognosis in survivors after ischemic stroke. AF was reported to increase the annual risk of cardiovascular events by 5-fold [1,2]. In efforts to prevent cardiovascular events due to AF, researchers have focused on the identification of patients at high risk of developing cardiovascular events [3]. Several studies have suggested that atherosclerosis is associated with both the development and the outcome of AF [4]. For example, among the components of the $CHAD_2DS_2$-VASc score, age, hypertension, diabetes, history of stroke/transient ischemic attack, and vascular disease are known to be the important risk factors for atherosclerosis [5,6].

Carotid atherosclerosis $\geq 50\%$ in patients with AF is well known to be an independent risk factor for future ischemic stroke and vascular events [7–9]. However, the prognostic implication of carotid atherosclerosis < 50% is not well known. Carotid ultrasonography can easily detect mild carotid atherosclerosis through measurements of the carotid intima media thickness (IMT) and carotid plaque thickness [8–10]. However, little is known about the prognostic impact of the number of carotid plaques on the outcome of patients with AF. In this regard, we evaluated the association between the total carotid plaque number (TPN) and long-term prognosis in ischemic stroke patients with AF.

2. Materials and Methods

2.1. Study Population

This is a hospital-based observational study in ischemic stroke patients who were prospectively registered to a stroke registry from January 2007 to December 2013 in Severance Hospital, Seoul, South Korea. [11]. The registry enrolled consecutive patients with acute ischemic stroke within 7 days of onset. During admission, all patients were evaluated with brain magnetic resonance imaging and/or computed tomography, as well as cerebral angiography (magnetic resonance angiography, computed tomography angiography, or digital subtraction angiography). Systemic evaluation included 12-lead electrocardiography (ECG), chest radiography, standard blood tests, lipid profile, and continuous ECG monitoring during stay in the stroke unit. Specific evaluation for finding the cardioembolic source, such as transthoracic echocardiography, transesophageal echocardiography, and 24-h Holter monitoring was done.

The stroke subtypes according to the Trial of ORG 10172 in Acute Stroke Treatment (TOAST) classification [12] and the presence of angiographic abnormalities were prospectively determined using neuroradiologist reports and the consensus of stroke specialists in weekly stroke conferences, and prospectively entered into a computerized database.

This study was approved by the institutional review board of Severance Hospital, Yonsei University Health System, which waived the requirement for informed consent from patients owing to the retrospective nature of the analysis.

2.2. Clinical Variables

We collected data on demographics and risk factors of stroke including hypertension, diabetes, hyperlipidemia, coronary artery disease, peripheral artery disease, history of stroke, transient ischemic accident or thromboembolism, and smoking habit. Hypertension was defined as a systolic blood pressure of ≥ 140 mmHg or a diastolic blood pressure of ≥ 90 mmHg, or any history of anti-hypertensive agent use. Diabetes was defined as fasting glucose level ≥ 7.0 mmol/L, random blood glucose level ≥ 11.0 mmol/L, glycated hemoglobin ≥ 6.5%, or a history of oral hypoglycemic agent or insulin use. Hyperlipidemia was defined as serum total cholesterol ≥ 6.21 mmol/L, low-density lipoprotein cholesterol ≥ 4.14 mmol/L, or any history of use of lipid-lowering agents after a diagnosis of hyperlipidemia. AF was diagnosed on the basis of the findings of routine ECG, Holter monitoring, or continuous ECG monitoring on the current admission or before admission. Paroxysmal AF was also considered the presence of AF. Congestive heart failure was determined from the history of heart failure diagnosis, treatment with loop diuretics, and ejection fraction ≤35% on echocardiography. Coronary artery occlusive disease (CAOD) was defined as any history of unstable angina, myocardial infarction, and CAOD. Peripheral artery occlusive disease was defined as any history of a diagnosis of peripheral artery disease at any hospital regardless of the presence or absence of intervention or medication for peripheral artery disease. Patients were considered current smokers if they had smoked any cigarettes within 1 year before admission. Medication history including anti-coagulant, anti-platelet, anti-hypertensive, and lipid-lowering agent use was collected. Laboratory data were also obtained for complete blood count, lipid profile, blood urea nitrogen level, and creatinine level. The severity of stroke was determined using the National Institute Health Stroke Scale (NIHSS) score at admission.

2.3. Carotid Artery Assessment

Carotid artery plaques were assessed using B-mode ultrasound (iU22 ultrasound system; Philips, Bothell, WA, USA) with a 3-9-MHz multifrequency linear array transducer. All measurements were done in a semi-dark room by two trained ultrasonographers. Bilateral longitudinal and transverse images of the common carotid arteries (CCAs) and internal carotid arteries (ICAs) were always obtained and the presence of plaque was decided after comparison of longitudinal and transverse images. The IMT in the CCAs was defined as the distance of the interface between the lumen-intima and the media-adventitia. The far wall of the carotid artery was visualized bilaterally in the CCAs (20–50 mm proximal to the bifurcation of blood flow), carotid bulb (0–20 mm proximal to the bifurcation of blood flow), and internal and external carotid arteries (0–20 mm distal to the bifurcation of blood flow). At 20, 25, and 30 mm proximal to the bifurcation of blood flow, IMT was bilaterally measured at the far wall of the CCAs during end-diastole, and calculated as the mean value for each patient. According to the Mannheim criteria [13], carotid plaque was defined as a focal structure encroaching into the arterial lumen by at least 0.5 mm, > 50% of surrounding IMT values, or thickness ≥ 1.5 mm above the distance of the interface between the lumen-intima and the media-adventitia.

The thickness of each plaque in the carotid arteries in the whole scanned area was also bilaterally measured. The TPN was determined by simply counting (bilaterally) the number of plaques in proximal ICAs and CCAs. The best cutoff values for TPN were determined using the Contal and O'Quigley method, which calculates the maximum hazard ratio (HR) based on log-rank statistics [14].

2.4. Follow-Up and Outcomes

After discharge, each patient was followed up with regularly at 3 months, 1 year, and yearly thereafter. At each follow-up visit, medical information including occurrence of any cardiovascular events, newly detected vascular risk factors, lifestyle modification after stroke, and re-admission to another hospital was obtained via face-to-face interviews with neurologists or through clinical research associates in the outpatient clinic. When the patients missed a scheduled visit, we obtained the information from the patients or their proxy through a telephone interview with a structured questionnaire [15]. In addition, we also obtained mortality data based on death certificates from the Korean National Statistical Office (http://www.kostat.go.kr).

The primary end point was major adverse cardiovascular events (MACE; cardiovascular mortality, non-cardiovascular mortality, and occurrence of non-fatal stroke or myocardial infarction). Cardiovascular mortality was defined as any mortality due to stroke, myocardial infarction, other cardiac disease, or unobserved sudden death. The secondary outcome was all-cause mortality. The censoring date was December 31, 2013.

2.5. Statistical Analysis

The data were presented as mean ± standard deviation or medians (interquartile range [IQR]), as appropriate. Differences between the two groups were compared with the chi-square test, Fisher's exact test, Student's *t*-test, and the Mann–Whitney U-test, as appropriate. Survival analysis was conducted, and survival curves were plotted using Kaplan–Meier analysis. The difference of survival time between groups was analyzed using a log-rank test. To determine the independent predictor of MACE and all-cause mortality, Cox proportional hazard regression analysis was used, and HR and 95% confidence interval (CI) values were summarized. Cox proportional hazard regression analysis was conducted with adjustments for age, sex, initial NIHSS score, and variables with $p < 0.1$ in the univariate analysis.

To evaluate the added value of carotid plaque burden for the prognosis of ischemic stroke caused by AF, we constructed the model incorporating variables in the CHA_2DS_2-VAS_c score and other variables associated with carotid plaque burden such as IMT, maximal carotid plaque thickness, and TPN. We compared the following five models: (1) CHA_2DS_2-VAS_c score variables alone; (2) addition of IMT; (3) addition of maximal carotid plaque thickness; (4) addition of TPN; and (5) addition of IMT, maximal carotid plaque thickness, and TPN. For internal validation of the newly developed model, time-dependent receiver-operating characteristic curves and areas under the curve (AUCs) were determined based on Heagerty's incident / dynamic AUCs during the median follow-up time [16]. A boot strapping method with 1000 re-samplings for calculating the 95% CI and the difference between the c-indices of each model was applied [17]. All tests were two-sided, and $p < 0.05$ was considered statistically significant. Statistical analysis was performed using R software, version 3.1.3 (R Foundation of Statistical Computing, Vienna, Austria).

3. Results

3.1. Patients' Characteristics

A total of 3727 consecutive ischemic stroke/transient ischemic attack patients were enrolled during the study period. After the exclusion of 2896 patients without AF, a total of 831 patients with AF remained. Among them, 150 patients without carotid ultrasonography and 76 patients with valvular heart disease were excluded. Patients who had > 50% stenosis in the intracranial or extracranial arteries ($n = 143$), complex aortic atheroma (≥ 4 mm or mobile atheroma) ($n = 6$), lacunar infarction ($n = 50$), and other rare etiologies ($n = 14$) according to the TOAST classification were also excluded. Finally, a total of 392 patients were analyzed (Figure 1).

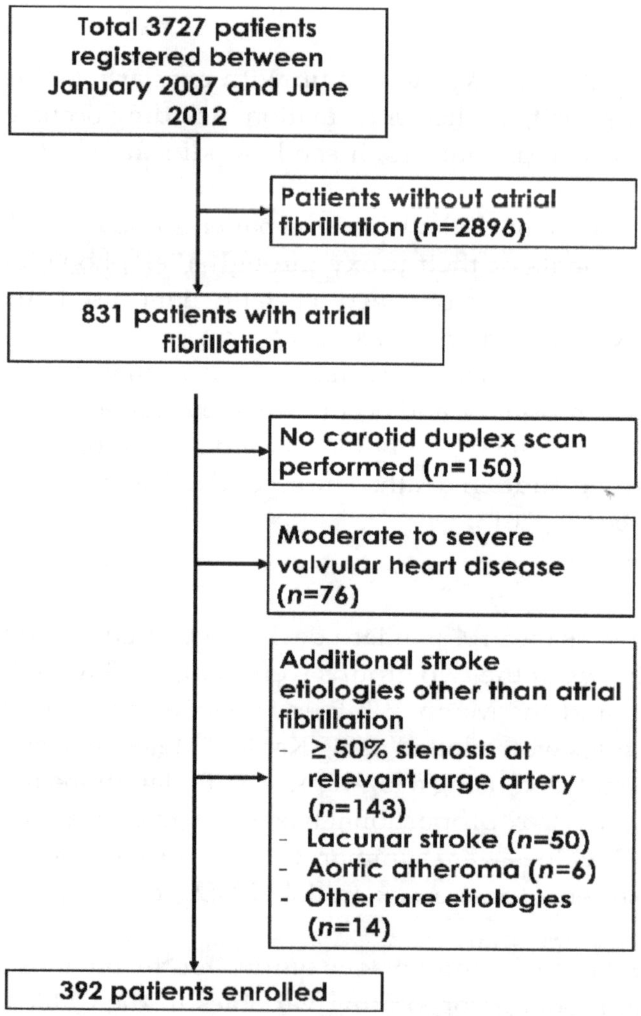

Figure 1. Flow sheet for study patients' selection.

The baseline characteristics of the enrolled patients are summarized in Table 1. The mean age of the total enrolled patients was 69.2 ± 10.3 years, and 225 (57.5%) patients were men. The median NIHSS score at admission was 5.5 (IQR 2–13). Before admission, 88 (22.4%) patients were taking oral anticoagulants. Carotid plaques were found in 343 (87.5%) patients. The median TPN was 3 (IQR 2–6). The median IMT and plaque thickness was 0.8 (IQR 0.7–0.9) and 2.1 (IQR 1.7–2.9), respectively. The inter-rater reliability based on the intraclass correlation coefficient (ICC) between ultrasonographers for carotid duplex sonography parameters was excellent, as follows: TPN (ICC: 0.983, $p < 0.001$), IMT (ICC: 0.966, $p < 0.001$), and maximal plaque thickness (ICC: 0.892, $p = 0.001$). In case of disagreement between ultrasonographers regarding parameters of the carotid duplex sonography, any disagreement was resolved by consensus. Following the Contal and O'Quigley method, the patients were categorized into two groups according to the best cutoff values for TPN (TPN ≤ 4 vs. TPN ≥ 5). The TPN ≤ 4 group consisted of 239 (71.0%) patients, and the TPN ≥ 5 group comprised 153 (39.0%) patients. Patients in the TPN ≥ 5 group were older and more likely to have hypertension, CAOD, statin use, or anti-hypertensive drug use. In addition, the TPN ≥ 5 group had higher IMT (0.9 ± 0.2 vs. 0.8 ± 0.2, $p < 0.001$) and larger maximal plaque thickness (3.0 ± 0.9 vs. 1.7 ± 1.1, $p < 0.001$) than the TPN ≤ 4 group.

Table 1. Clinical characteristics of study patients according to the total carotid plaque number (TPN).

	TPN ≤ 4 (*N* = 239)	TPN ≥ 5 (*N* = 153)	*P* Value
Demographics			
Age, years	66.4 ± 10.5	73.5 ± 8.4	< 0.001
Sex, men	134 (56.1)	91 (59.5)	0.575
Initial NIHSS score	5 (2–13)	6 (2–13)	0.639
Risk factors			
Hypertension	155 (64.9)	126 (82.4)	< 0.001
Diabetes mellitus	53 (22.2)	46 (30.1)	0.102
Smoking	38 (15.9)	23 (15.0)	0.930
Hyperlipidemia	38 (15.9)	37 (24.2)	0.057
PAOD	5 (2.1)	7 (4.6)	0.275
CAOD	47 (19.7)	50 (32.7)	0.005
CHF	33 (13.8)	21 (13.7)	1.000
Laboratory findings			
Hemoglobin, g/dL	14.1 ± 2.1	13.5 ± 1.5	0.001
White blood cell, × 10^9/L	8202.7 ± 2827.0	7830.1 ± 2939.5	0.211
Platelet, × 10^9/L	225.6 ± 69.9	224.6 ± 70.0	0.885
Blood urea nitrogen, mmol/L	17.4 ± 6.3	18.8 ± 9.6	0.190
Creatinine, μmol/L	1.0 ± 0.8	1.3 ± 1.6	0.128
Total cholesterol, mmol/L	170.8 ± 35.8	167.2 ± 39.4	0.361
Triglyceride, mmol/L	96.2 ± 50.2	89.5 ± 45.3	0.184
HDL-cholesterol, mmol/L	45.0 ± 11.5	44.8 ± 11.9	0.865
LDL-cholesterol, mmol/L	106.5 ± 32.3	103.6 ± 35.7	0.399
Premorbid medication			
Antiplatelet agent	98 (41.0)	76 (49.7)	0.114
Anticoagulants	60 (25.1)	28 (18.3)	0.147
Statin	36 (15.1)	44 (28.8)	0.002
Antihypertensive agent	93 (38.9)	81 (52.9)	0.009
Carotid duplex measurement			
IMT, mm	0.8 ± 0.2	0.9 ± 0.2	< 0.001
Maximal plaque thickness, mm	1.7 ± 1.1	3.0 ± 0.9	< 0.001
Total plaque number, n	2 (1–3)	7 (5–10.5)	< 0.001

Data are shown as n (%), mean ± SD, or median (IQR). SD, standard deviation; IQR, interquartile range; NIHSS, National Institute of Health Stroke Scale; PAOD, peripheral artery occlusive disease; CAOD, coronary artery occlusive disease; CHF, congestive heart failure;; HDL, high density lipoprotein; LDL, low density lipoprotein; IMT, intimal medial thickness.

3.2. Outcome

The mean follow-up period was 2.42 ± 1.83 years. During the follow-up, a total of 113 (28.8%) MACE occurred in 60 (25.1%) patients of the TPN ≤ 4 group and in 53 (34.6%) patients of the TPN ≥ 5 group. In Kaplan–Meier analysis, the TPN ≥ 5 group showed a higher MACE rate than the TPN ≤ 4 group (log-rank test, $p < 0.001$) (Figure 2A). Multivariate Cox proportional regression analysis showed that the TPN ≥ 5 group had a significantly higher MACE rate than the TPN ≤ 4 group after adjusting for age, sex, and variables with $p < 0.1$ in univariate analysis (adjusted hazard ratio [HR], 1.50; 95% CI, 1.01–2.21; $p < 0.05$) (Table 2).

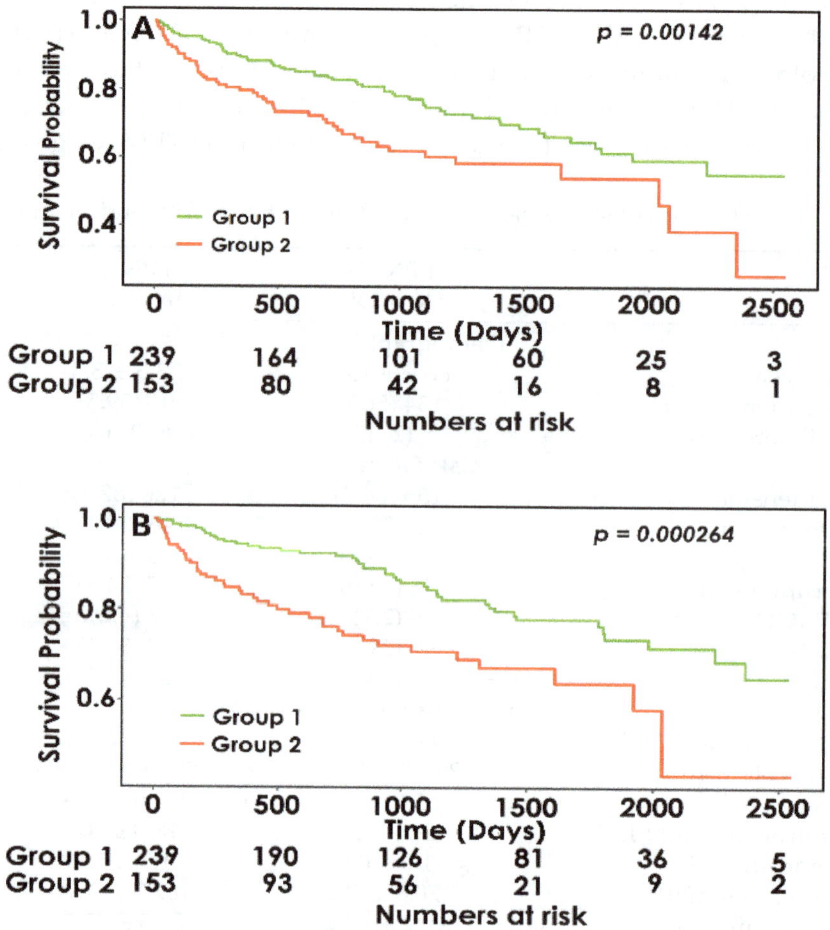

Figure 2. Kaplan–Meier analysis for (**A**) major adverse cardiovascular event (MACE); (**B**) all-cause mortality according to the total carotid plaque number (TPN).

In terms of all-cause mortality, 88 (22.4%) patients had died during the follow up period. In Kaplan–Meier curve analysis, the TPN ≥ 5 group showed a higher mortality rate than the TPN ≤ 4 group (log-rank test, $p < 0.001$) (Figure 2B). In multivariate Cox proportional regression analysis after adjusting for age, sex, and variables with $p < 0.10$ in univariate analysis, patients in the TPN ≥ 5 group showed an increased risk of all-cause mortality (adjusted HR, 2.69; 95% CI, 1.40–5.17; $p < 0.05$) compared with patients in the TPN ≤ 4 group (Table 2).

Table 2. Unadjusted and adjusted hazard ratio for MACE and all-cause mortality according to the total carotid number of plaque.

	MACE				All-Cause Mortality			
	Univariate Analysis		Multivariate Analysis		Univariate Analysis		Multivariate Analysis	
	HR (95% CI)	*P* Value	HR (95% CI)	*P* Value	HR (95% CI)	*P* Value	HR (95% CI)	*P* Value
Demographics								
Age	1.05 (1.03–1.07)	0.000	1.04 (1.01–1.06)	0.002	1.07 (1.05–1.10)	0.000	1.05 (1.02–1.08)	0.003
Sex	0.66 (0.45–0.95)	0.027	1.03 (0.67–1.59)	0.887	0.66 (0.43–1.00)	0.051	0.95 (0.49–1.84)	0.874
Initial NIHSS score	1.06 (1.03–1.08)	0.000	1.05 (1.02–1.08)	0.001	1.07 (1.04–1.00)	0.446	1.07 (1.03–1.11)	0.000
Risk factors								
Hypertension	1.32 (0.86–2.04)	0.208			1.21 (0.74–1.96)	0.446		
Diabetes mellitus	1.02 (0.66–1.56)	0.933			1.10 (0.68–1.78)	0.106		
Smoking	1.18 (0.72–1.93)	0.512			1.16 (0.66–2.02)	0.603		
PAOD	1.70 (0.69–4.18)	0.247			2.68 (1.08–6.65)	0.033	1.25 (0.36–4.41)	0.727
CAOD	1.51 (1.01–2.26)	0.046	1.14 (0.75–1.75)	0.532	1.74 (1.11–2.73)	0.016	1.18 (0.64–2.16)	0.588
CHF	1.66(1.05–2.61)	0.029	1.22 (0.76–1.97)	0.411	2.31 (1.43–3.72)	0.001	1.72 (0.83–3.57)	0.148
Laboratory findings								
Hemoglobin	0.88 (0.80–0.95)	0.002	0.91 (0.82–1.01)	0.909	0.86 (0.79–0.94)	0.001	0.94 (0.79–1.11)	0.466
White blood cell	1.00 (1.00–1.00)	0.831			1.00 (1.00–1.00)	0.836		
Platelet	1.00 (1.00–1.00)	0.361			1.00 (0.99–1.00)	0.040	1.00 (0.99–1.00)	0.998
BUN	1.02 (0.99–1.05)	0.157			1.03 (1.01–1.06)	0.018	1.01 (0.98–1.05)	0.590
Creatinine	1.05 (0.88–1.24)	0.600			1.08 (0.91–1.28)	0.371		
Total cholesterol	1.00 (0.99–1.00)	0.089			0.99 (0.99–1.00)	0.067		
Triglyceride	1.00 (1.00–1.00)	0.929	1.00 (0.99–1.01)	0.184	1.00 (1.00–1.00)	0.974		
HDL–cholesterol	1.00 (0.98–1.01)	0.844			1.00 (0.98–1.02)	0.987		
LDL–cholesterol	0.99 (0.99–1.00)	0.071	1.00 (0.99–1.00)	0.234	0.99 (0.99–1.00)	0.051		
Premorbid medication								
Antiplatelet agent	1.03 (0.71–1.49)	0.867			1.02 (0.67–1.56)	0.916		
Anticoagulants	0.78 (0.49–1.23)	0.288			0.83(0.50–1.40)	0.494		
Statin	1.41 (0.92–2.16)	0.117			1.28 (0.78–2.11)	0.330		
Antihypertensive agent	1.45 (0.99–2.13)	0.056			1.75 (1.13–2.70)	0.011	1.73 (0.89–3.38)	0.106
Total plaque number								
TPN ≤ 4 (reference)	1		1		1		1	
TPN ≥ 5	1.82 (1.25–2.64)	0.002	1.50 (1.01–2.21)	0.044	2.16 (1.41–3.29)	< 0.001	2.69 (1.40–5.17)	0.003

MACE, major adverse cardiovascular events; HR, hazard ratio; CI, confidential interval; National Institute of Health Stroke Scale; PAOD, peripheral artery occlusive disease; CAOD, coronary artery occlusive disease; CHF, congestive heart failure; BUN, blood urea nitrogen; HDL, high density lipoprotein; LDL, low density lipoprotein; IMT, intimal medial thickness.

3.3. *Prognostic Utility of Carotid Plaque Burden on Ischemic Stroke Caused by AF*

During the median follow-up period, the c-indices of Heagerty's incident/dynamic AUC of each model were calculated (Table 3 and Supplementary Figure S1). The baseline model consisted of age, sex, congestive heart failure, diabetes mellitus, CAOD, and peripheral artery occlusive disease, which are the same variables of the $CHAD_2DS_2$-VASc score. The c-index for the baseline model was 0.651 (95% CI, 0.605–0.705) in MACE and 0.712 (95% CI, 0.658–0.766) in all-cause mortality. In model 5, including of all parameters of carotid plaque burden including TPN, maximal plaque thickness, and IMT improved prognostic utility that with the $CHAD_2DS_2$-VASc score alone in MACE (c-index, 0.686, 95% CI, 0.638–0.737, $p = 0.045$) and all-cause mortality (c-index, 0.734, 95% CI (0.686–0.786, $p = 0.025$).

Table 3. C-indices of Heagerty's incident/dynamic AUC for predicting MACE and all-cause mortality

	MACE			All–Cause Mortality		
	c–Index (95% CI)	Difference	*P*–Value	c–Index	Difference	*P*–Value
Model 1 *	0.651 (0.605–0.705)	Reference		0.696 (0.647–0.753)	Reference	
Model 2 †	0.661 (0.613–0.714)	0.010 (−0.005–0.033)	0.267	0.712 (0.658–0.766)	0.016 (−0.005–0.046)	0.218
Model 3 ‡	0.672 (0.626–0.726)	0.020 (0.001–0.049)	0.214	0.716 (0.670–0.769)	0.019 (0.001–0.045)	0.113
Model 4 §	0.657 (0.609–0.710)	0.006 (0–0.022)	0.317	0.701 (0.651–0.756)	0.005 (−0.001–0.021)	0.405
Model 5 ‖	0.686 (0.638–0.737)	0.034 (0.006–0.071)	0.045	0.734 (0.686–0.786)	0.038 (0.006–0.075)	0.025

AUC, area under the curve; MACE, major adverse cardiovascular events; CI, confidence interval. * Model 1: CHA_2DS_2-VAS_c variables (age, sex, hypertension, diabetes mellitus, congestive heart failure, coronary artery occlusive disease, peripheral artery occlusive disease) † Model 2: Model 1 plus carotid intima medial thickness; ‡ Model 3: Model 1 plus total number of plaque; § Model 4: Model 1 plus maximal thickness of plaque; || Model 5: Model 1 plus carotid intima medial thickness plus maximal plaque thickness plus total number of plaque.

4. Discussion

The present study revealed that carotid plaque burden of < 50% carotid stenosis was a strong prognostic marker in patients with AF. Among the parameters of carotid plaque burden, TPN is easily counted during carotid ultrasonography examination. It showed an impact on the outcome of ischemic stroke patients with AF. Moreover, the carotid plaque burden improved the predictive value of the $CHAD_2DS_2$-VASc score in predicting cardiovascular events and mortality in ischemic stroke patients with AF.

AF is the most common cause of cardioembolic stroke. Patients with AF had markedly reduced survival compared with those without AF. In the Framingham Heart Study, the risk factor-adjusted odds ratio for death was 1.5 and 1.9 in men and women, respectively [18]. Patients with AF frequently have concomitant cerebral atherosclerosis (20–50% of cases) [19,20]. It is well known that atherosclerosis is a systemic disorder that plays an important role in the prognosis of patients with AF [4]. It can be assumed that patients with AF are more likely to have additional atherosclerotic burden and may have poor prognosis. We previously reported that patients who have both large artery atherosclerosis (>50% atherosclerotic stenosis in the relevant artery) and cardioembolism showed higher cardiovascular mortality than patients with a single cause of either large artery atherosclerosis or cardioembolism [21]. Thus, it can be inferred that concomitant carotid atherosclerosis with AF is associated with the development of cardiovascular events despite the presence of < 50% stenosis.

To date, little is known about the impact of < 50% atherosclerotic stenosis of the carotid artery on the outcome of ischemic stroke patients with AF. The presence of large artery atherosclerosis can be screened using luminography including computed tomography angiography, magnetic resonance angiography, or digital subtraction angiography. However, arterial wall changes including small plaques or increased IMT in the carotid artery cannot be detected using luminography. Carotid ultrasonography is a noninvasive imaging examination that can easily and accurately evaluate carotid plaques and IMT in the arterial lumen.

We found that the TPN ≥ 5 group had a 1.5-fold higher MACE rate than the TPN ≤ 4 group after adjustments. Moreover, considering all parameters of carotid plaque burden, including TPN, maximal plaque thickness, and IMT, contributed to the improvement of the risk stratification of ischemic stroke patients with AF over that with the $CHAD_2DS_2$-VASc risk score alone. The components of the $CHAD_2DS_2$-VASc score are clinical variables including old age, hypertension, diabetes, and vascular disease. These variables are also well-known risk factors for atherosclerosis [6]. Therefore, adding the carotid plaque burden to the model improves the risk prediction.

In line with our findings, cohort studies including non-stroke patients also reported similar results. In ARAPACIS (Atrial Fibrillation Registry for Ankle-brachial Index Prevalence Assessment: Collaborative Italian Study), a prospective nationwide observational cohort study in patients with non-valvular AF, the investigators reported that carotid plaque detection improves the predictive value of the $CHAD_2DS_2$-VASc score in patients with AF [22]. The ARIC (Atherosclerosis Risk in Communities) study investigators also reported that carotid IMT and the presence of carotid plaque are associated with an increased risk of ischemic stroke in patients with AF. The addition of carotid IMT and carotid plaque to the model provided an incremental predictive value for the risk of stroke over the $CHAD_2DS_2$-VASc score alone in adults with AF who had no prior ischemic stroke. Although we reached similar findings, a difference of the present study from the two cohort studies is that we enrolled only ischemic stroke patients with AF. Another difference is that we adopted TPN because this variable can be easily and acutely measured on routine carotid ultrasonography [10].

Currently, the method for the secondary prevention of ischemic stroke caused by AF is anticoagulation with a vitamin K antagonist or a direct oral anticoagulant (DOAC) [23]. However, vitamin K antagonists can prevent only 67% of future ischemic stroke events and DOAC did not show superiority over vitamin K antagonists [24,25]. Identification of high-risk patients for future events despite anticoagulation treatment is important. Carotid atherosclerosis and atherosclerotic burden can be easily detected using carotid duplex ultrasonography. Although TPN is less accurate and operator-dependent method than quantification measurement of carotid plaque such as total plaque area [26,27], TPN can be easily counted and may be helpful in identifying high risk patients in daily clinical practice. Our study has several limitations. First, unstable plaque morphology and hypoechoic plaque are associated with an increased risk of ischemic stroke; however, we did not analyze the characteristics of individual plaques. Nevertheless, unstable carotid plaque is known to be prevalent in advanced carotid atherosclerosis, and our study did not include patients with >50% stenosis in an intracranial or extracranial artery. Thus, the influence of the morphologic feature of carotid plaques may be little. Second, carotid duplex ultrasonography was conducted by two ultrasonographers; however, the measurement agreement between them was high. Third, potential selection bias may exist. To minimize selection bias, we recruited consecutive ischemic stroke patients with AF.

5. Conclusions

In conclusion, TPN is an important risk predictor in ischemic stroke patients with AF. In addition, considering all parameters of carotid plaque burden including TPN, maximal plaque thickness, and IMT may contribute to improving the risk prediction in ischemic stroke patients with AF, compared with the prediction with the clinical variables of $CHAD_2DS_2$-VASc score alone. These findings suggest that carotid ultrasonography may be useful in reclassifying these patients.

Author Contributions: Conceptualization, H.P. and H.S.N.; Methodology, Y.D.K., and J.Y.; Formal analysis, M.H., H.S.L., and J.K.C.; Investigation, H.P., Y.D.K., and J.Y.; Writing—original draft preparation, H.P and H.S.N.; Writing—review and editing, H.P., J.H.H., and H.S.N.; Supervision, H.P., M.H., Y.D.K., J.Y., H.S.L., J.K.C., J.H.H., and H.S.N. Read and approved the final manuscript, all authors.

Acknowledgments: We thank Junghye Choi, BS, for her efforts in data collection.

References

1. Schnabel, R.B.; Yin, X.; Gona, P.; Larson, M.G.; Beiser, A.S.; McManus, D.D.; Newton-Chen, C.; Lubitz, S.A.; Magnani, J.W.; Ellinor, P.T.; et al. 50 year trends in atrial fibrillation prevalence, incidence, risk factors, and mortality in the framingham heart study: A cohort study. *Lancet* **2015**, *386*, 154–162. [CrossRef]
2. Wolf, P.A.; Mitchell, J.B.; Baker, C.S.; Kannel, W.B.; D'Agostino, R.B. Impact of atrial fibrillation on mortality, stroke, and medical costs. *Arch. Intern. Med.* **1998**, *158*, 229–234. [CrossRef]
3. Lau, D.H.; Nattel, S.; Kalman, J.M.; Sanders, P. Modifiable risk factors and atrial fibrillation. *Circulation* **2017**, *136*, 583–596. [CrossRef]
4. Bekwelem, W.; Jensen, P.N.; Norby, F.L.; Soliman, E.Z.; Agarwal, S.K.; Lip, G.Y.; Pan, W.; Folsom, A.R.; Longstreth, W.T., Jr.; Alonso, A.; et al. Carotid atherosclerosis and stroke in atrial fibrillation: The atherosclerosis risk in communities study. *Stroke* **2016**, *47*, 1643–1646. [CrossRef] [PubMed]
5. European Heart Rhythm Association; European Association for Cardio-Thoracic Surgery; Camm, A.J.; Kirchhof, P.; Lip, G.Y.; Schotten, U.; Savelieva, I.; Ernst, S.; van Gelder, I.C.; Al-Attar, N.; et al. Guidelines for the management of atrial fibrillation: The task force for the management of atrial fibrillation of the European Society of Cardiology (ESC). *Eur. Heart J.* **2010**, *31*, 2369–2429. [PubMed]
6. Cha, M.J.; Kim, Y.D.; Nam, H.S.; Kim, J.; Lee, D.H.; Heo, J.H. Stroke mechanism in patients with non-valvular atrial fibrillation according to the $CHADS_2$ and $CHAD_2DS_2$-VASc score. *Eur. J. Neurol.* **2012**, *19*, 473–479. [CrossRef]
7. Nagai, Y.; Kitagawa, K.; Sakaguchi, M.; Shimizu, Y.; Hashimoto, H.; Yamagami, H.; Narita, M.; Ohtsuki, T.; Hori, M.; Matsumoto, M. Significance of earlier carotid atherosclerosis for stroke subtypes. *Stroke* **2001**, *32*, 1780–1785. [CrossRef]
8. Steinvil, A.; Sadeh, B.; Bornstein, N.M.; Havakuk, O.; Greenberg, S.; Arbel, Y.; Konigstein, M.; Finkelstein, A.; Banai, S.; Halkin, A. Impact of carotid atherosclerosis on the risk of adverse cardiac events in patients with and without coronary disease. *Stroke* **2014**, *45*, 2311–2317. [CrossRef] [PubMed]
9. Störk, S.; van den Beld, A.W.; von Schacky, C.; Angermann, C.E.; Lamberts, S.W.; Grobbee, D.E.; Bots, M.L. Carotid artery plaque burden, stiffness, and mortality risk in elderly men: A prospective, population-based cohort study. *Circulation* **2004**, *110*, 344–348. [CrossRef] [PubMed]
10. Maeda, S.; Sawayama, Y.; Furusyo, N.; Shigematsu, M.; Hayashi, J. The association between fatal vascular events and risk factors for carotid atherosclerosis in patients on maintenance hemodialysis: Plaque number of dialytic atherosclerosis study. *Atherosclerosis* **2009**, *204*, 549–555. [CrossRef] [PubMed]
11. Lee, B.I.; Nam, H.S.; Heo, J.H.; Kim, D.I. Yonsei stroke registry. Analysis of 1,000 patients with acute cerebral infarctions. *Cerebrovasc. Dis.* **2001**, *12*, 145–151. [CrossRef] [PubMed]
12. Adams, H.P., Jr.; Bendixen, B.H.; Kappelle, L.J.; Biller, J.; Love, B.B.; Gordon, D.L.; Marsh, E.E. Classification of subtype of acute ischemic stroke. Definitions for use in a multicenter clinical trial. Toast. Trial of org 10172 in acute stroke treatment. *Stroke* **1993**, *24*, 35–41. [CrossRef] [PubMed]
13. Touboul, P.J.; Hennerici, M.G.; Meairs, S.; Adams, H.; Amarenco, P.; Bornstein, N.; Csiba, L.; Desvarieux, M.; Ebrahim, S.; Hernadez, R.H.; et al. Mannheim carotid intima-media thickness and plaque consensus (2004–2006–2011). An update on behalf of the advisory board of the 3rd, 4th and 5th watching the risk symposia, at the 13th, 15th and 20th european stroke conferences, Mannheim, Germany, 2004, Brussels, Belgium, 2006, and Hamburg, Germany, 2011. *Cerebrovasc. Dis.* **2012**, *34*, 290–296. [PubMed]
14. Contal, C.; O'Quigley, J. An application of changepoint methods in studying the effect of age on survival in breast cancer. *Comput. Stat. Data Anal.* **1999**, *30*, 253–270. [CrossRef]
15. Yoo, J.; Song, D.; Baek, J.H.; Kim, K.; Kim, J.; Song, T.J.; Lee, H.S.; Choi, D.; Kim, Y.D.; Nam, H.S.; et al. Poor long-term outcomes in stroke patients with asymptomatic coronary artery disease in heart CT. *Atherosclerosi* **2017**, *265*, 7–13. [CrossRef]

16. Heagerty, P.J.; Zheng, Y. Survival model predictive accuracy and ROC curves. *Biometrics* **2005**, *61*, 92–105. [CrossRef]
17. Uno, H.; Cai, T.; Pencina, M.J.; D'Agostino, R.B.; Wei, L. On the C-statistics for evaluating overall adequacy of risk prediction procedures with censored survival data. *Stat. Med.* **2011**, *30*, 1105–1117. [CrossRef] [PubMed
18. Benjamin, E.J.; Wolf, P.A.; D'Agostino, R.B.; Silbershatz, H.; Kannel, W.B.; Levy, D. Impact of atrial fibrillation on the risk of death: The framingham heart study. *Circulation* **1998**, *98*, 946–952. [CrossRef] [PubMed]
19. Chang, Y.J.; Ryu, S.J.; Lin, S.K. Carotid artery stenosis in ischemic stroke patients with nonvalvular atrial fibrillation. *Cerebrovasc. Dis.* **2002**, *13*, 16–20. [CrossRef]
20. Kanter, M.C.; Tegeler, C.H.; Pearce, L.A.; Weinberger, J.; Feinberg, W.M.; Anderson, D.C.; Gomez, C.R.; Rothrock, J.F.; Helgason, C.M.; Hart, R.G.; et al. Carotid stenosis in patients with atrial fibrillation. Prevalence, risk factors, and relationship to stroke in the Stroke Prevention in Atrial Fibrillation Study. *Arch. Intern. Med.* **1994**, *154*, 1372–1377. [CrossRef] [PubMed]
21. Kim, Y.D.; Cha, M.J.; Kim, J.; Lee, D.H.; Lee, H.S.; Nam, C.M.; Nam, H.S.; Heo, J.H. Long-term mortality in patients with coexisting potential causes of ischemic stroke. *Int. J. Stroke* **2015**, *10*, 541–546. [CrossRef] [PubMed]
22. Basili, S.; Loffredo, L.; Pastori, D.; Proietti, M.; Farcomeni, A.; Vestri, A.R.; Pignatelli, P.; Daví, G.; Hiatt, W.R.; Lip, G.Y.H.; et al. Carotid plaque detection improves the predictive value of cha2ds2-vasc score in patients with non-valvular atrial fibrillation: The ARAPACIS study. *Int. J. Cardiol.* **2017**, *231*, 143–149. [CrossRef [PubMed]
23. Kirchhof, P.; Benussi, S.; Kotecha, D.; Ahlsson, A.; Atar, D.; Casadei, B.; Castella, M.; Diener, H.-C.; Heidbuchel, H.; Hendriks, J.; et al. 2016 ESC guidelines for the management of atrial fibrillation developed in collaboration with EACTS. *Eur. Heart J.* **2016**, *37*, 2893–2962. [CrossRef] [PubMed]
24. Hart, R.G.; Pearce, L.A.; Aguilar, M.I. Meta-analysis: Antithrombotic therapy to prevent stroke in patients who have nonvalvular atrial fibrillation. *Ann. Intern. Med.* **2007**, *146*, 857–867. [CrossRef] [PubMed]]
25. Lip, G.Y.; Lane, D.A. Stroke prevention in atrial fibrillation: A systematic review. *JAMA* **2015**, *313*, 1950–1962. [CrossRef]
26. Mitchel, C.; Korcarz, C.E.; Genper, A.D.; Kaufman, J.D.; Post, W.; Tracy, R.; Gassett, A.J.; Ma, N.; McClelland, R.L.; Stein, J.H. Ultrasound carotid plaque features, cardiovascular disease risk factors and events: The Multi-Ethnic Study of Atherosclerosis. *Atheroslcerosis* **2018**, *276*, 195–202. [CrossRef]
27. López-Melgar, B.; Fernández-Friera, L.; Sánchez-González, J.; Vilchez, J.P.; Cecconi, A.; Mateo, J.; Penãlvo, J.L.; Oliva, B.; García-Ruiz, J.M.; Kauffman, S.; et al. Accurate quantification of atherosclerotic plaque volume by 3D vascular ultrasound using the volumetric linear array method. *Atherosclerosis* **2016**, *248*, 230–237. [CrossRef]

2

Etiology of Ischemic Strokes of Patients with Atrial Fibrillation and Therapy with Anticoagulants

Jan C. Purrucker [1,*], Kyra Hölscher [1], Jennifer Kollmer [2] and Peter A. Ringleb [1]

1 Department of Neurology, Heidelberg University Hospital, 69120 Heidelberg, Germany; hoelscher@stud.uni-heidelberg.de (K.H.); Peter.Arthur.Ringleb@med.uni-heidelberg.de (P.A.R.)
2 Department of Neuroradiology, Heidelberg University Hospital, 69120 Heidelberg, Germany; jennifer.kollmer@med.uni-heidelberg.de
* Correspondence: jan.purrucker@med.uni-heidelberg.de

Abstract: Background: Reducing the number of ischemic strokes in patients with atrial fibrillation despite oral anticoagulation remains an important, yet largely unsolved challenge. Therefore, we assessed the etiology of ischemic strokes despite anticoagulation with vitamin K antagonists (VKA) or non-VKA oral anticoagulants (NOACs). Methods: Patients with known atrial fibrillation (AF), treatment with VKA or NOAC, and acute ischemic stroke admitted between 2015 and 2018 (1st half) were identified from the hospital database. Brain imaging data were independently reviewed. An integrated etiologic classification according to the ASCOD system was made. Medication errors (admission INR <2.0 in the VKA- or NOAC-specific concentration <10 ng/mL) or dosage/dosing errors were also analyzed. Results: Of 3610 patients screened, $n = 341$ were included (VKA, $n = 127$; NOAC, $n = 214$). An overall increasing rate of OAC-associated stroke per year was observed. In 95.3% of patients with adequate diagnostic work-up ($n = 321/337$), at least one additional potential, uncertain, or unlikely non-cardiac cause of stroke was identified. More patients in the VKA than in the NOAC group had a medication error (81/127, 63.8% vs. 102/205, 49.8%; $p = 0.013$). Conclusions: Stroke risk factors despite atrial fibrillation were highly prevalent. Although less common with NOACs than VKAs, medication errors are still frequent.

Keywords: anticoagulant drugs; cerebral stroke; vitamin K antagonist; antithrombins; factor Xa inhibitors

1. Introduction

Oral anticoagulation effectively reduces the risk of ischemic stroke in patients suffering from non-valvular atrial fibrillation (AF) compared to placebo or platelet inhibition [1,2]. Interestingly, while non-vitamin K antagonist oral anticoagulants (NOAC) have been shown to reduce the relative risk of intracerebral hemorrhage compared to vitamin K antagonists (VKA) by 50%, the relative risk of ischemic stroke despite oral anticoagulation has remained largely unchanged [3]. Indeed, a significant proportion of patients experience ischemic stroke while receiving oral anticoagulation therapy; in the primary prevention subgroup analyses of the randomized-control-trials comparing NOACs with VKA in AF patients, 0.7% to 1.3% of the patients suffered from an ischemic stroke per year, while in the secondary prevention cohorts, the percentage of patients developing at least a second ischemic stroke/transient ischemic attack was 1.8% to 2.3% per year [4–7]. Notably, in the primary prevention analyses, ischemic strokes occurred 2.1 to 10.1 times more often than hemorrhagic strokes and 2.2 to 27.4 times more often in the secondary prevention cohorts [4–7]. Recently, a pooled analysis underlined that patients with AF and oral anticoagulation before stroke were at a higher risk of recurrent stroke than patients without anticoagulation [8]. Thus, reducing the number of recurrent ischemic strokes in patients with AF despite oral anticoagulation remains an important, yet largely unsolved challenge. Data deciphering the causes of ischemic strokes despite oral anticoagulation remain scarce, however.

Herein, we aim to provide a more profound understanding of the etiology of ischemic strokes despite oral anticoagulation in order to inform clinical practice as well as future interventional studies to address the unmet need of further reducing recurrent stroke events in patients with AF who receive oral anticoagulation.

2. Experimental Section

2.1. Patient Cohort Description, and Patient Involvement

Consecutive patients with acute ischemic stroke (ICD-10 I63.x) admitted to the certified Stroke Unit or NeuroIntensive Care Unit of the Heidelberg University Hospital between 2015 and 2018 (1st half) were screened. Inclusion criteria for further data analysis were age ≥ 18 years, known non-valvular AF (paroxysmal, persistent, or permanent), and therapy with oral anticoagulation (VKA or NOAC (i.e., dabigatran, rivaroxaban, apixaban or edoxaban)) at the time of stroke onset. Patients were excluded in case of early palliative care orders, known presence of additional, high cardio-embolic risks besides AF, or insufficient quality or availability of source data. Furthermore, patients with documented pause of OAC >3 days before the index stroke, recent start of OAC <3 days before stroke, or bridging-therapy (administration of low-molecular-weight heparin) were also excluded. The research questions were developed due to the daily demanding questions of patients regarding the reasons why they were suffering from stroke despite taking oral anticoagulation. Results will be disseminated within the patient council of our Department of Neurology, Heidelberg University Hospital. Approval was obtained from the ethics committee of the Medical Faculty of Heidelberg, Germany, before beginning this study (S-525/2018). Informed consent of individual participants was waived due to the observational retrospective design of this study according to local and EU data regulations.

2.2. Data Acquisition

Information about medical history, stroke severity and course, performance, and results of both diagnostic and imaging and treatment modalities were extracted from the digital hospital archive. All diagnostic and treatment decisions were made during routine care. Diagnostic evaluation and treatment were administered in accordance with international and national guidelines, as well as with local standard operating procedures (available in German at https://www.klinikum.uni-heidelberg.de/neurologische-klinik/neurologie-und-poliklinik/ueber-uns/downloads). Briefly, during emergency assessment, patients receive a brain CT or MRI; if large-vessel occlusion is suspected or recanalization therapy planned (i.e., intravenous thrombolysis and/or endovascular therapy), CT or MR angiography is conducted. CT/MRI perfusion is performed in selected cases only. During the 24- to ≥72-h acute stroke diagnostics and therapy, additional follow-up CT or MRI procedures, extra- and transcranial Doppler/duplex sonography, continuous ECG and blood pressure monitoring, and echocardiography (transthoracic or transesophageal) are initiated. Routine laboratory results of non-specific coagulation tests (activated partial thromboplastin time (aPTT), international normalized ratio (INR), and thrombin time) as well drug-specific tests (anti-factor Xa or hemoclot assay) and platelet counts obtained at admission are collected. As a cut-off to differentiate between lower than expected NOAC concentrations, the level is set at 30 ng/mL following considerations previously published in Drouet et al. [9], and we use a lower cut-off of 10 ng/mL for sensitivity analyses, both of which are applicable to all NOACs. Renal function is assessed according to creatinine levels and the estimated glomerular filtration rate is electronically calculated (eGFR) according to the Chronic Kidney Disease Epidemiology Collaboration (CKD-EPI) equation, or if not available, the Modification of Diet in Renal Disease (MDRD) equation. Routine laboratory testing also includes measurement of the glycated hemoglobin (HBa1c) and a lipid profile. If indicated, a CSF analysis is performed, as is vasculitis screening (anti-nuclear antibodies, anti-double-stranded DNA, anti-neutrophil cytoplasmic antibodies, cardiolipin antibodies, C3c and C4 complement, and lupus anticoagulants).

2.3. Imaging Analysis

Brain CT or 3T MRI examinations were performed as part of local routine testing. Images were reviewed by a board-certified neuroradiologist (JK) and independently cross-checked by a board-certified neurologist (JP). Readers were blinded to all patient characteristics except for admission date. Lacuna was defined as a subcortical infarct smaller than or equal to 1.5 cm (≤2.0 cm on MRI diffusion images) in the largest dimension and in the distribution of the small, penetrating cerebral arteries, and with a fluid attenuated inversion recovery sequence (FLAIR) rim hyperintensity and parenchymal void (in follow-up) [10]. Acute infarcts were considered potentially non-embolic only if a lacuna or a small singular subcortical infarct was observed and there was a sign of small-vessel disease. White-matter changes were evaluated according to the Fazekas score (from 0 (no hyperintensity) to 3 (irregular periventricular hyperintensity extending into the deep white matter or large confluent lesions)) [11]. There was a good interrater correlation (0.7, 95% CI 0.61–0.72). For the analyses, the arithmetic mean of each of the of the two raters' assessment was used.

2.4. Etiologic Classification

By integrating all diagnostic results, including the independent image analysis and clinical syndrome, one etiology or competing etiologies of the current stroke were classified according to ASCOD phenotyping (A: atherosclerosis; S: small-vessel disease; C: cardiac pathology; O: other causes; and D: dissection) [12]. Within ASCOD, the likelihood that every potential disease is causal for the stroke is graded in a 3(+2)-step system (1, potentially causal; 2, uncertain causality; 3 unlikely causal link; 0, disease is absent; 9, insufficient work-up to grade the disease). As all patients included in the current study had AF, we set C = 1 *a priori*, but investigated to determine any further cardio-embolic sources. Owing to the fact that a clinical syndrome suggesting a deep branch artery stroke was allowed to be classified as an uncertain potential cause in small-vessel disease without evidence on CT or MRI of a recent infarct (ASCOD, S2), acute stroke symptoms were classified according to the Oxford Community Stroke Project Classification [13]. Pure motor stroke, pure sensory stroke, sensorimotor stroke, and ataxic hemiparesis were considered as a lacunar syndrome.

2.5. Data Analysis

The distribution of continuous data is described as mean (SD) or median (interquartile ranges); for categorical data, absolute and relative frequencies (count and percentage) are reported. The Kolmogorov–Smirnov test was used to ascertain distribution of data. To compare proportions of demographic and clinical characteristics between patients with VKA and NOAC, the Fisher exact test was used. To compare continuous variables, the t-test or the non-parametric Mann–Whitney test was used, according to the skewness of the data. Admission time stamps were grouped to four time-intervals (0–6, 6–12, 12–18, and 18–24 h) for comparing drug-specific concentration levels. The intraclass correlation co-efficient was calculated to evaluate the reliability of the two raters' scorings (two-way mixed, single-measure, or absolute agreement). All statistical tests are descriptive and no adjustment for multiple comparisons was made. Tests were 2-sided, and a $p < 0.05$ is regarded as significant. Analyses were conducted using IBM SPSS Statistics, version 25 and 26 (IBM Corp., Armonk, NY, USA).

3. Results

Of 3610 patients suffering from acute ischemic stroke and admitted during the 3.5-year study period, $n = 506$ patients with AF plus therapy with oral anticoagulation were identified. After excluding $n = 107$ patients, mainly because of known pause of oral anticoagulation >3 days, and further excluding $n = 14$ patients with additional, high cardio-embolic risks (mechanical heart valve or assist devices) and $n = 44$ patients who did not receive a full diagnostic work-up due to palliative care decisions, $n = 341$ patients were included in the analyses (VKA, $n = 127$ (37%), and NOAC, $n = 214$ (63%)) (see Figure 1 for patient in-/exclusion flow chart). Patients and case characteristics were well balanced between VKA- and NOAC-treated patients (see Table 1 for full patient details). Approximately half of the NOAC patients were treated with low-dose NOAC prescriptions (49.2%, Table 1). Concomitant antiplatelet therapy was prescribed more often in the NOAC than in the VKA group (10.3% vs. 2.4%, $p = 0.009$). While a total of 115 patients (33.7%) received endovascular therapy (EVT), with no difference between the VKA and NOAC group, fewer patients in the NOAC group were treated with intravenous thrombolysis (IVT, VKA 22.8% vs. NOAC, 7.5%, $p < 0.001$).

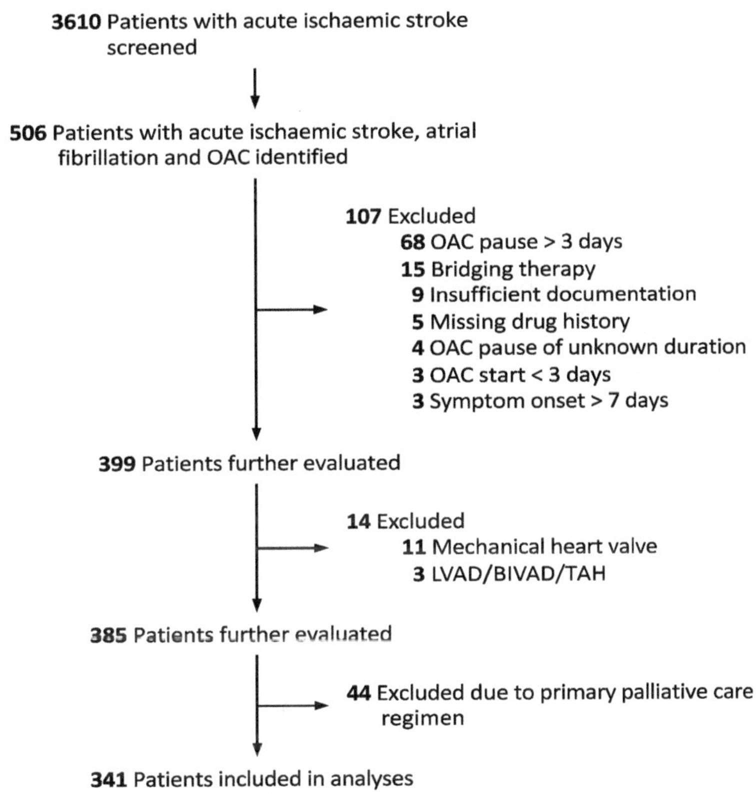

Figure 1. Flow chart of study population. OAC, oral anticoagulation; LVAD, left ventricular assist device; BIVAD, biventricular assist device; TAH, total artificial heart.

Table 1. Patients and case characteristics ($n = 341$).

	VKA ($n = 127$)	NOAC ($n = 214$)	p-Value
Age, mean (SD)	79.4 (8.0)	77.9 (8.9)	0.119
Women	57 (44.9)	102 (47.7)	0.654
NOAC			-
Apixaban	-	65 (30.4)	
Dabigatran	-	34 (15.9)	
Edoxaban	-	14 (6.5)	
Rivaroxaban	-	101 (47.2)	
Low-dose NOAC	-	97/197 (49.2)	
Phenprocoumon	125 (98.4)	-	
Concomitant antiplatelet therapy	3 (2.4)	22 (10.3)	0.009
Comorbidities			
Arterial hypertension	112 (88.2)	195 (91.1)	0.455
Diabetes mellitus	47 (37.0)	71 (33.2)	0.482
Hyperlipidemia	51 (40.2)	67 (31.3)	0.101
Ischemic heart disease	46 (36.2)	75 (35.0)	0.907

Table 1. *Cont.*

	VKA (n = 127)	NOAC (n = 214)	p-Value
Myocardial infarction	19 (15.0)	30 (14.0)	0.873
Peripheral artery disease	16 (12.6)	22 (10.3)	0.594
Stroke/TIA	39 (30.7)	81 (37.9)	0.198
Bleeding	6 (4.7)	14 (6.5)	0.635
Smoking	14 (11.0)	34 (15.9)	0.26
Malignancy, active	4 (3.3)	12 (5.9)	0.428
Renal function at admission			
GFR; mean (SD)	66.5 (22.3)	68.2 (20.3)	0.471
GFR < 50 mL/min	26 (20.5)	43 (20.1)	>0.99
GFR < 30 mL/min	9 (7.1)	8 (3.7)	0.201
Lipid levels, serum, mg/dl mmol/L			
HDL cholesterol	41 (34–51) 1.1 (0.9–1.3)	44 (35–52) 1.1 (0.9–1.3)	0.409
LDL cholesterol	90 (68–112) 2.3 (1.8–2.9)	97 (71–118) 2.5 (1.8–3.1)	0.202
LDL cholesterol ≥ 70 mg/dl (≥1.8 mmol/L)	89/120 (74.2)	161/204 (78.9)	0.34
Triglycerides	104 (72–129)	97 (71–128)	0.355
Onset (last-seen-well in case exact onset is unknown) to admission *, hours	3.7 (2.0–8.4)	3.5 (1.5–7.0)	0.445
Functional status			
Pre-stroke mRS	2 (1–3)	2 (1–3)	0.943
mRS at admission	4 (3–4)	3 (2–4)	0.251
mRS at discharge	3 (2–4)	3 (2–4)	0.799
NIHSS at admission	7 (3–17)	3 (3–16)	0.758
Imaging modality			
CT	123 (96.9)	210 (98.1)	0.477
MRI	32 (25.2)	54 (25.2)	>0.99
Large-vessel occlusion	61 (48.0)	109 (50.9)	0.654
IVT	29 (22.8)	16 (7.5)	<0.001
EVT	41 (32.3)	74 (34.6)	0.723
CAS	0 (0)	4 (1.9)	0.301
CEA	1 (0.8)	7 (3.3)	0.266

Data are median (IQR) or n (%) if not indicated otherwise. * exact onset or last-seen-well documented in n = 100 (VKA), and n = 148 (NOAC) cases. GFR, glomerular filtration rate; HDL, high-density lipoprotein; LDL, low-density lipoprotein; mRS, modified Rankin scale; NIHSS, National Institute of Health Stroke Scale; CT, computed tomography; MRI, magnet resonance imaging; IVT, intravenous thrombolysis; EVT, endovascular therapy; CAS, carotid artery stenting; CEA, carotid endarterectomy; VKA, vitamin K antagonist; NOAC, non-VKA oral anticoagulant.

3.1. *Time Trends*

While the absolute number of patients under VKA therapy suffering from an acute ischemic stroke decreased, a steeper increase in NOAC-treated patients was observed from 2015 to 2018, leading to an overall increase in OAC-associated ischemic strokes. The relative increase in NOAC-treated patients was independent of the admission type (external referral vs. direct admission), indicating a general trend (Figure 2).

3.2. *Coagulation Status*

A subtherapeutic INR <2.0 at admission was observed in 63.8% (n = 81) of the VKA-treated patients and an INR <1.8 in 52.8% (n = 67). INR values >3.0 were observed in 6.3% (n = 8). Those VKA patients with INR <2.0 had a median GFR of 75 mL/min (IQR 52–85), i.e., within the licensed GFR range for an alternative therapy with NOACs. For 88.3% (n = 189) of the patients with prescribed NOAC therapy, NOAC-specific quantitative coagulation testing was available at admission. NOAC concentrations ≤10 ng/mL were found in 22.9% (n = 49) and concentrations ≤30 ng/mL in 29.9% (n = 64) of the NOAC-treated patients. In a sensitivity analysis, performed due to the more rapid on- and offset of NOACs compared to VKA, we limited the analysis to patients admitted within a maximum of 12 h since "last-seen-well" (87.5% of $n = 248$ patients with clear documented "last-seen-well"). There was no difference in the fraction of patients with NOAC concentrations ≤10 ng/mL ($p = 0.514$), or ≤30 ng/mL ($p > 0.99$) respectively, between patients admitted within >12 h after "last-seen-well" and <12 h. In patients admitted in longer-time-windows, NOAC-specific tests were performed less frequently. Measured NOAC concentrations also did not differ between admission time intervals ($p = 0.193$). However, concentrations ≤10 ng/mL were determined in more patients receiving once-daily dosing than in patients with twice-daily dosing regimens (77.6% vs. 22.4%, $p < 0.001$).

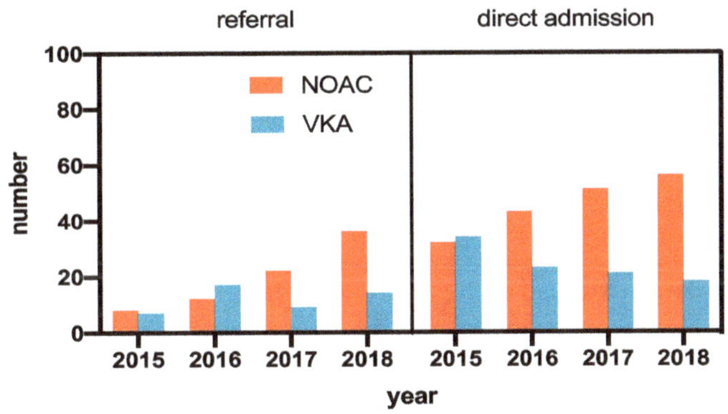

Figure 2. Admission time trend of patients with acute ischemic stroke and known AF and oral anticoagulation. VKA, vitamin K antagonist; NOAC, non-VKA oral anticoagulant. For 2018, data were extrapolated from the first half of the year.

3.3. Dosage Errors

In a total of 58 patients (31%) from the NOAC group for whom full documented medication schedules were available ($n = 187$, 87.4%), pre-stroke dosage errors were encountered. Of the 58 patients, $n = 13$ (22.4%) received a non-licensed dosage according to the most recent prescription labelling for prevention of stroke or systemic embolism in AF: OD instead of BD prescription, dabigatran $n = 4$, apixaban, $n = 4$; rivaroxaban was prescribed at 10 mg OD in $n = 3$ patients, and in one patient, 2.5 mg BD in combination with aspirin 100 mg per day was prescribed. In addition, one patient received a dose of 15 mg rivaroxaban BD (i.e., a higher than indicated dose) due to failure to reduce the dosage 21 days after a pulmonary embolism two months before stroke. Furthermore, in 45 patients, a heterogeneous pattern of further dosing errors was observed, mainly due to underdosing. Rivaroxaban-treated patients were more often underdosed ($n = 23/86$, 26.7%,) than patients receiving the factor Xa inhibitors apixaban ($n = 9/59$, 15.3%) and edoxaban ($n = 1/14$, 7.1%). A potential underdose was observed in $n = 4$ patients under dabigatran treatment (low dose despite age 75–80 years and GFR > 50 mL/min). In contrast, overdosing was observed less frequently among all patients (rivaroxaban, $n = 5$ and edoxaban, $n = 2$). Of patients without dosage errors and admission within 12 h of last-seen-well, 23.9% had NOAC levels ≤10 ng/mL at admission, indicating potential non-intake.

3.4. Medication Errors

The composite 'medication error' of either laboratory-based evidence of insufficient anticoagulation (here defined as INR < 2.0 in the VKA- or drug-specific concentration <10 ng/mL in the NOAC-group, respectively) and/or dosage or dosing errors was observed in 183/332 patients (55.1%), with more medication errors in the VKA (81/127, 63.8%) than in the NOAC group (102/205, 49.8%; $p = 0.013$).

3.5. Etiologic Classification of OAC-Associated Strokes

A cardiac source of embolism without any further non-cardiac cause of embolism or thrombosis (ASCOD: C =1, ASOD = 0) was found in 16 patients (4.7%; $n = 4$ VKA, $n = 12$ NOAC). In the remaining 95.3% of patients with an adequate diagnostic work-up ($n = 321/337$), there was at least one additional

(a) potential, (b) uncertain, or (c) unlikely non-cardiac cause of stroke. Table 2 summarizes these causes. Briefly, a potentially atherosclerotic cause of stroke was considered (ASCOD: A = 1) in numerically fewer VKA- than NOAC-treated patients (VKA, 10.2% vs. NOAC, 16.5%, $p = 0.147$). Small-vessel disease was considered potentially causal (ASCOD: S = 1) in 16 patients (4.7%; $n = 3$ VKA, $n = 13$ NOAC, $p = 0.148$), and potentially causal or cause uncertain in 76 patients (22.3%) (Table 2). A rare, potentially causal disease (ASCOD: O = 1) was not found in any of the VKA- but was found in $n = 2$ of the NOAC-treated patients (polycythemia/thrombocythemia); neither of these two patients had been co-treated with antiplatelet agents at the time of stroke. An ipsilateral dissection was observed in $n = 2$ of the NOAC patients but in none of the VKA patients. Figure 3 provides a visualization of the ASCOD categorization, including the relative fraction of patients with present 'medication error' with regard to each ASCOD category. No incidence of a 'medication error' was found in 24/48 (50%) patients with a potentially atherosclerotic cause (ASCOD: A = 1) or in 8/16 patients (50%) with potentially causal small-vessel disease (ASCOD: S = 1).

Table 2. Etiologic classification.

Disease (Causality)	VKA ($n = 127$)	NOAC ($n = 214$)	p
Cardiac pathology (potential)	127	214	-
Atherosclerosis (potential)	13/125 (10.4)	35/212 (16.5)	0.147
Atherosclerosis (potential or uncertain)	19/125 (15.2)	42/212 (19.8)	0.309
Small-vessel disease (potential)	3 (2.4)	13 (6.1)	0.184
Small-vessel disease (potential or uncertain)	21 (16.5)	55 (25.7)	0.059
Other causes (potential)	0 (0)	2 (0.9)	0.531
Dissection (potential)	0 (0)	2 (0.9)	0.531
Insufficient work-up (N9)	2 (1.6)	2 (0.9)	0.63

Data are n (%). ASCOD, A: atherosclerosis; S: small-vessel disease; O: other causes; D: dissection. The category C (cardiac pathology) was set to potential (1) in all patients due to the known atrial fibrillation. Presence of any further disease category (in any grade) was allowed in all categories but N9. N9 = insufficient work-up in ≥1 of the ASCOD categories. VKA, vitamin K antagonist; NOAC, non-VKA oral anticoagulant.

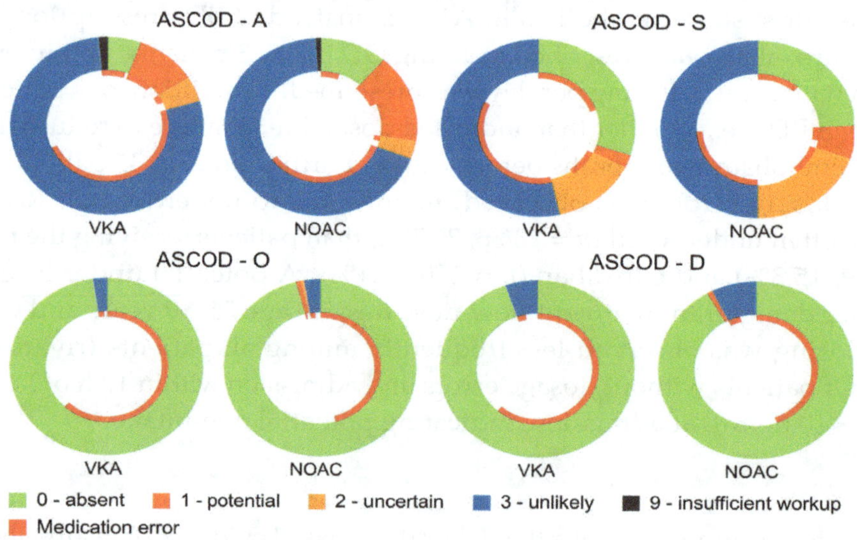

Figure 3. Visualization of the ASCOD categorization, including the relative fraction of patients with present 'medication error' with regard to each ASCOD category (inner red circle). Medication error was defined as either laboratory-based evidence of insufficient anticoagulation (here defined as INR < 2.0 in the VKA-, or drug-specific concentration < 10 ng/mL in the NOAC-group, respectively) and/or dosage or dosing errors. ASCOD, A: atherosclerosis; S: small-vessel disease; O: other causes; D: dissection. The category C (cardiac pathology) was set to 1 in all patients due to the known atrial fibrillation and, thus, is not presented. VKA, vitamin K antagonist; NOAC, non-VKA oral anticoagulant.

4. Discussion

Our study investigated different etiologies of stroke in patients with known AF despite oral anticoagulation and reveals two major findings: (1) medication errors are observed in more than half of the patients, and (2) relevant non-cardiac causes of stroke are prevalent in up to one-fifth of the patients.

Low rates of anticoagulation due to practical concerns like, for example, the requirement of frequent routine INR monitoring to adjust the dosing schemes, were among the reasons triggering the development of NOACs. In patients treated with VKA, we observed INR below the therapeutic range (<2.0) in 64%. Since it has been previously shown that the relative benefit of NOACs over VKA, in terms of the reduction of vascular events, and mortality is increasing at centers with poor INR control compared to good control [14], a stringent INR monitoring, as well as early considerations to switch to NOACs if the INR is not achieving the therapeutic range, is recommended [15]. In contrast to VKA, routine monitoring is still not recommended in NOACs [9]. Indeed, according to our data, potential medication errors are reduced with NOACs compared to VKA in patients who suffer from stroke, despite oral anticoagulation, but continue to occur in approximately 50%.

Approximately one-fifth of the patients without formal dosage-error had even very low NOAC-levels (≤10 ng/mL), and actual non-intake of the prescribed medication must be assumed as the most probable reason for this finding. Further reasons for medication errors include a tendency to use lower than indicated doses, especially due to failures to adjust dosage according to current renal function. Rivaroxaban, the factor Xa inhibitor with the most variable available doses in different indications [16], was the NOAC showing the highest rate of medication errors. Another study recently reported a rate of up to 65% of patients with Factor Xa inhibitor treatment having received an inappropriate dose regimen before stroke [17]. Furthermore, lower plasma levels at admissions were associated with greater stroke severity [17,18]. Although different available doses principally enhance the possibility to better tailor individual medications, our data underline the growing need to educate prescribing physicians. Software-based systems might, by integrating diagnoses, weight, and GFR/creatinine levels, support physicians.

We also observed that therapy with NOACs given on a once-daily dosing regimen led to a 3.5-fold relative increase in low (≤10 ng/mL) specific NOAC concentrations at admission compared to NOACs given twice daily. It is known that the peak-to-trough variability is larger for once-daily dosing; furthermore, single omitted doses lead to a greater decrease in plasma levels in a once-daily vs. a twice-daily regimen [19]. As it is extremely difficult in practice to manage patient adherence more closely, the broad implementation of smart tools reminding patients to take their drugs is important (reminder packaging) [20]. Data from larger population-based registries will help to gain more insight into the potential risks of once-daily regimens for NOACs with short half-lives, especially in patients with healthy kidneys.

Due to the observational nature of our study, we cannot prove that medication errors caused the ischemic stroke event in individual patients or determine the level to which a concurrent risk factor contributed to the stroke. However, in 50% of the patients with a potentially atherosclerotic cause or relevant small-vessel disease, no medication error was detected. Risk factors such as arterial hypertension, diabetes, and chronic heart failure (i.e., risk factors for both atherosclerotic and small-vessel disease) further increase the risk of stroke in patients with AF, and thus, were integrated in the commonly used $CHA_2DS2VASc$ score [21]. Currently available data cannot determine whether adding a low-dose antiplatelet to a NOAC would be beneficial or not in preventing recurrent stroke in patients with significant atherosclerosis and AF [22,23], a therapeutic option that warrants examination in a randomized clinical trial.

To make full use of stroke prevention, lowering low-density lipoprotein (LDL) levels should also be kept in focus. Current LDL level targets were only reached in a minority in our study, with 77% of the patients having LDL cholesterol levels ≥70 mg/dl (≥1.8 mmol/L), which is the recommended upper threshold according to recent guidelines for patients at high risk [24,25].

As a strength of our study, NOAC plasma levels at administration were available for 88% of patients from routine clinical testing; therefore, reliance on medication history alone was not necessary to determine potential medication errors. Due to the different pharmacokinetics of NOACs compared to VKA, it is impossible to extrapolate the actual level at the time of stroke-onset from a single measured value later on. Acknowledging the rapid on- and offset of NOACs, we performed a sensitivity analysis by limiting the analysis to those patients who were admitted within 12 h of last-seen-well before, but could not find any difference in the fraction of patients with low NOAC levels compared to patients arriving in later time-windows. This reflects a previously shown high variability of NOAC concentrations, even when similar intervals since last intakes are compared [26].

While we classified all our study data based on the existence of a potential cardiac etiology due to AF irrespective of medication status (as suggested by the ASCOD classification), this was handled differently in another observational study on stroke patients receiving NOAC [27].

Our study also has some limitations. We did not co-register current use of lipid-lowering therapies, such as statins, which might have pleiotropic effects in addition to the mechanistic function of lowering LDL [28]. Due to the observational nature of our study, all data are hypothesis-generating, but might help to inform future interventional trials. We did not include a matched cohort of non-stroke patients because the comprehensive work-up at the level done in stroke patients to unveil even less common cardiovascular diseases is not performed routinely in other diseases. While we observed a continuous increase in ischemic strokes despite NOAC therapy and a stabilizing rate of VKA-associated strokes, a population-based analysis would be necessary to elucidate the potential underlying reasons for this trend. An increase in oral anticoagulation therapies, in general, with preferred primary use of NOACs, and consequently increasing stroke rates would correspond with results from registries [29].

5. Conclusions

Medication errors in patients with AF suffering from ischemic strokes despite therapy with oral anticoagulants are still common, despite the introduction of NOACs. Concurrent risk factors, such as atherosclerotic disease and hypercholesterinemia are not treated adequately. Interventional trials need to determine whether better patient education, e.g., in conjunction with smart devices to increase therapy adherence, as well as a more stringent follow-up of these patients with AF to optimize concurrent risk factor treatment would be sufficient to reduce the risk of stroke in these high-risk group.

Author Contributions: Conceptualization, J.C.P.; Formal analysis, J.C.P., K.H. and J.K.; Investigation, K.H. and J.K.; Methodology, J.C.P. and P.A.R.; Supervision, J.C.P.; Validation, J.C.P., K.H. and J.K.; Visualization, J.C.P.; Writing—original draft, J.C.P.; Writing—review & editing, J.C.P., K.H., J.K. and P.A.R. All authors have read and agreed to the published version of the manuscript.

Acknowledgments: The authors acknowledge Sherryl Sundell for language editing.

References

1. Hart, R.G.; Pearce, L.A.; Aguilar, M.I. Meta-analysis: Antithrombotic therapy to prevent stroke in patients who have nonvalvular atrial fibrillation. *Ann. Intern. Med.* **2007**, *146*, 857–867. [CrossRef] [PubMed]
2. Connolly, S.J.; Eikelboom, J.; Joyner, C.; Diener, H.C.; Hart, R.; Golitsyn, S.; Flaker, G.; Avezum, A.; Hohnloser, S.H.; Diaz, R.; et al. Apixaban in patients with atrial fibrillation. *N. Engl. J. Med.* **2011**, *364*, 806–817. [CrossRef] [PubMed]
3. Ruff, C.T.; Giugliano, R.P.; Braunwald, E.; Hoffman, E.B.; Deenadayalu, N.; Ezekowitz, M.D.; Camm, A.J.; Weitz, J.I.; Lewis, B.S.; Parkhomenko, A.; et al. Comparison of the efficacy and safety of new oral anticoagulants with warfarin in patients with atrial fibrillation: A meta-analysis of randomised trials. *Lancet* **2014**, *383*, 955–962. [CrossRef]
4. Diener, H.C.; Connolly, S.J.; Ezekowitz, M.D.; Wallentin, L.; Reilly, P.A.; Yang, S.; Xavier, D.; Di Pasquale, G.; Yusuf, S.; RE-LY Study Group. Dabigatran compared with warfarin in patients with atrial fibrillation and

previous transient ischaemic attack or stroke: A subgroup analysis of the RE-LY trial. *Lancet Neurol.* **2010**, *9*, 1157–1163. [CrossRef]

5. Hankey, G.J.; Patel, M.R.; Stevens, S.R.; Becker, R.C.; Breithardt, G.; Carolei, A.; Diener, H.C.; Donnan, G.A.; Halperin, J.L.; Mahaffey, K.W.; et al. Rivaroxaban compared with warfarin in patients with atrial fibrillation and previous stroke or transient ischaemic attack: A subgroup analysis of ROCKET AF. *Lancet Neurol.* **2012**, *11*, 315–322. [CrossRef]
6. Easton, J.D.; Lopes, R.D.; Bahit, M.C.; Wojdyla, D.M.; Granger, C.B.; Wallentin, L.; Alings, M.; Goto, S.; Lewis, B.S.; Rosenqvist, M.; et al. Apixaban compared with warfarin in patients with atrial fibrillation and previous stroke or transient ischaemic attack: A subgroup analysis of the ARISTOTLE trial. *Lancet Neurol.* **2012**, *11*, 503–511. [CrossRef]
7. Rost, N.S.; Giugliano, R.P.; Ruff, C.T.; Murphy, S.A.; Crompton, A.E.; Norden, A.D.; Silverman, S.; Singhal, A.B.; Nicolau, J.C.; SomaRaju, B.; et al. Outcomes With Edoxaban Versus Warfarin in Patients With Previous Cerebrovascular Events: Findings From ENGAGE AF-TIMI 48 (Effective Anticoagulation With Factor Xa Next Generation in Atrial Fibrillation-Thrombolysis in Myocardial Infarction 48). *Stroke* **2016**, *47*, 2075–2082. [CrossRef]
8. Seiffge, D.J.; De Marchis, G.M.; Koga, M.; Paciaroni, M.; Wilson, D.; Cappellari, M.; Macha Md, K.; Tsivgoulis, G.; Ambler, G.; Arihiro, S.; et al. Ischemic Stroke despite Oral Anticoagulant Therapy in Patients with Atrial Fibrillation. *Ann. Neurol.* **2020**. [CrossRef]
9. Drouet, L.; Bal Dit Sollier, C.; Steiner, T.; Purrucker, J. Measuring non-vitamin K antagonist oral anticoagulant levels: When is it appropriate and which methods should be used? *Int. J. Stroke* **2016**, *11*, 748–758. [CrossRef]
10. Wardlaw, J.M.; Smith, E.E.; Biessels, G.J.; Cordonnier, C.; Fazekas, F.; Frayne, R.; Lindley, R.I.; O'Brien, J.T.; Barkhof, F.; Benavente, O.R.; et al. Neuroimaging standards for research into small vessel disease and its contribution to ageing and neurodegeneration. *Lancet Neurol.* **2013**, *12*, 822–838. [CrossRef]
11. Fazekas, F.; Chawluk, J.B.; Alavi, A.; Hurtig, H.I.; Zimmerman, R.A. MR signal abnormalities at 1.5 T in Alzheimer's dementia and normal aging. *AJR Am. J. Roentgenol.* **1987**, *149*, 351–356. [CrossRef] [PubMed]
12. Amarenco, P.; Bogousslavsky, J.; Caplan, L.R.; Donnan, G.A.; Wolf, M.E.; Hennerici, M.G. The ASCOD phenotyping of ischemic stroke (Updated ASCO Phenotyping). *Cerebrovasc. Dis.* **2013**, *36*, 1–5. [CrossRef] [PubMed]
13. Bamford, J.; Sandercock, P.; Dennis, M.; Burn, J.; Warlow, C. Classification and natural history of clinically identifiable subtypes of cerebral infarction. *Lancet* **1991**, *337*, 1521–1526. [CrossRef]
14. Wallentin, L.; Yusuf, S.; Ezekowitz, M.D.; Alings, M.; Flather, M.; Franzosi, M.G.; Pais, P.; Dans, A.; Eikelboom, J.; Oldgren, J.; et al. Efficacy and safety of dabigatran compared with warfarin at different levels of international normalised ratio control for stroke prevention in atrial fibrillation: An analysis of the RE-LY trial. *Lancet* **2010**, *376*, 975–983. [CrossRef]
15. Hindricks, G.; Potpara, T.; Dagres, N.; Arbelo, E.; Bax, J.J.; Blomstrom-Lundqvist, C.; Boriani, G.; Castella, M.; Dan, G.A.; Dilaveris, P.E.; et al. 2020 ESC Guidelines for the diagnosis and management of atrial fibrillation developed in collaboration with the European Association of Cardio-Thoracic Surgery (EACTS). *Eur. Heart J.* **2020**. [CrossRef]
16. European Medicines Agency. *European Public Assessment Report (EPAR) for Xarelto*; European Medicines Agency: Amsterdam, The Netherland, 2019.
17. Stoll, S.; Macha, K.; Marsch, A.; Gerner, S.T.; Siedler, G.; Frohlich, K.; Volbers, B.; Strasser, E.F.; Schwab, S.; Kallmunzer, B. Ischemic stroke and dose adjustment of oral Factor Xa inhibitors in patients with atrial fibrillation. *J. Neurol.* **2020**, *267*, 1–6. [CrossRef]
18. Macha, K.; Marsch, A.; Siedler, G.; Breuer, L.; Strasser, E.F.; Engelhorn, T.; Schwab, S.; Kallmunzer, B. Cerebral Ischemia in Patients on Direct Oral Anticoagulants. *Stroke* **2019**, *50*, 873–879. [CrossRef]
19. Vrijens, B.; Heidbuchel, H. Non-vitamin K antagonist oral anticoagulants: Considerations on once- vs. twice-daily regimens and their potential impact on medication adherence. *Europace* **2015**, *17*, 514–523. [CrossRef]
20. Costa, E.; Giardini, A.; Savin, M.; Menditto, E.; Lehane, E.; Laosa, O.; Pecorelli, S.; Monaco, A.; Marengoni, A. Interventional tools to improve medication adherence: Review of literature. *Patient Prefer Adherence* **2015**, *9*, 1303–1314. [CrossRef]

3

Mortality Prediction of the CHA2DS2-VASc Score, the HAS-BLED Score, and their Combination in Anticoagulated Patients with Atrial Fibrillation

Doralisa Morrone [1,†], Sonja Kroep [2,†], Fabrizio Ricci [3,4], Giulia Renda [3], Giuseppe Patti [5], Paulus Kirchhof [6,7], Ling-Hsiang Chuang [2], Ben van Hout [2,8] and Raffaele De Caterina [1,4,*]

1 Division of Cardiology, Department of Surgical, Medical and Molecular Pathology and Critical Care Medicine, University of Pisa, 50124 Pisa, Italy; doralisa.morrone@unipi.it
2 Pharmerit—An OPEN Health Company, 3068 AV Rotterdam, The Netherlands; skroep@pharmerit.com (S.K.); ling-hsiang.chuang@york.ac.uk (L.-H.C.); bvanhout@pharmerit.com (B.v.H.)
3 Institute of Cardiology and Center of Excellence on Aging, G. d'Annunzio University, 66100 Chieti-Pescara, Italy; fabrizioricci@hotmail.it (F.R.); grenda@unich.it (G.R.)
4 Fondazione VillaSerena per la Ricerca, Città Sant'Angelo, 65013 Pescara, Italy
5 Department of Thoracic and Cardiovascular Diseases, University of Eastern Piedmont, 28100 Novara, Italy; giuseppe.patti@uniupo.it
6 University of Birmingham Institute of Cardiovascular Sciences, University of Birmingham, UHB and SWBH NHS Trusts, Birmingham B15 2TT, UK; p.kirchhof@bham.ac.uk
7 Heart and Vascular Center, Hamburg University, 20251 Hamburg, Germany
8 School of Health and Related Research (ScHARR), The University of Sheffield, Sheffield S10 2TN, UK
* Correspondence: raffaele.decaterina@unipi.it
† These authors share first authorship.

Abstract: Background and Objectives: Atrial fibrillation (AF) is associated with increased mortality, predictors of which are poorly characterized. We investigated the predictive power of the commonly used CHA_2DS_2-VASc score (congestive heart failure, hypertension, age $\geq$ 75 years [doubled], diabetes, stroke/transient ischemic attack/thromboembolism [doubled], vascular disease [prior myocardial infarction, peripheral artery disease, or aortic plaque], age 65–75 years, sex category [female]), the HAS-BLED score (hypertension, abnormal renal/liver function, stroke, bleeding history or predisposition, labile international normalized ratio [INR], elderly [age $\geq$ 65 years], drugs/alcohol concomitantly), and their combination for mortality in AF patients. Methods: The PREvention oF thromboembolic events—European Registry in Atrial Fibrillation (PREFER in AF) was a prospective registry including AF patients across seven European countries. We used logistic regression to analyze the relationship between the CHA_2DS_2-VASc and HAS-BLED scores and outcomes, including mortality, at one year. We evaluated the performance of logistic regression models by discrimination measures (C-index and DeLong test) and calibration measures (Hosmer and Lemeshow goodness-of-fit and integrated discrimination improvement (IDI), with bootstrap techniques for internal validation. Results: In 5209 AF patients with complete information on both scores, average one-year mortality was 3.1%. We found strong gradients between stroke/systemic embolic events (SSE), major bleeding and—specifically—mortality for both CHA_2DS_2-VASc and HAS-BLED scores, with a similar C-statistic for event prediction. The predictive power of the models with both scores combined, removing overlapping components, was significantly enhanced ($p < 0.01$) compared to models including either CHA_2DS_2-VASc or HAS-BLED alone: for mortality, C-statistic: 0.740, compared to 0.707 for CHA_2DS_2-VASc or 0.646 for HAS-BLED alone. IDI analyses supported the significant improvement for the combined score model compared to separate score models for all outcomes. Conclusions: Both the CHA_2DS_2-VASc and the HAS-BLED scores predict mortality similarly in patients with AF, and a combination of their components increases prediction significantly. Such combination may be useful for investigational and—possibly—also clinical purposes.

Keywords: atrial fibrillation; morbidity; mortality; risk scores; CHA_2DS_2-VASc score; HAS-BLED score

1. Introduction

Atrial fibrillation (AF) is common, and is associated not only with high incidences of stroke, thromboembolism and disabilities, but also with significant mortality [1,2]. Treatment guidelines recommend considering both thromboembolic and bleeding risks when prescribing anticoagulation for stroke prevention in AF [1,2]. The CHA_2DS_2-VASc score (congestive heart failure, hypertension, age ≥ 75 years [doubled], diabetes, stroke/transient ischemic attack/thromboembolism [doubled], vascular disease [prior myocardial infarction, peripheral artery disease, or aortic plaque], age 65–75 years, sex category [female]) has been developed as a clinical risk score in patients with AF to predict the risk of stroke [3], and is now adopted in most widely used guidelines to assess such risk [1,2]. In some studies, the CHA_2DS_2-VASc score has also been used beyond its original purpose and disease populations. The score has been shown to predict outcomes broader than ischemic stroke, for instance thromboembolic events and death, in non-AF patient populations, such as patients with ischemic heart disease [4], diabetes [5], heart failure [6], in non-AF community patients [7], or in unselected patients [8]. The HAS-BLED score (hypertension, abnormal renal/liver function, stroke, bleeding history or predisposition, labile international normalized ratio [INR], elderly [age ≥ 65 years], drugs/alcohol concomitantly) was developed to predict bleeding amongst AF patients [9]. It is still widely used, although now de-emphasized due the lesser relevance of bleeding considerations in isolation to determine therapy for AF [1,2].

Due to the overlapping risk factors between CHA_2DS_2-VASc and HAS-BLED scores, both appear to predict adverse events of any kind. The compared performances of the two scores and their potential combination for the prediction of mortality have not been previously evaluated, and might be of interest due to the wide adoption of these scores. The aim of the current study was to investigate such predictive power in patients with AF.

2. Methods

Individual patient data were pooled from the PREvention oF thromboembolic events—European Registry in Atrial Fibrillation (PREFER in AF), a prospective registry of 7243 AF patients from 461 hospitals and 7 European countries (Austria, France, Germany, Italy, Spain, Switzerland, and the United Kingdom) conducted between January 2012 and January 2013, with 1-year follow-up. Details of the PREFER in AF Registry, including main findings at enrolment and definitions used, have been published [10]. For the purpose of this study, we focused on the following outcomes: ischemic stroke and or systemic embolic events (SEE), major bleeding and all-cause mortality.

2.1. Registry Data and Patients' Population

Patients were included in the PREFER in AF registry if they were at least 18 years of age, gave written informed consent for participation, and had a history of AF documented by electrocardiography or by an implanted pacemaker or defibrillator within the preceding 12 months. Patients were consecutively enrolled with no explicit exclusion criteria in order to avoid selection biases. Patients' characteristics, including demographic and clinical data, information on risk factors and treatment strategies, were collected at baseline and entered into an electronic case-report form with on-site verification of source data in approximately 5% of the sites. The study management was overseen by a scientific Steering Committee, as published [10]. Baseline data were collected between January 2012 and January 2013. A total of 7243 patients were enrolled in 461 centers from seven European countries (Austria, France, Germany, Italy, Spain, Switzerland, and the U.K.). For regional comparisons, Austria, Switzerland, and Germany were combined into one pre-specified region labelled "DACH". Forty-two percent of enrolling physicians were office-based, and 53% were hospital-based; 89% were cardiologists. After baseline inclusion, patients were followed-up for one year, recording information on clinical events, clinical characteristics, patterns of prescriptions and patients' adherence to guidelines, quality of life and treatment satisfaction.

One year after the baseline enrolment, patients underwent a follow-up visit (12 ± 2 months after baseline visit). As for the baseline visit, all data were captured through an electronic case report form (eCRF) including a wide range of plausibility checks for the entered variables. In addition, on-site source data verification was performed in approximately 5% of the sites. The study management was executed through a contract research organization (SSS International Clinical Research GmbH, Munich, Germany). The study management was overseen by a scientific steering committee. Considered variables were the same as the enrollment visit, including demographic data, data about AF incidence and type, heart rate and symptoms, risk factors and comorbidities, thromboembolic risk evaluated by $CHADS_2$ and CHA_2DS_2-VASc score, bleeding risk from the HAS-BLED score, history of significant clinical events and hospitalizations, treatment for AF, and anticoagulation quality evaluated by the last 3 INR values prior to follow-up visit.

Patients who completed both CHA_2DS_2-VASc and HAS-BLED risk scores at baseline and at the one-year follow-up were included in the current study. The CHA_2DS_2-VASc score ranges between 0 and 9, with a higher score indicating a higher risk of stroke. HAS-BLED also ranges between 0 and 9, with a higher score indicating a higher risk of bleeding. For the purpose of this analysis, the CHA_2DS_2-VASc and HAS-BLED risk scores at study entry were used. For the analysis of their combination, overlapping components were used only once. Because of some differences in the definition of hypertension (blood pressure consistently above 140/90 mmHg or treated hypertension on medication in the CHA_2DS_2-VASc score [3]; uncontrolled, >160 mmHg systolic in the HAS-BLED score [9]), the more inclusive definition of hypertension in the CHA_2DS_2-VASc score was retained for the combination score, in this case therefore ranging between 0 and 12. Sensitivity analyses were conducted to assess whether medication type had an effect on the model performance.

2.2. *Outcomes*

The combined endpoint of ischemic stroke and/or SEE was defined as ischemic stroke, transient ischemic attack (TIA) ("a small ischemic stroke"), arterial embolism, venous thromboembolic event, or pulmonary thromboembolism event during the follow-up. Major bleeding was defined, according to the definition of the International Society on Thrombosis and Haemostasis (ISTH), as gastrointestinal bleeding, intracerebral bleeding, or other life-threatening or major bleeding occurring during the follow-up [11]. Estimates of death rates relied on spontaneous reporting. Data were extracted from the comments section of the electronic case-report form and then verified with each site to gain more information about their validity.

2.3. *Statistical Methods*

Descriptive statistics are presented here as frequencies and percentages (n, %) for categorical variables, and as means and standard deviations (SDs) for continuous variables. The difference in baseline characteristics between the study sample and non-study sample were tested, using the Chi-squared test, the rank sum test, or the *t*-test as appropriate.

Logistic regression was used to separately analyze the relationships between the three outcome events (i.e., stroke/SSE, major bleeding and mortality) and the CHA_2DS_2-VASc and HAS-BLED scores. For each outcome, five analyses were conducted, evaluating different sets of explanatory variables. The first two analyses evaluated the predictive power of the CHA_2DS_2-VASc scores. One analysis included the total risk score as a continuous explanatory variable (ranging from 0 to 9), while the second analysis evaluated the individual items of the CHA_2DS_2-VASc score [3] as explanatory variables, which were treated as dichotomous variables [i.e., congestive heart failure (or left ventricular systolic dysfunction), hypertension: blood pressure consistently above 140/90 mmHg (or treated hypertension on medication), age: ≥75 years, age 65–74 years, diabetes mellitus, prior stroke or transient ischemic attack or thromboembolism, vascular disease (i.e., peripheral artery disease, myocardial infarction, aortic plaque), female sex]. The third and fourth analyses considered the HAS-BLED score [9], with one analysis including the total risk score only as a continuous exploratory variable (ranging from 0–9), and a second analysis considering individual components of the HAS-BLED scores [9] as dichotomous variables (i.e., hypertension, abnormal renal/liver function, stroke, bleeding history or predisposition, labile international normalized ratio, age $\geq$ 65 years, drugs/alcohol concomitantly). For the final analysis, the combination of individual items of the CHA_2DS_2-VASc and HAS-BLED scores were used as explanatory variables (dichotomously) rather than a combination of the total score, excluding double reporting of overlapping risk items. The confidence intervals of the coefficients for each logistic regression model were corrected for bias and skewness in the distribution of the bootstrap estimates, for which the average was taken over 100 repetitions, obtained by bootstrap with resampling.

The performance of each model was evaluated by discrimination and calibration [12]. To evaluate discrimination, we used the C-index (area under the curve, AUC) using bootstrap to obtain bias-corrected standard errors, after which the null-hypothesis of no differences between the C-indexes of the models was tested using the Wald test. In addition, we evaluated the integrated discrimination improvement (IDI) [13]. We assessed calibration, referring to the agreement between observed number of events and predicted probability of the occurrence of these events [14], using the Hosmer and Lemeshow goodness-of-fit test.

We performed all analyses with the STATA statistical software (StataCorp. 2017. Release 15. College Station, TX, USA).

3. Results

3.1. Patient Characteristics

In the original PREFER in AF population, of the 7243 patients, age (mean $\pm$ SD) was 71.5 $\pm$ 11 years, 60.1% were male, and the CHA_2DS_2VASc score was 3.4 $\pm$ 1.8. Thirty percent of the patients had paroxysmal, 24.0% persistent, 7.2% long-standing persistent, and 38.8% permanent AF. Oral anticoagulation (OAC) was used in most patients: 4799 patients (66.3%) received a vitamin K antagonist (VKA) as mono-therapy, 720 patients (9.9%) a combination of VKA and antiplatelet agents (AP), and 442 patients (6.1%) received a new oral anticoagulant drugs (NOAC). AP alone was given in 808 patients (11.2%) and there was no antithrombotic therapy in 474 patients (6.5%). Amongst 5209 patients who had complete information for both the CHA_2DS_2VASc and HAS-BLED scores at baseline, the mean age was 71.8 $\pm$ 10.5 years; 3145 subjects (60.4%) were male. This subsample of 5209 patients was representative of the whole sample population published in the registry [10] across a wide spectrum of baseline variables, including comorbidities. Patients' characteristics at baseline are shown in Table 1. Stroke risk was high (mean CHA_2DS_2VASc total score of 3.4 $\pm$ 1.8), with a total score ranging between 2 and 5 in the majority of patients (>70%). Bleeding risk had a total score ranging from 1 to 3 in >80% of cases, and a mean HAS-BLED total score of 2.0 $\pm$ 1.1. There was a different representation of the type of AF: permanent AF was found more frequently, accounting for 2070 patients (40%); long-standing persistent AF was the least represented category, with only 391 patients (7.52%); and paroxysmal and persistent AF accounted for 1499 and 1239 patients (29% vs. 24%), respectively. In terms of treatment, the majority of patients (3548, 68%) were on treatment with a vitamin K antagonist (VKA) at baseline, and with a small number (305 patients, 6%) taking a non-vitamin K antagonist oral anticoagulant (NOAC).

Table 1. Patients' characteristics at baseline.

		n	%
Patients		5209	100.0
Age, mean (SD)		71.76	
Male gender		3145	60.4
Country			
	France	1264	24.3
	DACH	543	10.4
	Italy	1088	20.9
	Spain	1399	26.9
	UK	915	17.6
Education			
	Primary school	2500	48.0
	Secondary school	1651	31.7
	University or above	726	13.9
	Missing	332	6.4
AF Type			
	Paroxysmal	1499	28.8
	Persistent	1239	23.8
	Long-standing persistent	391	7.5
	Permanent	2070	39.7
	MIssing	10	0.2
Medication at Baseline Visit			
	NOAC	305	5.9
	VKA	3548	68.1
	Antiplatelet	540	10.4
	VKA+Antiplatelet	539	10.4
	Neither NOAC nor VKA nor Antiplatelet	277	5.3
Medication at Follow-up visits			
	NOAC	637	12.2
	VKA	3284	63.0
	Antiplatelet	389	7.5
	VKA + Antiplatelet	306	5.9
	Neither NOAC nor VKA nor Antiplatelet	593	11.4
	0	233	4.5
	1	517	9.9
	2	823	15.8
	3	1138	21.9
	4	1176	22.6
	5	722	13.9
	6	376	7.2
	7	151	2.9
	8	63	1.2
	9	10	0.2
HAS-BLED			
	0	425	8.2
	1	1264	24.3
	2	1841	35.3
	3	1173	22.6
	4	396	7.6

Table 1. *Cont.*

	n	%
5	94	1.8
6	14	0.3
7	2	0.0
Additional comorbities		
	5209	100.0
Congestive heart failure	1546	29.7
Hypertension	3726	71.5
Diabetes mellitus	1181	22.7
Stroke/TIA	832	16.0
Vascular disease	1177	22.6
Renal function	696	13.4
Liver function	103	2.0
Stroke	475	9.1
Bleeding	244	4.7
Labile INR	692	13.3
Drug	1387	26.6
Alcohol	130	2.5

Abbreviations: SD = standard deviation; DACH = Germany, Austria, and Switzerland; AF = atrial fibrillation; NOAC = non-vitamin K antagonist oral anticoagulant; VKA = vitamin K antagonist; CHA2DS2-VASc = congestive heart failure, hypertension, age 75 years [doubled], diabetes, stroke/transient ischemic attack/thromboembolism [doubled], vascular disease [prior myocardial infarction, peripheral artery disease, or aortic plaque], age 65–75 years, sex category [female]; HAS-BLED = hypertension, abnormal renal/liver function, stroke, bleeding history or predisposition, labile international normalized ratio [INR], elderly [age ≥ 65 years], drugs/alcohol concomitantly; TIA = transient ischemic attack.

The majority of the non-study sample (n = 2034 patients, excluded when no risk scores were available) had similar baseline characteristics as patients included in the study sample, with the exception of chronic kidney disease (CKD), AF type at baseline, treatment with NOAC/VKA/antiplatelet agents, and age. CKD was more prevalent in the study sample compared to the non-study sample (study vs. non-study sample: 13.8% vs. 11.2%), while paroxysmal AF was more prevalent in the non-study sample (study vs. non-study sample: 28.8% vs. 33.0%). Patients were older in the study sample (study vs. non-study sample: 71.8 vs. 70.7 years). Finally, baseline treatment of VKA was more prevalent in the study sample, while NOAC and antiplatelet baseline treatment were more prevalent in the non-study sample.

3.2. *Outcome Distributions*

Rates of stroke/SEE and major bleeding at the one-year follow-up were 2.3% (122 patients) and 2.9% (149 patients), respectively. At one year, 3.1% of patients died (160 out of 5209). The percentage of patients with the examined outcomes (i.e., stroke/SSE, major bleeding, and death) in each risk score category of CHA_2DS_2VASc and HAS-BLED, respectively, are shown in Figures 1 and 2. There was a strong gradient between the outcome frequency and risk scores: overall, higher risk scores were both positively correlated with the occurred outcomes. However, there were very few events in the highest score category, with only 10 patients having a CHA_2DS_2-VASc total score of 9, and only 2 patients with a HAS-BLED total score of 7 (none reported a HAS-BLED total score of 8 or 9).

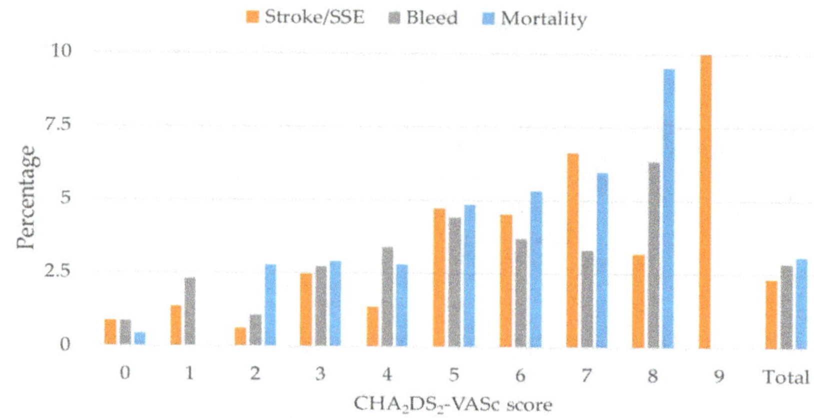

Figure 1. Outcomes (stroke/systemic embolic events (SSE), bleeding and mortality) by CHA_2DS_2-VASc risk score in the present study.

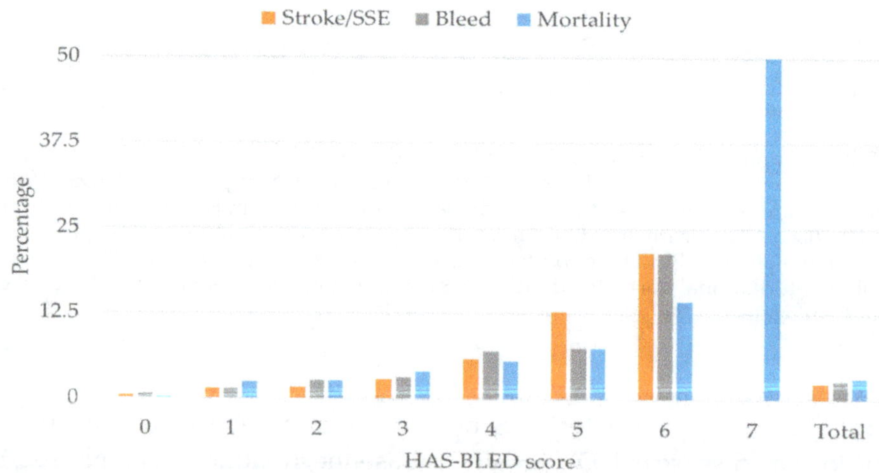

Figure 2. Outcomes (stroke/systemic embolic events (SSE), bleeding and mortality) by HAS-BLED risk score in the present study.

3.3. *Logistic Regression Analysis Results*

3.3.1. CHA_2DS_2-VASc Risk Score

The predictive values of the CHA_2DS_2-VASc risk score for each outcome event are shown in Table S1.

Amongst the models including only the total risk score of CHA_2DS_2-VASc as an explanatory variable, only the model predicting major bleeding had a good fit (p-value > 0.05), as indicated by the Hosmer–Lemeshow goodness-of-fit test (p = 0.014, 0.269 and 0.039 for stroke/SSE, major bleeding, and mortality, respectively). As suggested by the C-statistic, the predictive ability was highest for the model predicting stroke/SSE (0.584; 95% CI 0.536–0.637), followed by the model predicting mortality (0.559; 95% 0.513–0.604) and the model predicting major bleeding (0.520; 95% CI 0.478–0.567).

The models with individual components of the CHA_2DS_2VASc risk score presented a better fit according to the Hosmer–Lemeshow goodness-of-fit test (with the exception of the model predicting mortality) and an improved predictive ability compared to the model based on the total score alone. Components of the scores assessed here and showing a statistically significant coefficient were different across models predicting different outcomes. For instance, for predicting mortality, congestive heart failure, hypertension, age >75 years, and diabetes mellitus were statistically significant, whereas in predicting stroke/SSE, only the terms congestive heart failure and stroke/TIA had a statistically significant coefficient.

3.3.2. HAS-BLED Risk Score

For the models including only the total risk score of HAS-BLED as an explanatory variable, all models had a good fit (p-value > 0.05), as indicated by the Hosmer–Lemeshow goodness-of-fit test ($p = 0.432$, 0.594 and 0.250 for stroke/SSE, major bleeding, and mortality, respectively). Evaluating the models with individual components, the Hosmer–Lemeshow goodness-of-fit test indicated a good fit for all models as well (Table S2). The models with individual components were all compared to models with total scores (C-statistics were significantly improved, $p < 0.05$ for all models). However, items with statistically significant coefficients varied depending on the outcome of interest; for instance, history of bleeding was statistically significant for predicting major bleeding but was not statistically significant for predicting mortality or stroke/SSE (Table S2).

3.3.3. CHA_2DS_2-VASc and HAS-BLED Combined

Combining the individual components of the CHA_2DS_2VASc and HAS-BLED risk scores with the exclusion of duplicated items generated the most favorable predictive results. All models had a good fit, indicated by the lowest value of the Hosmer goodness-of-fit test (p-value > 0.05) with a C-statistic of 0.731 (95% CI 0.681–0.778), 0.702 (95% CI 0.659–0.747) and 0.740 (95% CI 0.699–0.780) for stroke/SSE, major bleeding, and mortality, respectively (Table 2). For predicting stroke/SSE, statistically significant items included congestive heart failure, stroke/TIA, abnormal liver function, labile INR, and drugs; for predicting major bleeding, statistically significant items included age >75 years, vascular disease, abnormal renal and liver function, bleeding and alcohol consumption; and for predicting mortality, statistically significant items included congestive heart failure, hypertension, age >75 years, abnormal renal and liver function.

The predictive performance of the models combining the CHA_2DS_2VASc and HAS-BLED components compared to the CHA_2DS_2-VASc individual component models alone was enhanced for the prediction of all outcomes (Table 3 and Figure 3). For mortality, the C-statistic showed a significant improvement (0.707 vs. 0.740, $p = 0.005$). Although the improvement in sensitivity was small, it was significant (IDI: 1.79%; $p < 0.001$). Similar results were demonstrated in models predicting stroke and major bleeding, with the largest improvements demonstrated in the model predicting stroke/SSE.

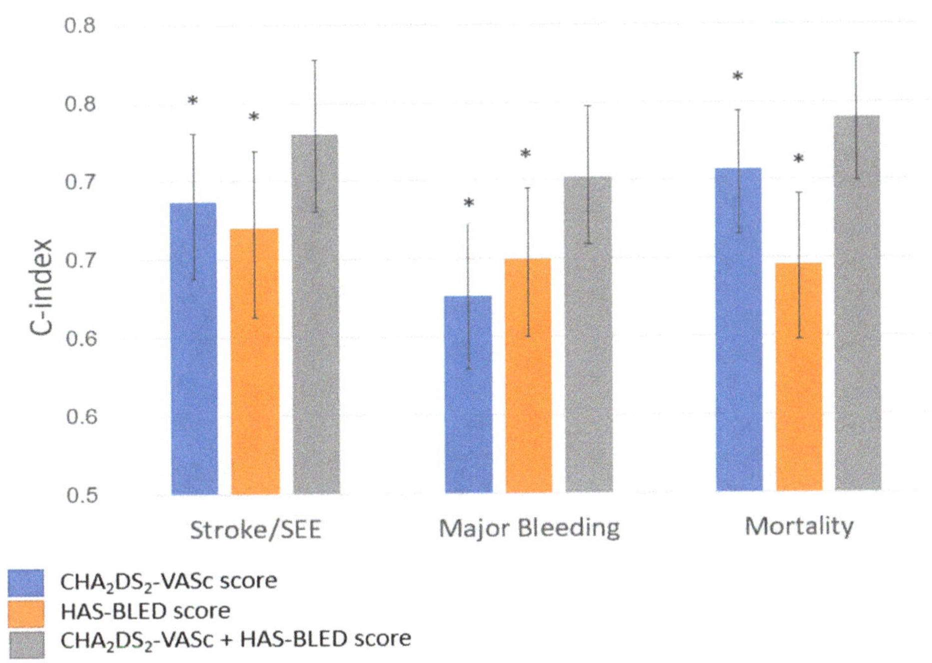

Figure 3. C-index of logistic models by outcome and predictor items risk scores; * denotes a C-index of the specific score significantly different (p-value < 0.05) from C-index of the combined score.

Table 2. Logit regression results with CHA2DS2-VASc and HAS-BLED combined.

	Coefficient	*p*-Value	Bias	95% CI (Bias-Corrected)		Log-Likelihood	Homes-LEWESHOW	C-Statistic	95% CI (Bias-Corrected)	
						−522.351	1.000	0.731	0.681	0.778
Stroke/Systemic Embolic Events										
Congestive heart failure	0.643	0.002	0.015	0.234	1.038					
Hypertension	−0.082	0.714	−0.016	−0.467	0.362					
Age >75 years	0.534	0.089	0.023	−0.059	1.190					
Diabetes mellitus	0.053	0.811	−0.026	−0.403	0.446					
Stroke/transient ischemic attack	1.017	0.000	0.011	0.625	1.308					
Vascular disease	−0.344	0.144	0.017	−0.840	0.071					
Age 65 to 74 years	0.037	0.917	0.022	−0.634	0.576					
Sex category	0.283	0.218	0.003	−0.231	0.648					
Abnormal renal function	−0.193	0.522	−0.016	−0.926	0.327					
Abnormal liver function	1.014	0.010	−0.041	0.087	1.686					
Bleeding	0.375	0.345	−0.117	−0.282	1.019					
Labile INR	0.920	0.000	−0.004	0.460	1.237					
Drug	0.872	0.000	−0.024	0.494	1.312					
Alcohol	0.690	0.183	−0.020	−0.502	1.551					
Constant	-5.079	0.000	−0.059	-5.740	−4.328					
Major bleeding						−628.686	0.999	0.702	0.659	0.747
Congestive heart failure	−0.138	0.487	−0.005	−0.581	0.221					
Hypertension	0.030	0.887	0.011	−0.353	0.472					
Age >75 years	0.661	0.015	0.035	0.066	1.119					
Diabetes mellitus	−0.134	0.498	−0.037	−0.579	0.216					
Stroke/transient ischemic attack	−0.136	0.582	0.022	−0.546	0.388					
Vascular disease	0.637	0.001	−0.015	0.299	1.069					
Age 65 to 74 years	−0.107	0.708	0.020	−0.618	0.368					
Sex category	0.035	0.868	−0.016	−0.305	0.453					
Abnormal renal function	0.541	0.006	0.032	0.264	1.002					
Abnormal liver function	0.890	0.022	−0.045	−0.005	1.654					
Bleeding	1.425	0.000	0.018	0.947	1.804					

Table 2. *Cont.*

		Coefficient	*p*-Value	Bias	95% CI (Bias-Corrected)		Log-Likelihood	Homes-LEWESHOW	C-Statistic	95% CI (Bias-Corrected)	
	Labile INR	0.417	0.059	0.007	0.119	0.937					
	Drug	0.219	0.263	−0.013	−0.043	0.677					
	Alcohol	0.904	0.023	−0.077	0.174	1.527					
	Constant	−4.428	0.000	−0.051	−4.976	−3.905					
Mortality							−649.047	0.233	0.740	0.699	0.780
	Congestive heart failure	0.802	0.000	0.001	0.365	1.075					
	Hypertension	−0.453	0.013	0.015	−0.811	−0.129					
	Age >75 years	1.051	0.000	0.032	0.460	1.476					
	Diabetes mellitus	0.246	0.222	−0.022	−0.119	0.684					
	Stroke/transient ischemic attack	0.070	0.743	0.013	−0.432	0.399					
	Vascular disease	0.082	0.705	−0.028	−0.335	0.459					
	Age 65 to 74 years	0.229	0.522	0.041	−0.627	0.825					
	Sex category	0.010	0.958	−0.032	−0.365	0.333					
	Abnormal renal function	0.969	0.000	0.032	0.481	1.269					
	Abnormal liver function	1.003	0.001	−0.032	0.399	1.602					
	Bleeding	0.420	0.152	−0.047	−0.229	0.829					
	Labile INR	0.111	0.661	−0.009	−0.411	0.539					
	Drug	0.259	0.178	0.003	−0.080	0.593					
	Alcohol	0.126	0.812	−0.120	−0.918	0.945					
	Constant	−4.625	0.000	−0.061	−5.200	−4.130					

Abbreviations: CHA_2DS_2-VASc = congestive heart failure, hypertension, age ≥75 years [doubled], diabetes, stroke/transient ischemic attack/thromboembolism [doubled], vascular disease [prior myocardial infarction, peripheral artery disease, or aortic plaque], age 65–74 years, sex category [female]; HAS-BLED = hypertension, abnormal renal/liver function, stroke, bleeding history or predisposition, labile international normalized ratio [INR], elderly [age ≥65 years], drugs/alcohol concomitantly.

Table 3. Evaluation of the predictive ability of the prediction models for the detection of stroke/SSE, major bleeding and mortality using C-index and integrated discrimination improvement indices.

Outcome		C-Statistic	95% CI (Bias-Corrected)		*p*-Value	IDI, %	*p*-Value
Stroke/SSE							
	CHA_2DS_2-VASc	0.687	0.638	0.730	REF		
	CHA_2DS_2-VASc + HAS-BLED	0.731	0.681	0.778	0.010	3.11	0.000
	HAS-BLED	0.670	0.613	0.719	REF		
	CHA_2DS_2-VASc + HAS-BLED	0.731	0.681	0.778	0.001	1.46	0.000
Major bleeding							
	CHA_2DS_2-VASc	0.626	0.579	0.672	REF	2.11	0.000
	CHA_2DS_2-VASc + HAS-BLED	0.702	0.659	0.747	0.000		
	HAS-BLED	0.650	0.600	0.698	REF	0.88	0.000
	CHA_2DS_2-VASc + HAS-BLED	0.702	0.659	0.747	0.002		
Mortality							
	CHA_2DS_2-VASc	0.707	0.666	0.744	REF		
	CHA_2DS_2-VASc + HAS-BLED	0.740	0.700	0.779	0.005	1.79	0.000
	HAS-BLED	0.646	0.598	0.691	REF		
	CHA_2DS_2-VASc + HAS-BLED	0.740	0.700	0.779	0.000	1.26	0.000

Abbreviations: SSE: Systemic Embolic Events; REF; reference model; IDI, integrated discriminating improvement index; CHA2DS2-VASc=congestive heart failure, hypertension, age ≥75 years [doubled], diabetes, stroke/transient ischemic attack/thromboembolism [doubled], vascular disease [prior myocardial infarction, peripheral artery disease, or aortic plaque], age 65–74 years, sex category [female]; HAS-BLED=hypertension, abnormal renal/liver function, stroke, bleeding history or predisposition, labile international normalized ratio [INR], elderly [age ≥65 years], drugs/alcohol concomitantly.

The improvement of the models with the CHA_2DS_2VASc and HAS-BLED combined components over the HAS-BLED individual component models alone was significant in all models in terms of C-statistic and IDI (Table 3 and Figure 3). Moreover, we found small but significant improvement in sensitivity for all outcomes

We found no heterogeneity in analyzing data restricted to patients on NOACs (Table S3). Details on the analyses broken down for AF type (paroxysmal, persistent, long-standing persistent, permanent) are reported in Table S4. We found numerical improvements of the C-statistic in all types of AF, although the achievement of statistically significant improvements was limited by the limitations of sample sizes.

4. Discussion

This study has three new major interesting findings: 1. Mortality was higher than the occurrence of stroke/SSE in the patient population of this nearly-contemporary registry with mostly anticoagulated AF patients; 2. Both the CHA_2DS_2VASc and the HAS-BLED risk scores were reasonably good predictors of stroke/SSE and major bleeding, but they were also good predictors of mortality; 3. A combination of items included in the two scores significantly improved prediction of death. These results may have practical implications for the prediction of adverse events in patients with AF.

AF is the most common type of heart rhythm disorder and is associated with a 1.5- to 1.9-fold higher risk of death in part due to the strong association with thromboembolic events. Since data from the Framingham heart study, AF has been known to be an independent risk factor for stroke [15]: therefore a major management decision in AF is determining the risk of stroke and appropriate antithrombotic treatment weighted against the risk of serious bleeding. The CHA_2DS_2-VASc and HAS-BLED risk scores are the most widely used algorithms to determine the yearly thromboembolic risk and to predict bleeding [16]. They were developed to predict stroke/SSE and bleeding in non-anticoagulated patients, and not developed to predict mortality, which is yet a numerically relevant endpoint in AF even when the risk of stroke/SSE is abated by anticoagulation. Determining, therefore, the comparative performances of these scores in anticoagulated patients not only for stroke/SSE and bleeding, but also for mortality, is new and medically relevant.

4.1. *Previous Study Comparisons: Scores for Stroke vs. Scores for Bleeding*

Previous data from the AMADEUS trial data base in AF patients anticoagulated with either idraparinux or VKAs demonstrated that the $CHADS_2$ and CHA_2DS_2-VASc scores (used for stroke risk assessment) could be used to predict serious bleeding, comparing against a score—HAS-BLED—intended for bleeding assessment [17]. In a subsequent comparison of stroke risk scores ($CHADS_2$ and CHA_2DS_2-VASc) and three bleeding risk scores [HAS-BLED, Outcomes Registry for Better Informed Treatment of Atrial Fibrillation (ORBIT), and AnTicoagulation and Risk factors In Atrial fibrillation (ATRIA)] from a large administrative database of NOAC-treated patients in routine clinical practice, $CHADS_2$, CHA_2DS_2-VASc, HAS-BLED, ORBIT and ATRIA scores had similar performances in predicting major bleeding, highlighting that patients at a high risk of stroke are also at high risk of bleeding [18]. Thus, previous data concur with the present findings, indicating that current risk scores, also because of overlapping components, do not have a high discriminating capacity for stroke/SSE vs. bleeding events.

4.2. *Previous Studies for Mortality Prediction in Atrial Fibrillation*

We carried out a comprehensive literature search to investigate published articles regarding the prediction of death through clinical scores derived for AF. We retrieved 25 published articles referring to mortality prediction (Table S5), Whenever in AF, all these studies referred to anticoagulated patients, a setting different from the original one used to derive the CHA_2DS_2-VASc score [3]. In several instances, causes of death in AF appeared unrelated to thromboembolism or bleeding. For example, in anticoagulated AF patients with a median CHA_2DS_2-VASc score of 4, Gallego et al. showed that more deaths (4.5/100 patient-years) occurred for causes other than a thromboembolic (only 1.3 patient-years) or a hemorrhagic event (0.4 patient-years). Here, the HAS-BLED score, besides bleeding, predicted adverse events, including all-cause and cardiovascular mortality [19].

Several studies out of AF have shown that scores such as HAS-BLED [20] and CHA_2DS_2-VASc [4,5,21–23] predict adverse events other than stroke and bleeding, including death. Some previous studies, such as the one from the GARFIELD-AF registry [24], have reported a better prediction of events than the two above scores. Previous literature converges in demonstrating death as a numerically frequent outcome in anticoagulated AF patients, more than thromboembolic or bleeding events; and that scores are general markers of risk, including the risk of death. No previous report, however, has addressed the possibility of predicting risk through a combination of CHA_2DS_2-VASc and HAS-BLED. This would have medical relevance due to the current widespread adoption of these scores.

4.3. Added Value of the Present Study from the PREFER in AF Registry

The PREFER in AF registry informed on AF patient profiles in a real-world clinical context, helping to identify specific at-risk patient groups, including those with comorbidities that predispose them to thrombotic events. The current study deriving from that registry is the first that compares and combines a stroke risk score with a bleeding score in order to give the best predictive value on mortality. In line with previously published studies, our report shows strong gradients between the CHA_2DS_2-VASc and the HAS-BLED risk scores and outcomes examined (stroke/SSE, major bleeding and death). Here, the CHA_2DS_2-VASc score predicts mortality, in addition to stroke/SSE, better than the HAS-BLED. Our study also confirms the previous literature in showing that statistical predictions are in any case sub-optimal, in the light of the moderately good C-statistic. The risk of stroke/SSE and major bleeding in our study population is slightly higher than in other publications studying the PREFER in AF registry (see references listed in Table S5). This is likely due to the higher risk of the population included and perhaps also because of the compression of risk of stroke and major bleeding observed with the introduction of the NOACs. Our study, in particular, highlights the different weight of the individual components of both scores to predict future death: here, the hierarchy of predictive weight included congestive heart failure, hypertension, age >75 years, and diabetes among the CHA_2DS_2-VASc components; whereas hypertension, liver function and age >65 years were the strongest predictors of mortality in the HAS-BLED risk score. The different weight of individual components in risk prediction for various outcomes is evidently diluted when attributing similar weights (1 or 2 points at best) to the individual components. The usefulness of pursuing a better statistical prediction in spite of reduced practicality—the main advantage of these easy-to-use scores—remains, however, debatable. A novelty here, however, is that the combination of non-duplicated components of the two scores had the highest predictive power for mortality, confirming on the one hand that both ischemic and bleeding events can predict—and in part trigger—the frequent occurrence of death in anticoagulated AF; but also that such components predict triggers of death not easily attributed to thromboembolism or bleeding. The ability to predict such occurrences may allow the focusing on treatment of modifiable risk factors, in addition to only focusing on thrombosis and bleeding, in such populations. Because of the widespread use of the CHA_2DS_2-VASc and of the HAS-BLED risk score, a combination of their individual components—as shown here—might be useful to risk-stratify patients in epidemiological surveys and prospective trials, as well as, possibly, to better allocate incremental preventive measures.

5. Limitations

Although recruitment of consecutive patients at each center was mandatory in PREFER in AF, we cannot exclude biases in patient enrollment and selection, as well as in treatment decisions. Patients excluded from the study sample were fairly numerous; therefore, a limitation is the relatively frequent lack of reporting of risk scores/missing values in the overall registry. Overall, mean age of the study sample was slightly older than in the non-study sample, but the different distribution of other factors (more use of VKA and higher prevalence of CKD) suggests that patient cases included were perhaps more severe than patients excluded. Such considerations limit, in any case, the generalizability of the findings to the unselected PREFER in AF population. Moreover, mortality data could not exactly reflect real mortality, because data were extracted from the comments section of the electronic case-report forms, making death reporting potentially less accurate. However, we estimated that errors in this largely undisputed outcome are unlikely to be numerically relevant. The investigators' diligence on reporting adverse events was here indeed crucial for the accuracy of data collection. As for model analyses, there were a couple of limitations when evaluating predictive ability using discrimination and calibration measures. Our study was aimed at mainly investigating the predictive power of the CHA_2DS_2-VASc and HAS-BLED risk scores, as well as their combination, on mortality, especially compared to the separate risk scores, therefore no re-calibration of coefficients was conducted. We also deliberately did not venture in analyzing causes of death, likely unprecise and not sufficiently controlled in the registry. The relative shortness of the study follow-up is a further limit with a focus on mortality, but data presented here are the first focusing on this endpoint in anticoagulated patients in attempts at improving prediction with a combination of the two most widely used scores. Finally, at the time of the PREFER in AF registry, most patients with AF were treated with VKAs, which does not reflect the current prevalent treatment with NOACs. Whether such limitations affect current applicability of our findings is likely minor, considering the lack of a biologic plausibility (we do not suspect differences in risk prediction once adequate anticoagulation is ensured), and the reassuring results of our sensitivity analyses. The usefulness of the newly proposed combination score should be now, however, further tested in independent cohorts.

6. Conclusions

Mortality is an important component, so far insufficiently underscored, of the risk connected with AF. The CHA_2DS_2-VASc and the HAS-BLED scores both predict mortality in AF, and a combination of all their components increases prediction significantly. Such combination may be clinically useful. Until now, the main focus of research in AF has been stroke/SSE and bleeding. The availability of robust, real-world data to inform on patients' risk of death, now numerically more relevant than stroke/SEE in well-anticoagulated patients, will help to better identify strategies to further improve on AF outcomes.

Supplementary Materials:
Table S1. Logit regression result with CHA_2DS_2-VASc scores as explanatory variables; Table S2. Logit regression result with HAS-BLED scores as explanatory variables; Table S3. Comparison C-statistic in subjects treated with NOACs vs. total population CHA_2DS_2-VASc scores as explanatory variables; Table S4. Comparison C-statistic of the CHA_2DS_2-VASc score, the HAS-BLED score and their combination for Stroke/Systemic Embolic Events (SEE), Major Bleeding and Mortality, broken down according to the type of atrial fibrillation—paroxysmal, persistent, long-term persistent and permanent; Table S5: Previous studies of CHA_2DS_2-VASc and HAS-BLED scores to predict mortality; online Supplemental References.

Author Contributions: R.D.C., G.P. and P.K. contributed to the conception and design of the work. R.D.C., G.R., F.R., D.M., S.K., L.-H.C., and B.v.H. contributed to the acquisition, analysis and interpretation of the data for the work. D.M., R.D.C. and S.K. drafted the manuscript. G.R., G.P., P.K., F.R., L.-H.C., and B.v.H. critically revised the manuscript. All gave final approval and agree to be accountable for all aspects of work, ensuring integrity and accuracy. All authors have read and agreed to the published version of the manuscript.

Abbreviations

AF	Atrial fibrillation
ATRIA	AnTicoagulation and Risk factors In Atrial fibrillation
AUC	Area under the curve
$CHADS_2$	Congestive heart failure, hypertension, age ≥ 75 years, diabetes, stroke/transient ischemic attack/thromboembolism [doubled]
CHA_2DS_2-VASc	Congestive heart failure, hypertension, age ≥ 75 years [doubled], diabetes, stroke/transient ischemic attack/thromboembolism [doubled], vascular disease [prior myocardial infarction, peripheral artery disease, or aortic plaque], age 65–75 years, sex category [female]
CRUSADE	Can Rapid risk stratification of Unstable angina patients Suppress ADverse outcomes with Early implementation of the ACC/AHA guidelines
DACH	Germany (Deutschland), Austria, Switzerland (Confederatio Helvetica)
eCRF	Electronic case report form
GOF	Hosmer and Lemeshow goodness-of-fit test
GRACE	Global Registry of Acute Coronary Events
HAS-BLED	hypertension, abnormal renal/liver function, stroke, bleeding history or predisposition, labile international normalized ratio [INR], elderly [age ≥ 65 years], drugs/alcohol concomitantly
IDI	Integrated discrimination improvement
ISTH	International Society on Thrombosis and Haemostasis
NRI	Net reclassification improvement
NOAC	non-vitamin K antagonist oral anticoagulant
PREFER in AF	Prevention of Thromboembolic Events—European Registry in Atrial Fibrillation" study
SD	Standard deviation of the mean
SEE	Systemic embolic event
TIA	Transient ischemic attack
TIMI	Thrombolysis In Myocardial Infarction
VKA	Vitamin K antagonist

References

1. January, C.T.; Wann, L.S.; Calkins, H.; Chen, L.Y.; Cigarroa, J.E.; Cleveland, J.C., Jr.; Ellinor, P.T.; Ezekowitz, M.D.; Field, M.E.; Furie, K.L.; et al. 2019 AHA/ACC/HRS Focused Update of the 2014 AHA/ACC/HRS Guideline for the Management of Patients with Atrial Fibrillation: A Report of the American College of Cardiology/American Heart Association Task Force on Clinical Practice Guidelines and the Heart Rhythm Society. *J. Am. Coll. Cardiol.* **2019**, *74*, 104–132. [PubMed]
2. Hindricks, G.; Potpara, T.; Dagres, N.; Arbelo, E.; Bax, J.J.; Blomström-Lundqvist, C.; Boriani, G.; Castella, M.; Dan, G.-A.; Dilaveris, P.E.; et al. 2020 ESC Guidelines for the diagnosis and management of atrial fibrillation developed in collaboration with the European Association of Cardio-Thoracic Surgery (EACTS): The Task Force for the diagnosis and management of atrial fibrillation of the European Society of Cardiology (ESC) Developed with the special contribution of the European Heart Rhythm Association (EHRA) of the ESC. *Eur. Heart J.* **2020**. [CrossRef]
3. Olesen, J.B.; Lip, G.Y.; Hansen, M.L.; Hansen, P.R.; Tolstrup, J.S.; Lindhardsen, J.; Selmer, C.; Ahlehoff, O.; Olsen, A.M.; Gislason, G.H.; et al. Validation of risk stratification schemes for predicting stroke and thromboembolism in patients with atrial fibrillation: Nationwide cohort study. *BMJ* **2011**, *342*, d124. [CrossRef] [PubMed]
4. Renda, G.; Ricci, F.; Patti, G.; Aung, N.; Petersen, S.E.; Gallina, S.; Hamrefors, V.; Melander, O.; Sutton, R.; Engstrom, G.; et al. CHA2DS2VASc score and adverse outcomes in middle-aged individuals without atrial fibrillation. *Eur. J. Prev. Cardiol.* **2019**, *26*, 1987–1997. [CrossRef] [PubMed]
5. Angiolillo, D.J.; Patti, G.; Chan, K.T.; Han, Y.; Huang, W.C.; Yakovlev, A.; Paek, D.; Del Aguila, M.; Girotra, S.; Sibbing, D. De-escalation from ticagrelor to clopidogrel in acute coronary syndrome patients: A systematic review and meta-analysis. *J. Thromb. Thrombolysis* **2019**, *48*, 1–10. [CrossRef] [PubMed]
6. Melgaard, L.; Gorst-Rasmussen, A.; Lane, D.A.; Rasmussen, L.H.; Larsen, T.B.; Lip, G.Y. Assessment of the CHA2DS2-VASc score in predicting ischemic stroke, thromboembolism, and death in patients with heart failure with and without atrial fibrillation. *JAMA* **2015**, *314*, 1030–1038. [CrossRef] [PubMed]
7. Lip, G.Y.; Lin, H.J.; Chien, K.L.; Hsu, H.C.; Su, T.C.; Chen, M.F.; Lee, Y.T. Comparative assessment of published atrial fibrillation stroke risk stratification schemes for predicting stroke, in a non-atrial fibrillation population: The Chin-Shan Community Cohort Study. *Int. J. Cardiol.* **2013**, *168*, 414–419. [CrossRef]
8. Hrynkiewicz-Szymanska, A.; Dluzniewski, M.; Platek, A.E.; Szymanski, F.M.; Syska-Suminska, J.; Klos-Szadryn, A.; Glinka, M.; Strojek, M.; Kuciej, A.; Tomaszewska-Kiecana, M. Association of the CHADS2 and CHA 2DS 2-VASc scores with left atrial enlargement: A prospective cohort study of unselected atrial fibrillation patients. *J. Thromb. Thrombolysis* **2015**, *40*, 240–247. [CrossRef]
9. Pisters, R.; Lane, D.A.; Nieuwlaat, R.; de Vos, C.B.; Crijns, H.J.; Lip, G.Y. A novel user-friendly score (HAS-BLED) to assess 1-year risk of major bleeding in patients with atrial fibrillation: The Euro Heart Survey. *Chest* **2010**, *138*, 1093–1100. [CrossRef]
10. Kirchhof, P.; Ammentorp, B.; Darius, H.; De Caterina, R.; Le Heuzey, J.Y.; Schilling, R.J.; Schmitt, J.; Zamorano, J.L. Management of atrial fibrillation in seven European countries after the publication of the 2010 ESC Guidelines on atrial fibrillation: Primary results of the PREvention oF thromboemolic events—European Registry in Atrial Fibrillation (PREFER in AF). *Europaceschu* **2014**, *16*, 6–14. [CrossRef]
11. Schulman, S.; Kearon, C.; Subcommittee on Control of Anticoagulation of the Scientific Standardization Committee of the International Society on Thrombosis and Haemostasis. Definition of major bleeding in clinical investigations of antihemostatic medicinal products in non-surgical patients. *J. Thromb. Haemost.* **2005**, *3*, 692–694. [CrossRef] [PubMed]
12. Steyerberg, E.W.; Vickers, A.J.; Cook, N.R.; Gerds, T.; Gonen, M.; Obuchowski, N.; Pencina, M.J.; Kattan, M.W. Assessing the performance of prediction models: A framework for traditional and novel measures. *Epidemiology* **2010**, *21*, 128–138. [CrossRef] [PubMed]
13. van Smeden, M.; Moons, K.G.M. Event rate net reclassification index and the integrated discrimination improvement for studying incremental value of risk markers. *Stat. Med.* **2017**, *36*, 4495–4497. [CrossRef] [PubMed]
14. Nezic, D.G. Assessing the performance of risk prediction models. *Eur. J. Cardio-Thorac. Surg.* **2020**, *58*, 401. [CrossRef]

15. Wolf, P.A.; D'Agostino, R.B.; Belanger, A.J.; Kannel, W.B. Probability of stroke: A risk profile from the Framingham Study. *Stroke* **1991**, *22*, 312–318. [CrossRef]
16. Hauk, L. Newly Detected Atrial Fibrillation: AAFP Updates Guideline on Pharmacologic Management. *Am. Fam. Phys.* **2017**, *96*, 332–333.
17. Apostolakis, S.; Lane, D.A.; Buller, H.; Lip, G.Y. Comparison of the CHADS2, CHA2DS2-VASc and HAS-BLED scores for the prediction of clinically relevant bleeding in anticoagulated patients with atrial fibrillation: The AMADEUS trial. *Thromb. Haemost.* **2013**, *110*, 1074–1079. [CrossRef]
18. Yao, X.; Gersh, B.J.; Sangaralingham, L.R.; Kent, D.M.; Shah, N.D.; Abraham, N.S.; Noseworthy, P.A. Comparison of the CHA2DS2-VASc, CHADS2, HAS-BLED, ORBIT, and ATRIA risk scores in predicting non-vitamin K antagonist oral anticoagulants-associated bleeding in patients with atrial fibrillation. *Am. J. Cardiol.* **2017**, *120*, 1549–1556. [CrossRef]
19. Gallego, P.; Roldan, V.; Torregrosa, J.M.; Galvez, J.; Valdes, M.; Vicente, V.; Marin, F.; Lip, G.Y. Relation of the HAS-BLED bleeding risk score to major bleeding, cardiovascular events, and mortality in anticoagulated patients with atrial fibrillation. *Circ. Arrhythm. Electrophysiol.* **2012**, *5*, 312–318. [CrossRef]
20. Hsieh, M.J.; Lee, C.H.; Chen, C.C.; Chang, S.H.; Wang, C.Y.; Hsieh, I.C. Predictive performance of HAS-BLED risk score for long-term survival in patients with non-ST elevated myocardial infarction without atrial fibrillation. *J. Cardiol.* **2017**, *69*, 136–143. [CrossRef]
21. Onuk, T.; Karatas, M.B.; Ipek, G.; Gungor, B.; Akyuz, S.; Canga, Y.; Uzun, A.O.; Avci, I.I.; Osken, A.; Kasikcioglu, H.; et al. Higher CHA2DS2-VASc score is associated with increased mortality in acute pulmonary embolism. *Clin. Appl. Thromb. Hemost.* **2017**, *23*, 631–637. [CrossRef] [PubMed]
22. Paoletti Perini, A.; Bartolini, S.; Pieragnoli, P.; Ricciardi, G.; Perrotta, L.; Valleggi, A.; Vergaro, G.; Michelotti, F.; Boggian, G.; Sassone, B.; et al. CHADS2 and CHA2DS2-VASc scores to predict morbidity and mortality in heart failure patients candidates to cardiac resynchronization therapy. *Europace* **2014**, *16*, 71–80. [CrossRef] [PubMed]
23. Temizer, O.; Acar, B.; Yayla, C.; Unal, S.; Goktug Ertem, A.; Gucuk Ipek, E.; Canpolat, U.; Senturk, B.; Selcuk, H.; Selcuk, T. The association between CHA2DS2-VASc score and mortality in patients with heart failure with reduced ejection fraction. *Acta Cardiol. Sin.* **2017**, *33*, 429–435. [PubMed]
24. Fox, K.A.A.; Lucas, J.E.; Pieper, K.S.; Bassand, J.P.; Camm, A.J.; Fitzmaurice, D.A.; Goldhaber, S.Z.; Goto, S.; Haas, S.; Hacke, W.; et al. Improved risk stratification of patients with atrial fibrillation: An integrated GARFIELD-AF tool for the prediction of mortality, stroke and bleed in patients with and without anticoagulation. *BMJ Open* **2017**, *7*, e017157. [CrossRef]

4

Risk Factors, Co-Morbidities and Treatment of In-Hospital Patients with Atrial Fibrillation in Bulgaria

Stefan Naydenov [1,*], Nikolay Runev [1], Emil Manov [1], Daniela Vasileva [1], Yavor Rangelov [1] and Nadya Naydenova [2]

1 Department of Internal Diseases "Prof. St. Kirkovich", Medical University of Sofia, Sofia 1431, Bulgaria; nrunev@abv.bg (N.R.); doctor_emil_manov@abv.bg (E.M.); daniela.g.vasileva@gmail.com (D.V.); yavor.dok@abv.bg (Y.R.)

2 Clinic of Cardiology, UMHAT "St. Ekaterina", Medical University of Sofia, Sofia 1431, Bulgaria; nadma@abv.bg

* Correspondence: snaydenov@gmail.com

Abstract: Background and objectives: Atrial fibrillation (AF) is the most common arrhythmia worldwide and a major risk factor for cardiovascular complications. Our study aimed to investigate the prevalence, risk factors, demographics, co-morbidities and treatment of AF among in-hospital Bulgarian patients. Materials and Methods: A cross-sectional study including 1027 consecutive patients (n = 516, 50.2% males) with a mean age of 67.6 $\pm$ 11.3 years, hospitalized for any reason from 1 May until 31 December 2016 in one of the largest internal clinics in Bulgaria, was carried out. Results: Atrial fibrillation was diagnosed in 634 (61.7%) patients. The prevalence of modifiable AF risk factors was as follows: heart failure, 98.9%; arterial hypertension (HTN), 93.5%; valvular heart disease, 40.9%; chronic lung disease, 26.7%; type 2 diabetes mellitus, 24.9%; thyroid disease, 16.9%; and ischemic heart disease, 11.2%. Univariate logistic regression analysis identified the following risk factors with strongest impact on AF: left ventricular ejection fraction <40% (odds ratio (OR) = 1.951, 95% confidence interval (CI) 1.208–3.151), valvular heart disease (OR = 1.926, 95% CI 1.134–3.862), left ventricular ejection fraction 40–49% (OR = 1.743, 95% CI 1.248–3.017), HTN (OR = 1.653, 95% CI 1.092–3.458). History of ischemic stroke was present in 14.4% of the patients with AF. Oral antithrombotic drugs were prescribed to 85.7%: direct oral anticoagulants to 37.9%, vitamin K antagonists to 43.2%, and antiplatelets to 4.6%. Heart rate control medications and antiarrhythmics were prescribed to 75.4% and 40.2%, respectively. Conclusions: Atrial fibrillation was highly prevalent among our study population. Reduced and mid-range left ventricular ejection fraction, valvular heart disease, and HTN were the risk factors with the strongest association with AF. Although a large number of our AF patients were administered antithrombotic treatment, the prescription rate of oral anticoagulants should be further improved.

Keywords: atrial; fibrillation; in-hospital; embolic; risk; prevention

---

1. Introduction

Atrial fibrillation (AF) is the most common rhythm disorder among the general population [1–4]. The estimated number of AF patients worldwide is ~33.5 million, with higher incidence and prevalence in the developed countries [1–4]. The number of patients with this arrhythmia is expected to reach ~17 million in Europe by 2030, with >200,000 newly diagnosed patients annually [5–7].

Despite the better risk stratification and the new therapeutic strategies, a large number of AF patients continue to be at high risk for cardiovascular complications [1,3,8]. All-cause mortality is increased twice in females and 1.5-fold in males with AF compared to individuals in sinus rhythm after statistical adjustment for other risk factors [1,7]. While appropriate oral anticoagulation could decrease substantially the death rate due to ischemic stroke, other cardiovascular complications/events such as heart failure (HF) and sudden cardiac death are not sufficiently influenced even by the current therapeutic guidelines [1,8,9].

The huge medical, social and economic impact of AF gave us grounds to conduct an observational cross-sectional study among in-hospital patients, hospitalized for any reason in one of the largest internal clinics in Bulgaria, aiming to investigate: (1) The prevalence of AF; (2) Risk factors (RF) for occurrence of this arrhythmia, demographics and co-morbidities in AF patients; (3) Antiarrhythmic and rate control treatment; (4) Antithrombotic stroke prevention. Another reason for us to conduct this study was the lack of sufficient and reliable data about patients with AF from large national registries, clinical and/or epidemiological studies in Bulgaria.

2. Experimental Section

An observational cross-sectional study, including 1027 consecutive patients, of them 516 (50.2%) males, hospitalized for the period 1 May to 31 December 2016. The mean age of the study population was 67.6 ± 11.3 (24–92) years. The study was approved by the local ethics committee and conducted in accordance with the ethical standards, laid down in the 1964 Declaration of Helsinki and its later amendments, guidelines for good clinical practices, and local regulations (ethical approval number 124/09.03.2016). All participants signed an informed consent before enrollment in our study.

2.1. Patients' Selection

Patients meeting the following eligibility criteria were considered for enrolment in the study.

Inclusion criteria: All consenting patients hospitalized in our clinic for any reason except acute cerebrovascular accidents for the recruitment period.

Exclusion criteria: 1. Mentally disabled patients (irrespective of the reason) unable to understand or sign the written informed consent. 2. Patients unwilling to sign an informed consent for participation in our study for any reason.

Patients' information was collected in a structured questionnaire form including demographic characteristics, socio-economic data, medical history about complaints, RF, comorbidities and medical treatment. We gathered the necessary data directly from the patient's medical history and/or from the available medical documentation. The instrumental investigations included electrocardiography (ECG), transthoracic echocardiography, X-ray and the following laboratory parameters (fasting): full blood count with differential, K^+, Na^+, blood glucose, creatinine, uric acid, creatine kinase, troponin T, alanine and aspartate aminotransferase, total cholesterol, low-density and high-density cholesterol, triglycerides, prothrombin time activity, international normalization ratio, total protein and albumin, free thyroxine, thyroid-stimulating hormone. If patient's symptoms suggested HF, but the results from the physical examination, X-ray and echocardiography were inconclusive about presence of this syndrome, we examined also N-terminal pro b-type natriuretic peptide (NT-proBNP).

In patients with symptoms, signs and X-ray data for HF (+NT-proBNP examined in some of them) we applied the following echocardiographic criteria to establish the diagnosis "Heart failure with preserved ejection fraction" (HFpEF):

1. Left-ventricular ejection fraction $\geq$50%.
2. Presence of $\geq$3 of the following criteria:

- Septal e′ velocity $\leq$7 cm/s or lateral e′ velocity $\leq$10 cm/s;
- Average E/e′ $\geq$14;
- Tricuspid regurgitation velocity $\geq$2.8 m/s;
- Left atrial volume index $\geq$34 mL/m^2;
- Left ventricular mass index $\geq$115 g/m^2 for males and $\geq$95 g/m^2 for females;

- E acceleration >1900 cm/s;
- Isovolumetric relaxation time ≤65 ms;
- Deceleration time of the pulmonary venous diastolic velocity ≤220 ms.

All patients in sinus rhythm at admission and without previous history and/or medical documentation for AF episodes, were examined by 24-h Holter-ECG monitoring within 48 h of their hospitalization. Additional instrumental investigations were conducted when necessary (individual decision of the treating physician).

2.2. Statistical Analysis

The sample size of our study was defined by OpenEpi-free sample size calculator, available at: http://web1.sph.emory.edu/cdckms/sample%20size%202%20grps%20cohort.htm. The calculated minimal sample size needed for the study to be carried out was 1014 patients (statistical power set at 85%). The statistical analysis was performed by SPSS statistical package, version 19.0 (SPSS Inc., IBM Company, Chicago, IL, USA). The data were summarized by frequencies and percentages for categorical variables and by mean values and standard deviation for continuous ones. For comparison of categorical variables we used independent χ^2-test. The normality of distribution of continuous data was assessed by Shapiro-Wilk test. Analysis of variance (ANOVA) was used for comparison of parametric data. Logistic regression analysis was used to disclose risk factors for AF and ischemic stroke. All results were considered to be statistically significant for p-values <0.05.

3. Results

Atrial fibrillation was diagnosed in 634 (61.7%) of all patients in our study, of them 315 males (49.7%). Figure 1 and Tables 1 and 2 show the characteristics of the analyzed study population.

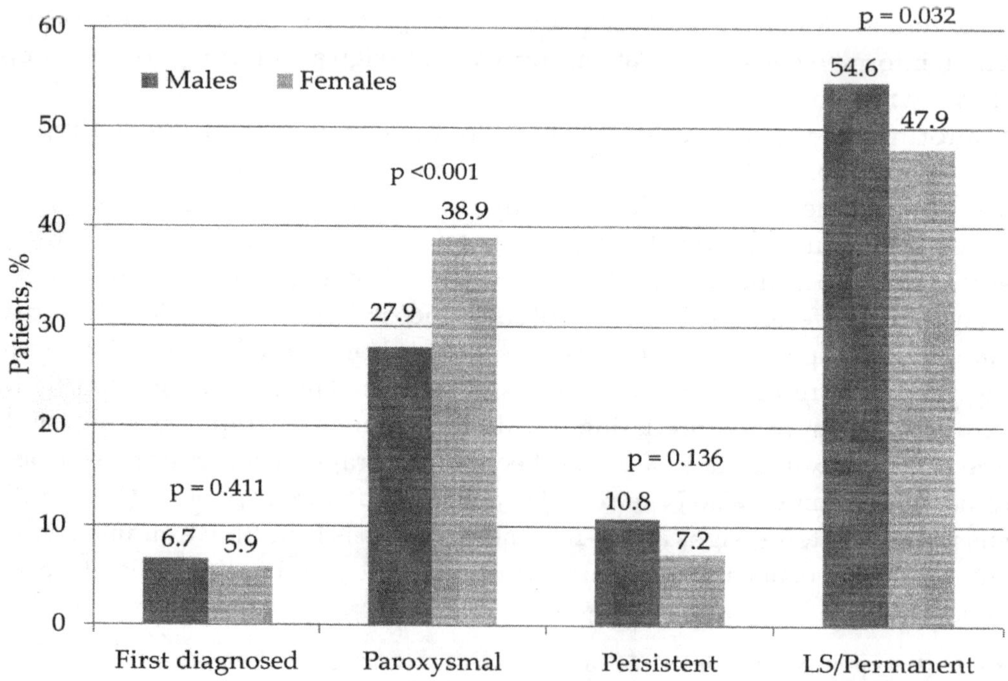

Figure 1. Gender differences in the types of AF; Independent χ^2-test was used for comparison of the prevalence of different AF types in both genders; AF—atrial fibrillation; LS—long-standing persistent; p—level of significance.

Table 1. Differences in age and prevalence of concomitant risk factors (RF) and diseases according to the presence and type of AF.

Risk Factors/Diseases	Sinus Rhythm $n = 393$	First Diagnosed AF $n = 40$	Paroxysmal AF $n = 212$	Persistent AF $n = 57$	LP/Permanent AF $n = 325$	p
Age, years	64.4 ± 11.0	67.2 ± 11.9	66.1 ± 12.8	68.4 ± 11.6	71.9 ± 8.6	<0.001
HTN, n (%)	381 (39.1)	38 (3.9)	200 (20.5)	56 (5.7)	299 (30.7)	0.394
IHD, n (%)	36 (33.6)	6 (5.6)	14 (13.1)	19 (17.8)	32 (29.9)	0.040
VHD *, n (%)	69 (21.0)	4 (1.2)	59 (18.5)	13 (4.0)	183 (55.8)	<0.001
Chronic lung disease, n (%)	116 (40.7)	13 (4.6)	70 (24.6)	18 (6.3)	68 (23.9)	<0.001
Type 2 DM, n (%)	119 (43.0)	7 (2.5)	45 (16.2)	12 (4.3)	94 (33.9)	0.112
Previous ischemic stroke, n (%)	32 (26.0)	3 (2.4)	24 (19.5)	8 (6.5)	56 (45.6)	0.014
Hypothyroidism, n (%)	41 (33.3)	5 (4.1)	39 (31.7)	8 (6.5)	30 (24.4)	0.068
Hyperthyroidism, n (%)	11 (31.4)	2 (5.7)	7 (20.0)	2 (5.7)	13 (37.1)	0.171

Age is presented as a mean value ± standard deviation; Independent χ^2-test was used for comparison of categorical variables and ANOVA for parametric variables; * Moderate to severe insufficiency or/and stenosis; AF—atrial fibrillation; CVD—cerebro-vascular disease; DM—diabetes mellitus; HTN—arterial hypertension; IHD—ischemic heart disease; p—level of significance. The p-value refers to the comparison of sinus rhythm versus each category of atrial fibrillation; RF—risk factors; VHD—valvular heart disease.

Table 2. Gender differences in age and prevalence of concomitant RF and diseases in patients with AF.

Risk Factors/Diseases	Males $n = 315$	Females $n = 319$	p
Age, years	68.2 ± 9.7	70.5 ± 12.2	<0.001
Heart rate , beats per minute	84.7 ± 10.8	87.6 ± 11.5	0.267
HTN, n (%)	301 (50.8)	292 (49.2)	0.440
IHD, n (%)	48 (68.6)	23 (32.4)	0.002
VHD *, n (%)	110 (42.5)	149 (57.5)	0.003
-Mitral valve, n (%)	52 (41.9)	72 (58.1)	0.010
-Aortic valve, n (%)	18 (58.1)	13 (41.9)	0.010
-Mitral and aortic valve, n (%)	17 (42.5)	23 (57.5)	0.042
- Prosthetic valve, n (%)	23 (35.9)	41 (64.1)	0.023
Chronic lung disease, n (%)	95 (56.2)	74 (43.8)	0.020
Type 2 DM, n (%)	85 (53.8)	73 (46.2)	0.032
Previous ischemic stroke, n (%)	45 (49.5)	46 (50.5)	0.624
Hypothyroidism, n (%)	15 (18.3)	67 (81.7)	<0.001
Hyperthyroidism, n (%)	9 (37.5)	15 (62.5)	0.020

Age and heart rate are presented as a mean value ± standard deviation; Independent χ^2-test was used for comparison of categorical variables and ANOVA for parametric variables; * Moderate to severe insufficiency or/and stenosis; AF—atrial fibrillation; DM—diabetes mellitus; HTN—arterial hypertension; IHD—ischemic heart disease; p—level of significance; RF—risk factors; VHD—valvular heart disease.

The mean heart rate of patients with first diagnosed AF at their disclosure (before application of rate control treatment) was 117.4 ± 14.6 beats per minute.

Heart failure was present in 627 (98.9%) patients with AF compared to 58 patients (14.8%) in sinus rhythm, $p < 0.001$. There was not significant gender difference in HF prevalence among AF patients: 311 males (49.6%) and 316 (50.4%) females, $p = 0.627$. In 74 (11.8%) of 627 AF patients with HF and 4 (6.9%) of 58 patients in sinus rhythm, HF was newly diagnosed after enrollment in our study, $p < 0.001$. Of all AF patients with HF, 40 (6.4%) had first diagnosed AF, 209 (33.3%)—paroxysmal, 55 (8.8%)—persistent and 323 (51.5%)—long-standing (LS)/permanent AF, $p < 0.001$. Third NYHA (New York Heart Association) class was most prevalent among AF patients—in 369 (58.9%), followed by II NYHA class—226 (36.0%), I NYHA class—21 (3.3%) and IV NYHA class—11 (1.8%), $p < 0.001$. There was not statistically significant gender difference regarding the NYHA class of AF population with HF.

The mean left ventricular ejection fraction (EF) of AF patients was 55.7 ± 11.4% compared to 59.6 ± 9.9% of patients in sinus rhythm, $p = 0.116$. The mean EF of patients with first diagnosed AF was 61.6 ± 8.6%, paroxysmal AF—59.9 ± 9.9%, persistent AF—57.6 ± 12.2%, LS/permanent AF—51.9 ± 11.7%, $p < 0.001$. Among the HF patients reduced left ventricular EF (HFrEF) <40% was found in 87 (13.9%), mid-range EF (HFmrEF) 40–49%—116 (18.5%) and HFpEF ≥50%—431 (68.7%), $p < 0.001$. There was not statistically significant difference by gender and type of AF regarding the sub-group analysis of EF groups. The association of different variables with AF is shown in Table 3.

Table 3. Conditions/co-morbidities, associated with AF.

Variable	OR	95% Confidence Interval for OR		*p*
		Lower Limit	Upper Limit	
EF < 40%	1.951	1.208	3.151	<0.001
VHD	1.926	1.134	3.862	0.010
EF 40–49%	1.743	1.248	3.017	<0.001
HTN	1.653	1.092	3.458	<0.001
Age ≥ 75 years	1.625	1.019	2.915	0.032
Age 65–74 years	1.426	1.008	2.084	0.020
IHD	1.395	1.040	1.873	0.026

Univariate logistic regression was used for assessment of the independent influence of different variables on the risk for development of AF. Prior independent χ^2-test was applied to identify categorical variables with statistically significant relationship to AF occurrence. These variables were entered into the univariate logistic regression model; AF—atrial fibrillation; EF—left ventricular ejection fraction; HTN—arterial hypertension; IHD—ischemic heart disease; OR—odds ratio for development of AF; *p*—level of significance; VHD—valvular heart disease.

The mean CHA_2DS_2-Vasc Score of AF patients, evaluating the risk for stroke and peripheral arterial embolic events was 3.83 ± 1.46 points (high risk): 3.43 ± 1.42 points for males and 4.13 ± 1.49 points for females, $p = 0.023$. The mean CHA_2DS_2-Vasc Score of patient with first diagnosed AF was 3.38 ± 1.40, paroxysmal AF—3.53 ± 1.53, persistent AF—3.32 ± 1.52, LS/permanent AF—4.08 ± 1.37 points, $p = 0.003$ for the last subgroup vs the others.

Among the 91 AF patients (14.4%) who had suffered ischemic stroke, 3 (3.3%) had first diagnosed AF, 24 (26.4%)-paroxysmal, 8 (8.8%)-persistent and 56 (61.5%)-LS/permanent AF, $p < 0.001$. The association of different variables with ischemic stroke is shown in Table 4.

Table 4. Conditions/co-morbidities, associated with ischemic stroke.

Variable	OR	95% Confidence Interval for OR		*p*
		Lower Limit	Upper Limit	
AF	1.793	1.151	2.792	<0.001
HTN	1.429	1.127	2.671	<0.001
Age ≥75 years	1.215	1.032	2.146	<0.001
Age 65–74 years	1.056	1.014	1.447	0.036

Univariate logistic regression was used for assessment of the independent influence of different variables on the risk of ischemic stroke. Prior independent χ^2-test was applied to identify categorical variables with statistically significant relationship to stroke occurrence. These variables were further entered into the univariate logistic regression model; AF—atrial fibrillation; EF—left ventricular ejection fraction; HTN—arterial hypertension; IHD—ischemic heart disease; OR—odds ratio for development of AF; *p*—level of significance; VHD—valvular heart disease.

The mean HAS-BLED Score of AF patients, evaluating the bleeding riskin anticoagulant treatment was 2.26 ± 0.97 points (moderate risk): 2.29 ± 1.01 points for males and 2.23 ± 0.93 points for females, $p = 0.431$. The mean HAS-BLED Score of patient with first diagnosed AF was 2.03 ± 0.80, paroxysmal AF—2.14 ± 1.02, persistent AF—2.16 ± 0.86, LS/permanent AF—2.39 ± 0.96 points, $p = 0.224$.

Oral antithrombotic treatment was prescribed to 543 (85.7%) of all AF patients: of them 265 (48.8%) males and 278 (51.2%) females, $p = 0.382$. Table 5 shows the prescription of different antithrombotics according to the type of AF.

Table 5. Antithrombotic treatment according to the type of AF.

	AF *n* (%)				
	First Diagnosed *n* (%)	**Paroxysmal** *n* (%)	**Persistent** *n* (%)	**LS/Permanent** *n* (%)	*p*
Treatment					
No	20 (50.0)	33 (15.6)	14 (24.6)	24 (7.4)	<0.001
DOACs	5 (12.5)	54 (25.5)	15 (26.3)	166 (51.1)	0.044
VKA	13 (32.5)	119 (56.1)	21 (36.8)	121 (37.2)	0.221
Antiplatelets	2 (5.0)	6 (2.8)	7 (12.3)	14 (4.3)	0.354
Total	40 (100)	212 (100)	57 (100)	325 (100)	

Independent χ^2-test was used for comparison of the presented categorical variables; AF—atrial fibrillation, LS—long-standing persistent, DOACs—direct oral anticoagulants (dabigatran, apixaban, rivaroxaban), *p*—level of significance; VKA—vitamin K antagonist.

The mean CHA2DS2-Vasc Score according to the oral antithrombotic treatment was: No treatment—3.6 ± 1.7 points, vitamin K antagonist (VKA)—3.9 ± 1.3 point, direct oral anticoagulants (DOACs)—3.3 ± 1.4, antiplatelets—4.0 ± 1.3 points; *p* no treatment/VKA = 0.009, *p* VKA/DOACs = 0.003, *p* DOACs/antiplatelet = 0.040; The mean HAS-BLED Score according to the oral antithrombotic treatment was: No treatment—2.2 ± 1.1 points, VKA—2.3 ± 0.9 points, DOACs—2.2 ± 0.8, antiplatelets—2.1 ± 1.0 points, $p = 0.156$.

Rate control treatment was administered to 478 (75.4%) AF patients: of them 232 (48.5%) males and 246 (51.5%) females, $p = 0.332$. Regarding the type of AF, rate control medication was administered to: first diagnosed—29 of 40 (72.5%), paroxysmal—133 of 212 (67.7%), persistent—37 of 57 (64.9%), LS/permanent—277 of 325 (85.2%), $p < 0.001$. Antiarrhythmic treatment was administered to 255 (40.2%): of them 128 (50.2%) males and 127 (49.8%) females, $p = 0.512$. Regarding the type of AF, antiarrhythmics were administered to: first diagnosed—22 of 40 (55.0%), paroxysmal—126 of 212 (59.4%), persistent—36 of 57 (63.2%), LS/permanent—71 of 325 (21.8%), $p < 0.001$. The drugs prescribed to our patients for rate and rhythm control are shown in Table 6.

Table 6. Medications, assigned to our patients for rate and rhythm control.

Medication	*n* (%)	*P*
Rate control		
Beta-blockers	379 (79.3)	
Calcium channel blockers	15 (3.1)	<0.0001
Digoxin *	84 (17.6)	
Total	478 (100)	
Rhythm control		
Amiodarone	111 (43.5)	
Propafenone	85 (33.3)	
Sotalol	47 (18.4)	0.03
Flecainide	12 (4.7)	
Total	255 (100)	

Independent χ^2-test was used for comparison of the presented categorical variables; *p*—level of significance; * Used only for acute heart rate control.

4. Discussion

The purpose of our study was to characterize AF in a "real-life" population of in-hospital patients, irrespective of the reason for which they were admitted. We found high prevalence of AF—more than

60% of all patients had at least 1 episode of this rhythm disorder. Our results differed significantly from published data of other hospital-based studies in which AF ranged from 2% to 27% [2–4,10]. These discrepancies might be attributed to some extent to the inclusion criteria–much broader for our study and also to the risk profile of the patients: advanced age and high prevalence of concomitant RF/diseases. Our results are important because a large number of hospital physicians meet in their daily clinical practice patients similar to ours.

Generally, we did not find statistically significant gender difference in AF prevalence, except for the paroxysmal AF, more prevalent in females. According to other studies AF was less common in women [1,4,11–14]. The mean age of our AF population was significantly higher (69.6 years) compared to patients in sinus rhythm (64.4 years), a finding confirmed also by other authors [1,10–13]. Previous studies demonstrated that age >65 years was a major and independent non-modifiable RF for AF [1–6]. Our logistic regression analysis also disclosed age as an important RF for this dysrhythmia: age 65–74 years increased the risk for AF by ~1.4 and age ≥75 years-by ~1.6.

We found HF and HTN to be the most prevalent modifiable RF for AF, followed by VHD, chronic lung diseases and type 2 DM. Regarding HF, almost 2/3 of our AF patients had HFpEF and the percentage of HFrEF was significantly lower (~14%) compared to data from other clinical studies [2–8,13]. The surprisingly high prevalence of HFpEF in our study could be explained by the advanced age of the AF population and the high presence of co-morbidities such as HTN, VHD, type 2 DM, IHD. However, our logistic regression analysis showed that reduced EF exerted strongest impact on the risk for development of AF, followed by moderate to severe VHD. Arterial hypertension was stated by other authors as the most significant modifiable RF for AF [1,12–19]. Despite the high prevalence among our AF population, HTN was the third most influential RF for AF in our study according to the logistic regression analysis.

The prevalence of AF in patients with chronic lung diseases in our study was similar to data, reported by other authors [1–5]. Our logistic regression analysis did not disclose these diseases as factors exerting statistically significant influence on the risk for AF occurrence, but other authors reported that some chronic lung diseases such as obstructive sleep apnea and chronic obstructive pulmonary disease increased the adjusted hazard ratio for AF development by 1.5 to 2.44 [1–5,7].

The prevalence of type 2 DM among our AF population was significantly higher compared to other surveys [1–7]. However, our analysis showed it did not exert significant impact on AF occurrence. The published data we found about the independent role of type 2 DM for AF development were contradictory: according to some researchers type 2 DM was not a risk factor for AF at all and according to others type 2 DM was a very strong and independent AF risk factor [1–4,13].

Surprisingly, IHD was less prevalent than expected among our AF population. Although regression analysis showed that this disease increased the risk for AF occurrence by ~1.4, this effect was much weaker than anticipated. Other clinical studies found much higher IHD prevalence among AF patients and myocardial ischemia was acknowledged by many as the second most important modifiable RF for AF after HTN [1–5].

We found high cardioembolic risk for all types of AF in our study (CHA2DS2-Vasc >3 points) and ~14% of our AF patients had suffered an ischemic stroke. Reiffel et al. reported that AF accounted for >15% of all strokes in the USA, 36% of strokes in people >80 years of age, and ~20% of cryptogenic strokes [15]. Our regression analysis disclosed AF as the strongest risk factor for ischemic stroke of all variables we analyzed, followed by HTN and age ≥75 years. According to published data that we found, HTN was the strongest predictor for ischemic stroke, followed by cerebrovascular atherosclerotic disease, diabetes, smoking and advanced age. Non-anticoagulated atrial fibrillation was considered by most authors as the fourth or fifth most important RF for ischemic stroke [4,8–11].

Oral antithrombotic treatment was prescribed to 85.7% of our AF patients with VKAs slightly more preferred to DOACs (43.2% vs. 37.9% respectively). Possible explanations for such physician's preference were the prevalence of VHD (i.e., valvular AF) in our study population and mostly the significantly higher cost of DOACs compared to VKAs in Bulgaria. The rate of oral anticoagulant treatment in AF patients, presented by other authors differs widely. Jain et al. reported that anticoagulant prescription in AF patients increased from 9% (1995–1998) to 30% (2011–2014) [20]. Weitz et al. found in their study that VKA prescription in AF decreased from 99% in 2010 to 67% by 2014 whereas DOACs administration increased to 33% [21]. The underuse of DOACs was not clinically justified even in terms of the bleeding risk. Large randomized clinical trials provided enough data proving the superiority of DOACs for embolic prevention and their more favorable bleeding-risk profile compared to VKAs [1,20,22].

Rate control treatment was prescribed to high percentage of our patients (~75%) with beta-blockers being the most preferred class. Digoxin had been applied only for acute heart rate control, when beta-blockers or verapamil did not have the necessary effect or in case of contraindications for their use. We tried to avoid chronic digoxin treatment because of reported data showing increased mortality in AF patients, treated continuously with this drug [23]. The clinical trials AFFIRM, RACE and HOT CAFÉ found that management of AF with the rhythm-control strategy offered no survival advantage over the rate-control strategy: the latter was associated with lower risk of adverse drug effects, reduced number of hospitalizations yearly and lower financial costs for patient's treatment [1,22–27]. In the AFFIRM trial, beta-blockers, applied alone or in combination with digoxin achieved target heart rate in ~70% of the patients and calcium channel blockers only in 54% [1]. The results from the RATAF study differed significantly from those in the AFFIRM trial-calcium channel antagonists had superiority to other drugs regarding 24-h heart rate control, reduction of frequency and severity of symptoms [1,25].

Antiarhythmic treatment was administered to 40% of our patients with amiodarone being the most used antiarrhythmic drug. The possible explanation was the high prevalence of patients with HF and/or structural heart changes in which most of the representatives of class I and class III antiarrhythmics (Vaughan Williams classification) are contraindicated [1]. The PREFER registry including >7000 patients from 7 European countries showed that the three most commonly administered antiarrhythmic drugs in AF patients were amiodarone (51%), flecainide (22%) and sotalol (12%) [23].

Study limitations: 1. The number of patients we included in our single-center study does not allow us to formulate general conclusions about the entire AF population in Bulgaria; 2. We analyzed only hospitalized patients with AF and our results should not be extrapolated to out-hospital patients. The comorbidities in hospitalized patients might differ significantly from out-hospital patients thus influencing the incidence, prevalence and other characteristics of AF. 3. We analyzed some major but not all concomitant RF and diseases in patients with AF.

5. Conclusions

Atrial fibrillation was highly prevalent among our study population. Reduced and mid-range left ventricular ejection fraction, valvular heart disease and HTN were the risk factors with the strongest association with AF. Although a large number of our AF patients were administered antithrombotic treatment, the prescription rate of oral anticoagulants should be further improved.

Author Contributions: S.N.: Concept of the study, resource provision, data collection and processing, analysis and interpretation of the results, literature search, manuscript writing, critical review of the manuscript, N.R.: Concept and design of the study, supervision of study performance, resource provision, data processing, analysis and interpretation of the results, manuscript writing, critical review of the manuscript, E.M.: Concept and design of the study, supervision of study performance, data collection, analysis and interpretation of the results, manuscript writing, critical review of the manuscript, D.V.: Patients' referral, data collection and processing, analysis and interpretation of the results, critical review of the manuscript, Y.R.: Design of the study, resource provision, patients' referral data collection and processing, critical review of the manuscript, N.N.: Resource provision, patients' referral, literature search, critical review of the manuscript.

References

1. Kirchhof, P.; Benussi, S.; Kotecha, D.; Ahlsson, A.; Atar, A.; Casadei, B.; Castella, M.; Diener, H.C.; Heidbuchel, H.; Hendriks, J. 2016 ESC Guidelines for the management of atrial fibrillation developed in collaboration with EACTS. *Eur. Heart J.* **2016**, *37*, 2893–2962. [CrossRef] [PubMed]
2. Chugh, S.; Havmoeller, R.; Narayanan, K.; Singh, D.; Rienstra, M.; Benjamin, E.J.; Gillum, R.F.; Kim, Y.H.; McAnulty, J.H.; Zheng, Z.J.; et al. Worldwide epidemiology of atrial fibrillation: A Global Burden of Disease 2010 Study. *Circulation* **2014**, *129*, 837–847. [CrossRef] [PubMed]
3. Colilla, S.; Crow, A.; Petkun, W.; Singer, D.; Simon, T.; Liu, X. Estimates of current and future incidence and prevalence of atrial fibrillation in the U.S. adult population. *Am. J. Cardiol.* **2013**, *112*, 1142–1147. [CrossRef] [PubMed]
4. Heeringa, J.; van der Kuip, D.; Hofman, A.; Kors, J.; van Herpen, G.; Stricker, B.H.C.; Stijnen, T.; Lip, G.Y.; Witteman, J.C. Prevalence, incidence and lifetime risk of atrial fibrillation: The Rotterdam study. *Eur. Heart J.* **2006**, *27*, 949–953. [CrossRef] [PubMed]
5. Krijthe, B.; Kunst, A.; Benjamin, E.; Lip, G.; Franco, O.; Hofman, A.; Witteman, J.C.; Stricker, B.H.; Heeringa, J. Projections on the number of individuals with atrial fibrillation in the European Union, from 2000 to 2060. *Eur. Heart J.* **2013**, *34*, 2746–2751. [CrossRef] [PubMed]
6. Runev, N.; Manov, E. Atrial fibrillation—Epidemiology and prognosis. *Bulg. Cardiol.* **2012**, *18*, 5–10.
7. Liao, K.; Chen, C. Incidence and risk factors of atrial fibrillation in Asian COPD patients. *Int. J. Chronic Obstr. Pulm. Dis.* **2017**, *12*, 2523–2530. [CrossRef] [PubMed]
8. Stewart, S.; Hart, C.; Hole, D.; McMurray, J. A population-based study of the long-term risks associated with atrial fibrillation: 20-year follow-up of the Renfrew/Paisley study. *Am. J. Med.* **2002**, *113*, 359–364. [CrossRef]
9. Lip, G.; Brechin, C.; Lane, D. The Global Burden of Atrial Fibrillation and Stroke. *Chest* **2012**, *142*, 1489–1498. [CrossRef] [PubMed]
10. Runev, N. Cardiovascular risk factors. In *Cardiology 2015*; Grigorov, M., Grigorov, V., Kitova, L., Eds.; Central Medical Library: Sofia, Bulgaria, 2015; pp. 69–73.
11. Runev, N.; Manov, E.; Naydenov, S.; Donova, T. Prevalence of cardiovascular risk factors in Bulgarian female population. *Eur. J. Prev. Cardiol.* **2014**, *22*, 103a.
12. Naydenov, S.; Dimchovski, E.; Vasileva, D.; Runev, N.; Manov, E.; Donova, T. Assessment of the risk factors in patients with atrial fibrillation. *Bulg. Cardiol.* **2014**, *20*, 29a.
13. Tadic, M.; Cuspidi, C. Type 2 diabetes mellitus and atrial fibrillation: From mechanisms to clinical practice. *Arch. Cardiovasc. Dis.* **2015**, *108*, 269–276. [CrossRef] [PubMed]
14. Runev, N.; Dimitrov, S. management of stroke prevention in Bulgarian patients with non-valvular atrial fibrillation (BUL-AF Survey). *Int. J. Cardiol.* **2015**, *187*, 683–685. [CrossRef] [PubMed]
15. Reiffel, J. Atrial fibrillation and stroke: Epidemiology. *Am. J. Med.* **2014**, *127*, 15–16. [CrossRef] [PubMed]
16. Naydenov, S.; Torbova, S.; Nikolov, F.; Naydenova, N. Abdominal obesity, arterial hypertension and diabetes mellitus in Bulgarian urban population. *Bulg. J. Cardiol.* **2013**, *2*, 15–24.
17. Milanova, M.; Naydenov, S.; Runev, N.; Manov, E. Impact of some modifiable cardiovascular risk factors on the early prognosis after acute myocardial infarction. *Acta Med. Mediterr.* **2017**, *33*, 821–825. [CrossRef]
18. Matveev, M.; Krasteva, V.; Naydenov, S.; Donova, T. Possibilities of signal-averaged orthogonal and vector electrocardiography for locating and size evaluation of acute myocardial infarction with ST-elevation. *Anatol. J. Cardiol.* **2007**, *7*, 193–197.
19. Ponikowski, P.; Voors, A.; Anker, S.; Bueno, H.; Cleland, J.; Coats, A.; Falk, V.; González-Juanatey, J.R.; Harjola, V.-P.; Mariell Jessup, E.A.J.; et al. 2016 ESC Guidelines for the diagnosis and treatment of acute and chronic heart failure: The Task Force for the diagnosis and treatment of acute and chronic heart failure of the European Society of Cardiology (ESC) Developed with the special contribution of the Heart Failure Association (HFA) of the ESC. *Eur. Heart J.* **2016**, *37*, 2129–2200. [CrossRef] [PubMed]
20. Jain, V.; Marshall, I.; Crichton, S.; McKevitt, C.; Rudd, A.; Wolfe, C. Trends in the prevalence and management of pre-stroke atrial fibrillation, the South London Stroke Register, 1995–2014. *PLoS ONE* **2017**, *12*, 0175980a. [CrossRef] [PubMed]
21. Weitz, J.; Semchuk, W.; Turpie, A.; Fisher, W.; Kong, C.; Ciaccia, A.; Cairns, J. Trends in Prescribing Oral Anticoagulants in Canada, 2008–2014. *Clin. Ther.* **2015**, *37*, 2506–2514. [CrossRef] [PubMed]

22. Katz, D.; Maddox, T.; Turakhia, M.; Gehi, A.; O'Brien, E.; Lubitz, S.; Turchin, A.; Doros, G.; Lei, L.; Varosy, P.; et al. Contemporary Trends in Oral Anticoagulant Prescription in Atrial Fibrillation Patients at Low to Moderate Risk of Stroke after Guideline-Recommended Change in Use of the CHADS2 to the CHA2DS2-VASc Score for Thromboembolic Risk Assessment: Analysis From the National Cardiovascular Data Registry's Outpatient Practice Innovation and Clinical Excellence Atrial Fibrillation Registry. *Circ. Cardiovasc. Qual. Outcomes* **2017**, *10*, e003476. [CrossRef] [PubMed]
23. Lopes, R.; Rordorf, R.; De Ferrari, G.; Leonardi, S.; Thomas, L.; Wojdyla, D.M.; Ridefelt, P.; Lawrence, J.H.; De Caterina, R.; Vinereanu, D.; et al. Digoxin and Mortality in Patients with Atrial Fibrillation. *J. Am. Coll. Cardiol.* **2018**, *71*, 1063–1074. [CrossRef] [PubMed]
24. Kirchhof, P.; Ammentorp, B.; Darius, H.; De Caterina, R.; Le Heuzey, J.; Schilling, R.; Schmitt, J.; Zamorano, J.L. Management of atrial fibrillation in seven European countries after the publication of the 2010 ESC Guidelines on atrial fibrillation: Primary results of the Prevention of thromboemolic events—European Registry in Atrial Fibrillation (PREFER in AF). *Europace* **2014**, *16*, 6–14. [CrossRef] [PubMed]
25. Kotecha, D.; Holmes, J.; Krum, H.; Altman, D.; Manzano, L.; Cleland, J.G.; Lip, G.Y.; Coats, A.J.; Andersson, B.; Kirchhof, P.; et al. Efficacy of beta blockers in patients with heart failure plus atrial fibrillation: An individual-patient data meta-analysis. *Lancet* **2014**, *384*, 2235–2243. [CrossRef]
26. Thrall, G.; Lane, D.; Carroll, D.; Lip, G. Quality of life in patients with atrial fibrillation: A systematic review. *Am. J. Med.* **2006**, *119*, 1–19. [CrossRef] [PubMed]
27. Hayward, C.; Patel, H.; Patel, K.; Di Mario, C.; Lyon, A.; Ahsan, S.; Rowland, E. The evolving landscape of oral anti-arrhythmic prescriptions for atrial fibrillation in England: 1998–2014. *Eur. Heart J. Cardiovasc. Pharmacother.* **2016**, *2*, 90–94. [CrossRef] [PubMed]

5

The Quality of Anticoagulation Therapy among Warfarin-Treated Patients with Atrial Fibrillation in a Primary Health Care Setting

Gediminas Urbonas [1,*], Leonas Valius [1], Gintarė Šakalytė [2], Kęstutis Petniūnas [1] and Inesa Petniūnienė [1]

1 Department of Family medicine, Medical Academy, Lithuanian University of Health Sciences, LT-50161 Kaunas, Lithuania; leonas.valius@fc.lsmuni.lt (L.V.); petniunaskestutis@gmail.com (K.P.); i.anulyte@gmail.com (I.P.)

2 Department of Cardiology, Medical Academy, Lithuanian University of Health Sciences, LT-50161 Kaunas, Lithuania; gintare.sakalyte@fc.lsmuni.lt

* Correspondence: gediminas.urbonas@fc.lsmuni.lt

Abstract: *Background and objectives:* Long-term therapy with oral anticoagulants is recommended for stroke prevention in patients with atrial fibrillation (AF). This study evaluated the quality of anticoagulation therapy among warfarin-treated AF patients in selected primary health care centres in Lithuania. *Materials and Methods*: This was a retrospective study conducted in nine primary health care centres in Lithuania. Existing medical records of randomly selected adult patients with AF who were treated with warfarin for at least 12 months were reviewed and analysed. Physicians' decisions to adjust warfarin dose were considered as consistent with the approved warfarin posology if warfarin dose was increased in case of international normalized ratio (INR) <2.0, decreased in case of INR >3.0 or unchanged in case of INR within 2.0 to 3.0. *Results:* The study population included 406 patients. The mean duration of treatment with warfarin was 5.4 years. The median number of INR measurements per patient per year was 8.0. More than half (57.3%) of available INR values were outside the target range, with 13.6% INR values being above 3.0 and 43.7% INR values—below 2.0. The median time in therapeutic range (TTR) was 40.0%; only 20% of patients had TTR of ≥65%. In about 40% of the cases with INR values outside the target range, no dose corrections were implemented. About 27% of decisions on warfarin dose adjustment were not consistent with the recommended warfarin posology. The median number of INR measurements was lower among patients living in urban areas, while the median TTR was significantly higher in urban patients than in rural patients. In the multivariate regression model, gender, HAS-BLED score and warfarin treatment duration were associated with a TTR of ≥65%. *Conclusions*: Anticoagulation control is suboptimal in routine clinical practice with a median TTR of 40%. Our findings suggest that there might be a room for improvement of anticoagulation control in primary care.

Keywords: atrial fibrillation; anticoagulation; INR; TTR; warfarin; primary care

1. Introduction

Atrial fibrillation (AF) is the most common disorder of heart rhythm. There were approximately 8.8 million adults with AF in the European Union in 2010 [1]. The prevalence of AF is increasing, mainly because of population aging, and it is estimated that the number of patients with AF will be doubled by 2060 [1]. Atrial fibrillation is associated with significant morbidities and mortality due to stroke and peripheral arterial embolism [2]. The risk of stroke is increased four- to five-fold in patients with AF [3].

Clinical guidelines for stroke prevention in patients with AF recommend long-term therapy with oral anticoagulants [4]. Despite the availability of a new class of anticoagulants, known as non-vitamin K oral anticoagulants (NOACs), the vitamin K antagonist (VKA), warfarin, remains the preferred anticoagulant for many patients [5]. The main reasons include lower warfarin price, contraindications and lower adherence to NOACs, as well as concerns for increased risk of myocardial infarction with NOACs [5]. Results from randomized controlled trials support the use of warfarin in patients with AF who are at moderate or high risk of stroke. Assuming a baseline risk of 45 strokes per 1000 patient-years, warfarin could prevent 30 strokes at the expense of only six additional major bleeds [6]. In patients with AF, adjusted-dose warfarin reduced stroke by approximately 60% compared with no treatment and by approximately 40% compared with antiplatelet therapy [7]. However, the use of warfarin is challenging because of its multiple interactions and narrow therapeutic index. Warfarin therapy requires continuous dose adjustment to maintain the international normalized ratio (INR) between 2.0 and 3.0. INR greater than 3.0 poses a higher risk of bleeding and INR less than 2.0 may increase a risk of thromboembolism [2,8]. It is recommended to determine INR at least weekly during initiation of warfarin therapy and at least monthly when anticoagulation is stable (INR in range) [4].

The time a patient spends within the therapeutic range (time in the therapeutic range; TTR) is accepted as a measure of anticoagulation quality. A 10% increase in time spent out of TTR is associated with a 29% increase in the risk of mortality, and 10 to 12% increase in the risk of an ischemic stroke and other thromboembolic events [9]. In the Global Anticoagulant Registry in the FIELD–Atrial Fibrillation (GARFIELD-AF) study, patients with TTR <65% had a 2.6-fold higher risk of stroke, 1.5-fold higher risk of major bleeding, and 2.4-fold higher risk of all-cause mortality [10]. A recent meta-analysis of 31 studies confirmed that increasing mean TTR is associated with a lower rate of both major bleeding and stroke/systemic embolism [11].

In this study, we aimed to evaluate the quality of anticoagulation therapy among warfarin-treated AF patients in selected primary health care centres (PHCCs) in Lithuania.

2. Materials and Methods

This was a retrospective study conducted in nine PHCCs (serving a total of 195,073 people) in Lithuania. The study was approved by the Ethics Committee of Lithuanian University of Health Sciences (issue number, BEC-LSMU(R)-21, 5 December 2016) and by the Kaunas Regional Biomedical Research Ethics Committee (issue number, BE-2-74, 8 October 2018). Six PHCCs were located in towns (Kaunas Dainava outpatient Clinic, Siauliai Central Outpatient Clinic, Kedainiai Primary Health Care Centre, Clinic of Family Medicine of Hospital of Lithuanian University of Health Sciences Kauno Klinikos, Saules Family Medicine Centre, Vita Longa Family Medicine Centre) and three PHCCs in rural areas (Kaltinenai Primary Health Care Centre, Rekyva Outpatient Clinic, Babtai Family Medicine Centre). Between January 2016 and January 2017, existing medical records of randomly selected adult patients with non-valvular AF who were treated with warfarin for at least 12 months were reviewed. In each PHCC, all patients with AF diagnosis (code I48 according to the International Classification of Diseases, 10th revision) were identified. Patients fulfilling inclusion criteria were selected in alphabetic order until the predefined number of patients was achieved in each PHCC. The data collected included details on health care centre (private or public), patient sociodemographic (gender, age, social status, residential area, distance to health care centre), concomitant medications with a potential of interaction with warfarin, risk factors for stroke and bleeding, INR results, warfarin treatment duration and warfarin dose (including dose corrections).

The HAS-BLED (Hypertension, Abnormal renal/liver function, Stroke, Bleeding history or predisposition, Labile INR, Elderly, Drugs/alcohol concomitantly) score was calculated by assigning 1 point each for the presence of arterial hypertension, renal or hepatic impairment, history of stroke, history of bleeding, labile INR, age $\geq$ 65 years, alcohol or drug abuse; 2 points were assigned if both renal and hepatic impairment or alcohol and drug abuse were presented. Patients were classified into two groups of bleeding risk according to the total HAS-BLED score: low risk (score ≤2) or high risk (score ≥3) [12].

The CHA2DS2-VASc (Congestive heart failure, Hypertension, Age ≥ 75 years, Diabetes, Stroke, Vascular disease, Age 65–74 years, Sex category) score was calculated by assigning 1 point each for the presence of heart failure, arterial hypertension, diabetes mellitus, vascular disease, age 65–74 years or female sex and 2 points for a history of stroke or transient ischemic attack or age ≥ 75 years [12].

Individual TTRs were determined by calculating the fraction of all INR values that were within the therapeutic range (i.e., the number of INRs in the range between 2.0 and 3.0 divided by the total number of INR tests). We stratified patients into two groups based on TTR level: TTR ≥65% (good control) and TTR <65% (poor control) (a cut-off value of <65% is used in the national conditions for reimbursement of NOACs in Lithuania as an indicator of poor anticoagulation control) [13].

Physicians' decisions to adjust warfarin dose were analysed. The decision was considered as consistent with the approved warfarin posology [14] if warfarin dose was increased in case of INR <2.0 or decreased in case of INR >3.0 or unchanged in case of INR within 2.0 to 3.0. The decision was considered as not consistent if warfarin dose was not changed in case of INR out of the target range (i.e., 2.0 to 3.0) or increased in case of INR >3.0 or decreased in case of INR <2.0.

Patients were grouped according their ability to work as follows: fully able to work (a person who has no restrictions to work because of age or a heath condition), retired (a person who left his or her job after reaching retirement age), disabled (a person unable to work because of a health condition) and not self-sufficient (a person unable to live without a permanent help of a caregiver).

Categorical data were presented as a count (n) and percentage (%). Continuous variables were presented as mean (standard deviation; SD) or median (interquartile range; IQR). We used the parametric Student *t*-test and nonparametric Mann-Whitney U for comparison of continuous variables between two independent samples. Spearman's rank correlation coefficient was used to assess correlation between CHA2DS2-VASc score and HAS-BLED score, and between the intensity of INR measurements and TTR. We conducted univariate and multivariate logistic analyses to identify factors that were independently associated with values of TTR ≥65.0%. The dependent variable was TTR (TTR <65.0% versus TTR ≥65.0%). The independent variables used in the univariate analysis were age, type of health care centre (private owned), gender (male), ability to work (retired, disabled, or not self-sufficient versus fully able to work), place of residence (rural), distance to health care centre, HAS-BLED score, CHA2DS2-VASc score, number of INR measurements per year, duration of warfarin treatment and use of medicines interacting with warfarin. Multivariate logistic regression was employed using the enter method, i.e., all variables that were significant in univariate analysis were entered into the equation at the same time. To build a final model, other variables were entered to test their contribution to the regression equation. Statistical differences were interpreted at 5% (two-sided) significance level. Data were analysed using the statistical software package SPSS version 20.

3. Results

The study population included 406 patients. Mean (SD) age of the patients was 75.2 (9.4) years, 55.7% were female and 70.9% were retired. The duration of treatment with warfarin ranged from 1 to 20 years. The mean treatment duration did not differ between males and females (5.2 (3.3) and 5.5 (4.0) years, respectively; $p = 0.934$). A total of 309 patients (76.1%) were taking concomitant medications with a known potential of interaction with warfarin. Baseline sociodemographic and clinical characteristics are summarized in Table 1.

The majority of patients (89.6%) had a high risk of stroke (CHA2DS2VASc score ≥3), and 63.5% of patients were at high risk of bleeding (HAS-BLED score ≥3) (Table 1). The HAS-BLED score and CHA2DS2-VASc score showed a moderate correlation (Spearman's rho: 0.476; $p < 0.001$).

Table 1. Sociodemographic and clinical characteristics of the study population.

Characteristics	
Type of health care centre	
private, n (%)	93 (22.9)
public, n (%)	313 (77.1)
Number of people served per health care centre, mean (SD [1])	21,674.8 (6792.2)
Age, mean (SD), years	75.2 (9.4)
Gender	
male, n (%)	180 (44.3)
female, n (%)	226 (55.7)
Place of residence	
rural, n (%)	75 (18.5)
urban, n (%)	331 (81.5)
Distance to healthcare centre, mean (SD), kilometres	3.50 (4.62)
Ability to work	
fully able to work, n (%)	34 (8.4)
retired, n (%)	288 (70.9)
disabled, n (%)	50 (12.3)
not self-sufficient, n (%)	34 (8.4)
Warfarin treatment duration, mean (SD), years	5.4 (3.7)
Concomitant medications with known potential to interact with warfarin	
strengthening the effect of warfarin, n (%)	183 (45.1)
lowering the effect of warfarin, n (%)	126 (31.0)
HAS-BLED [2]	
Total score, mean (SD)	2.85 (1.00)
Low bleeding risk (score $\leq$ 2), n (%)	146 (36.0)
High bleeding risk (score $\geq$ 3), n (%)	258 (63.5)
CHA2DS2-VASc [3] total score	
Mean (SD)	4.6 (1.6)
1, n (%)	7 (1.7)
2, n (%)	34 (8.4)
3, n (%)	45 (11.1)
4, n (%)	104 (25.6)
5, n (%)	106 (26.1)
6, n (%)	60 (14.8)
7, n (%)	31 (7.6)
8, n (%)	15 (3.7)
9, n (%)	3 (0.7)

[1] Standard deviation; [2] Hypertension, Abnormal renal/liver function, Stroke, Bleeding history or predisposition, Labile INR, Elderly, Drugs/alcohol concomitantly; [3] Congestive heart failure, Hypertension, Age $\geq$ 75 years, Diabetes, Stroke, Vascular disease, Age 65–74 years, Sex category.

The median (IQR) number of INR measurements per patient per year was 8.0 (6.0–10.0). More than half (57.3%) of available INR values were outside the target range, mostly below 2.0. The median TTR was 40.0%. Only 20% of patients had TTR ≥65%. Within one-year observational period, 31% of patients had at least two INR values below 1.5 (Table 2). The correlation between the number of INR measurements and TTR was insignificant (Spearman's rho: 0.089; $p = 0.074$).

The most common corrective actions taken by physicians were warfarin dose increases in the case of INR <2.0, and dose reductions in the case of INR >3.0. However, in about 40% of cases of INR outside the target range, no dose corrections were implemented (Table 2). There were 2423 (73.16%) decisions on warfarin dose adjustment consistent with the recommended warfarin posology and 889 (26.84%) inconsistent decisions. The proportion of decisions consistent with the recommended posology was significantly greater in PHCCs located in rural areas to compare to urban areas (77.8% versus 72.0%; chi square $p < 0.01$).

Table 2. Characteristics of anticoagulation control.

Characteristics	
International normalized ratio (INR)	
Total number of INR [1] measurements, n	3337
INR value, median (IQR [2])	2.2 (1.7–2.6)
INR within 2.0–3.0, n (%)	1424 (42.7)
INR <2.0, n (%)	1458 (43.7)
INR >3.0, n (%)	455 (13.6)
INR >8.0, n (%)	9 (0.3)
Patients with at least two INR values of <1.5	125 (30.8)
Time in therapeutic range (TTR)	
TTR [3], median (IQR), %	40.0 (25.0–60.0)
TTR <50%, n (%)	238 (58.6)
TTR 50–65%, n (%)	85 (20.9)
TTR ≥65%, n (%)	83 (20.4)
Warfarin dose adjustments	
INR <2.0	
Dose increased, n (%)	804 (55.8)
Dose decreased, n (%)	34 (2.4)
No dose correction, n (%)	602 (41.8)
INR >3.0	
Dose increased, n (%)	7 (1.6)
Dose decreased, n (%)	276 (61.1)
No dose correction, n (%)	169 (37.4)
TTR <65%	
Dose increased, n (%)	784 (29.6)
Dose decreased, n (%)	326 (12.3)
No dose correction, n (%)	1538 (58.1)
TTR ≥65%	
Dose increased, n (%)	56 (8.5)
Dose decreased, n (%)	37 (5.6)
No dose correction, n (%)	570 (86.0)

[1] International normalized ratio; [2] Interquartile range; [3] Time in therapeutic range.

The control of anticoagulation as expressed by the median number of INR measurements per patient was not significantly different between men and women, younger and older patients, among patients with different ability to work or bleeding risk (Table 3). Median TTR was significantly lower in patients with high bleeding risk (36.4%) as compared to low risk patients (55.6%) (Table 3). Among patients taking concomitant medicines that are known to increase the effect of warfarin, the median number of INR measurements was lower as compared to patients taking no medicines with a potential of interaction with warfarin. The median number of INR measurements was lower among patients living in urban areas, while no differences were observed in relation to distance to health care centre. In contrast, median TTR was significantly higher in urban patients than in rural patients (Table 3).

In the univariate analysis, higher HAS-BLED scores and CHA2DS2-VASc scores were significantly associated with lower odds ratios to attain TTR of ≥65.0% (Table 4). In the multivariate logistic analysis (Table 5), gender ($p = 0.041$), HAS-BLED score ($p < 0.001$) and duration of warfarin treatment ($p = 0.029$) were significantly associated with TTR of ≥65.0%. Male gender and higher HAS-BLED score were associated with decreased odds ratios of good anticoagulation. Each increase in HAS-BLED score by 1 point decreased the odd of having TTR of ≥65.0% by 0.42, whereas each additional year of warfarin treatment increased these odds ratio by 1.08.

Table 3. Comparison of anticoagulation control in patient subgroups.

Variable	INR [1] Measurements Per Patient		TTR [2]	
	Median (IQR [3])	*p* Value	Median (IQR)	*p* Value
Gender				
Men	8.0 (6.0–10.0)		40.0 (20.0–58.3)	
Women	8.0 (6.0–10.0)	0.807	40.0 (25.0–60.6)	0.360
Age				
<65 years	9.0 (6.3–10.0)		47.2 (28.9–66.7)	
≥65 years	8.0 (6.0–10.0)	0.316	40.0 (22.2–60.0)	0.172
HAS-BLED [4]				
Low bleeding risk	8.0 (6.0–10.0)		55.6 (33.3–71.4)	
High bleeding risk	8.0 (6.0–10.0)	0.520	36.4 (20.0–50.0)	<0.001
Concomitant medications with potential of interaction				
none	9.0 (6.0–11.0)		40.00(16.7–58.3)	
strengthening the effect of warfarin	7.0 (6.0–10.0)	0.048	40.0 (22.2–60.0)	0.559
lowering the effect of warfarin	8.0 (6.0–10.0)	0.066	33.3 (20.2–58.6)	0.658
both strengthing and/or lowering the effect of warfarin	8.0 (6.0–10.5)	0.499	41.7 (25.0–60.0)	0.317
Ability to work				
fully able to work	9.0 (6.8–11.0)		47.7 (26.7–62.5)	
retired	8.0 (6.0–10.0)	0.192	40.0 (22.2–60.0)	0.197
disabled	8.0 (7.0–10.3)	0.663	43.6 (25.0–60.0)	0.474
not self-sufficient person	9.0 (6.0–11.0)	0.757	47.2 (23.8–64.4)	0.920
Distance to health care centre				
<5 km	8.0 (6.0–10.0)		40.0 (25.0–60.0)	
≥5 km	9.0 (6.0–10.0)	0.755	41.7 (19.1–61.3)	0.751
Place of residence				
rural	10.0 (7.0–11.0)		33.3 (20.0–54.6)	
urban	8.0 (6.0–10.0)	<0.0001	41.7 (25.0–60.0)	0.040

[1] International normalized ratio; [2] time in therapeutic range; [3] interquartile range; [4] Hypertension, Abnormal renal/liver function, Stroke, Bleeding history or predisposition, Labile INR, Elderly, Drugs/alcohol concomitantly.

Table 4. Univariate logistic regression analysis for values of TTR ≥65.0%.

Variable	Odds Ratio	95% Confidence Interval	*p* Value
Age	0.98	0.96–1.01	0.163
Type of health care centre (private owned)	1.09	0.62–1.92	0.772
Gender (male)	0.74	0.45–1.22	0.236
Ability to work			
retired (versus fully able to work)	0.97	0.40–2.34	0.951
disabled (versus fully able to work)	0.96	0.33–2.85	0.947
not self-sufficient (versus fully able to work)	1.19	0.38–3.74	0.77
Place of residence (rural)	0.62	0.31–1.23	0.173
Distance to health care centre	0.97	0.91–1.04	0.419
HAS-BLED [1] score	0.46	0.35–0.61	<0.001
CHA2DS2-VASc [2] score	0.85	0.72–0.99	0.035
Number of INR measurements per year	0.96	0.87–1.05	0.346
Duration of warfarin treatment	1.06	0.99–1.12	0.090
Use of medicines interacting with warfarin (versus not using interacting medicine)	1.12	0.60–2.06	0.727

[1] Hypertension, Abnormal renal/liver function, Stroke, Bleeding history or predisposition, Labile INR, Elderly, Drugs/alcohol concomitantly; [2] Congestive heart failure, Hypertension, Age ≥ 75 years, Diabetes, Stroke, Vascular disease, Age 65–74 years, Sex category

Table 5. Multivariate logistic regression analysis for values of TTR ≥65.0%.

Variable	Odds Ratio	95% Confidence Interval	*p* Value
Gender (male)	0.57	0.33–0.98	0.041
HAS-BLED [1] score	0.42	0.31–0.57	<0.001
Duration of warfarin treatment	1.08	1.01–1.15	0.029

[1] Hypertension, Abnormal renal/liver function, Stroke, Bleeding history or predisposition, Labile INR, Elderly, Drugs/alcohol concomitantly.

4. Discussion

In our cohort of patients taking warfarin as an oral anticoagulant, only 20% of the patients had a TTR of ≥65%. Less than half (43%) of available INR values were within the therapeutic range of 2.0 to 3.0. Most of INR values out of the therapeutic range were due to inadequate anticoagulation (i.e., <2.0). We previously reported similar results in a smaller sample of patients [15]. Another Lithuanian study found that only 19% of the patients receiving anticoagulation therapy (mostly VKAs) were in the therapeutic range (INR value between 2.0 and 3.0) [16]. Although the population in that study was slightly different (i.e., patients with AF attending cardiologist consultation at the tertiary care centre), the most common reason of being outside therapeutic range was the same, i.e., INR <2.0. Other studies conducted in various countries also reported that patients outside the therapeutic INR range are mostly because of undercoagulation rather than overcoagulation [8,10,17]. It has been suggested that physicians might be reluctant to increase warfarin dose even in response to too low INR [17]. A specially designed retrospective study failed to identify the specific causes of over- and undercoagulation in patients on warfarin therapy. In that study, the common causes of undercoagulation included response to previous change in dosage (16.4%), noncompliance or dosing errors (16.3%) and initiation of therapy (15.6%). A combination of several factors (i.e., changes in drugs, medical condition, dietary vitamin K intake, alcohol use and activity level) accounted for only 15.1% of INRs below 2.0. The cause of undercoagulation remained unknown in 29.7% of INR values below 2.0 [18].

The quality of anticoagulation with VKAs, as measured by TTR, varies considerably between studies, study sites and countries [8,19–23]. Patients treated in specialist care setting have higher TTR compared to primary care [8,24,25]. Currently, there is no consensus whether a critical level of TTR exists below which anticoagulation therapy is ineffective. A post hoc analysis of a large randomized trial of oral anticoagulation therapy versus clopidogrel plus aspirin indicated a critical value for TTR of 65% [20]. In the GARFIELD-AF study, patients with TTR <65% had a 2.6-fold higher risk of stroke, 1.5-fold higher risk of major bleeding and 2.4-fold higher risk of all-cause mortality [10]. In a UK study, stroke risk in patients with TTR of ≥70% was reduced by 79% compared to patients with TTR <30% [26]. A retrospective, multicentre cohort study based on Swedish registries suggested that individual TTR should be maintained at ≥70% [27]. In a recent Finish nationwide study, outcomes in AF patients taking warfarin continued to improve with increasing TTR values up to TTR ≥ 80% [28]. In international guidelines, the recommended cut-off of TTR ranges from 60% to 70% [12,29–31]. The national conditions for reimbursement of NOACs in Lithuania allow a reassessment of warfarin-based anticoagulation therapies if TTR is <65% [12].

The only patient characteristics associated with TTR in our multivariate regression model were gender, HAS-BLED score and the duration of warfarin treatment. Several studies demonstrated that poor anticoagulation quality is associated with female gender [15,32,33] and anticoagulation quality is deteriorated over time [9,24,32,34]. In contrast to previously reported results [15,32,33], in our study, males had a higher risk of poor anticoagulation, suggesting that there could be some important confounding factors among male patients. It has been reported that patients' characteristics only explain 2–4% of the variation in individual's TTR in patients starting warfarin after the first diagnosis of AF or venous thromboembolism [35]. In patients with high quality TTR (≥70%) in an initial 6 months period on warfarin, patients' characteristics did not strongly predict TTR in the second 6 months period, although heart failure moderately increased the risk of TTR deterioration [36]. In the US Outcomes Registry for Better Informed Treatment of Atrial Fibrillation (ORBIT-AF study, renal dysfunction, advanced heart failure, frailty, prior valve surgery and higher risk for bleeding (ATRIA score) or stroke (CHA2DS2-VASc score) was significantly associated with lower TTR [23]. The Veterans AffaiRs Study to Improve Anticoagulation (VARIA) found that hospitalizations, alcohol abuse, substance abuse, cancer and dementia were particularly strong predictors of poor control and that patient-level predictors of anticoagulation control were different at the initiation of warfarin therapy than at the later periods [32]. People with higher warfarin awareness (i.e., patients' knowledge of warfarin's effect and food-drug interactions) had higher TTR levels [37,38].

The unexpected finding in our study was less intense INR monitoring in patients taking concomitant medicines that are known to increase the effect of warfarin. We had no information that could explain such results. However, it might be that such patients are taking more concomitant medicines because of more severe conditions, and therefore, they are not able to attend a physician's office for blood tests regularly.

In addition to patient-level characteristics, clinical skill in warfarin dosing decisions (i.e., extent to which warfarin dosing is consistent with a simple algorithm, which specified no dose change if the INR is in range and dose changes if the INR is out of range) has been shown to be an important determinant of TTR and the composite clinical outcome of stroke, systemic embolism and major bleeding [22]. We found that warfarin doses were not adjusted in about 40% cases of INR outside the target range. Nearly 30% of dose adjustment decisions were not consistent with the recommended warfarin posology. In addition, our patients had a median of 8.0 INR measurements per year, which is less than the number reimbursed by the National Health Insurance Fund (i.e., 12 INR measurements per year). INR monitoring may not be optimal for a variety of reasons, including too rare patients visits, requirements to receive a formal referral for a blood test, lack of patients' awareness of the importance of coagulation control, etc.

The findings of this study might implicate that possibilities for improvement of anticoagulation management exist in primary health care settings. However, we only analysed dose adjustment-related actions, which followed INR measurement and had no information on other factors (e.g., concomitant diseases) that might have determined physicians' decisions regarding warfarin dose adjustments. Of note, it is not recommended to adjust warfarin doses when single INR values are slightly out of range in patients with previously stable therapeutic INRs [39].

This study revealed that physicians working at rural PHCCs more frequently adjusted warfarin dose consistently with the recommended posology. Moreover, the INR monitoring was more intensive among patients living in rural areas, while no differences were observed in relation to distance to health care centre. Thus, rural PHCCs, which also served less people than urban PHCCs, seem to provide more optimal patient care. Despite anticoagulation management efforts, the median TTR in rural patients was significantly lower than in urban patients, implicating that patient-related factors might be important determinants of anticoagulation quality.

We found that patients at high bleeding risk (as assessed using HAS-BLED score) had lower TTR than patients at low risk. In addition, HAS-BLED score was significantly associated with having TTR of $\geq$65.0% in a multivariate logistic regression model. In the univariate analysis, CHA2DS2-VASc score was also associated with TTR of $\geq$65.0%. Other studies also reported that increased baseline bleeding and stroke risk is associated with poor INR control [40] or lower TTR [23]. It has been suggested that such paradox when higher risk patients appear to receive less optimal care may result from the negative impact of comorbidities on TTR either through poorer medication adherence or biological variation in clotting factors [34].

The results of this study should be interpreted with caution because of several limitations. First, this study has limitations of a retrospective observational design. Retrieved data depended on the accuracy and completeness of medical records available at PHCCs. Secondly, the selected PHCCs may not represent all Lithuanian PHCCs and whole population of warfarin-treated patients with AF; therefore, the generalizability of study findings is limited. In addition, we determined TTR using the fraction of INR's in range methodology, which is used in routine practice, whereas other published studies mostly used the Rosenthal linear interpolation method. However, the direct comparison of different methodologies used for measuring TTR did not distinguish the method that best reflects the quality of anticoagulation management [41].

5. Conclusions

This study confirmed that anticoagulation control is suboptimal in routine clinical practice with a median TTR of 40%. Although some of our findings suggest that there might be a room for improvement of anticoagulation control in primary care, a further nationwide study focusing on disease-, patient- and physician-related factors is needed to identify potential targets for actions.

Author Contributions: G.U. and L.V. conceived and designed the experiments; K.P. and I.P. performed the experiments; G.U. and G.Š. analysed the data; G.U., I.P. and G.Š. wrote the paper.

Acknowledgments: The authors thank Ligita Marozienė of UAB Biomapas (Lithuania) for providing medical writing support.

References

1. Krijthe, B.P.; Kunst, A.; Benjamin, E.J.; Lip, G.Y.; Franco, O.H.; Hofman, A.; Witteman, J.C.; Stricker, B.H.; Heeringa, J. Projections on the number of individuals with atrial fibrillation in the European Union, from 2000 to 2060. *Eur. Heart J.* **2013**, *34*, 2746–2751. [CrossRef] [PubMed]
2. Adlan, A.; Lip, G.Y. Preventative measures of stroke in patients with atrial fibrillation. *J. Atr. Fibrillation* **2012**, *4*, 399:1–399:13. [CrossRef]
3. McIntyre, W.F.; Healey, J. Stroke prevention for patients with atrial fibrillation: Beyond the guidelines. *J. Atr. Fibrillation* **2017**, *9*, 1475:1–1475:7. [CrossRef] [PubMed]
4. January, C.T.; Wann, L.S.; Alpert, J.S.; Calkins, H.; Cigarroa, J.E.; Cleveland, J.C., Jr.; Conti, J.B.; Ellinor, P.T.; Ezekowitz, M.D.; Field, M.E.; et al. 2014 AHA/ACC/HRS guideline for the management of patients with atrial fibrillation: A report of the American College of Cardiology/American Heart Association Task Force on Practice Guidelines and the Heart Rhythm Society. *J. Am. Coll. Cardiol.* **2014**, *64*. [CrossRef] [PubMed]
5. Burn, J.; Pirmohamed, M. Direct oral anticoagulants versus warfarin: Is new always better than the old? *Open Heart* **2018**, *5*, e000712:1–e000712:5. [CrossRef] [PubMed]
6. Segal, J.B.; McNamara, R.L.; Miller, M.R.; Kim, N.; Goodman, S.N.; Powe, N.R.; Robinson, K.A.; Bass, E.B. Prevention of thromboembolism in atrial fibrillation. A meta-analysis of trials of anticoagulants and antiplatelet drugs. *J. Gen. Intern Med.* **2000**, *15*, 56–67. [CrossRef]
7. Hart, R.G.; Pearce, L.A.; Aguilar, M.I. Meta-analysis: Antithrombotic therapy to prevent stroke in patients who have nonvalvular atrial fibrillation. *Ann. Intern Med.* **2007**, *146*, 857–867. [CrossRef] [PubMed]
8. Mearns, E.S.; White, C.M.; Kohn, C.G.; Hawthorne, J.; Song, J.S.; Meng, J.; Schein, J.R.; Raut, M.K.; Coleman, C.I. Quality of vitamin K antagonist control and outcomes in atrial fibrillation patients: A meta-analysis and meta-regression. *Thromb. J.* **2014**, *12*, 14:1–14:20. [CrossRef] [PubMed]
9. Jones, M.; McEwan, P.; Morgan, C.L.; Peters, J.R.; Goodfellow, J.; Currie, C.J. Evaluation of the pattern of treatment, level of anticoagulation control, and outcome of treatment with warfarin in patients with nonvalvar atrial fibrillation: A record linkage study in a large British population. *Heart* **2005**, *91*, 472–477. [CrossRef]
10. Haas, S.; Ten Cate, H.; Accetta, G.; Angchaisuksiri, P.; Bassand, J.P.; Camm, A.J.; Corbalan, R.; Darius, H.; Fitzmaurice, D.A.; Goldhaber, S.Z.; et al. Quality of vitamin K antagonist control and 1-year outcomes in patients with atrial fibrillation: A global perspective from the GARFIELD-AF registry. *PLoS ONE* **2016**, *11*, e0164076:1–e0164076:15. [CrossRef]
11. Vestergaard, A.S.; Skjøth, F.; Larsen, T.B.; Ehlers, L.H. The importance of mean time in therapeutic range for complication rates in warfarin therapy of patients with atrial fibrillation: A systematic review and meta-regression analysis. *PLoS ONE* **2017**, *12*, e0188482:1–e0188482:17. [CrossRef] [PubMed]
12. Kirchhof, P.; Benussi, S.; Kotecha, D.; Ahlsson, A.; Atar, D.; Casadei, B.; Castella, M.; Diener, H.C.; Heidbuchel, H.; Hendriks, J.; et al. 2016 ESC Guidelines for the management of atrial fibrillation developed in collaboration with EACTS. *Eur. J. Cardiothorac. Surg.* **2016**, *50*. [CrossRef] [PubMed]
13. Ministry of Health in The Republic of Lithuania. *Order No V-1389 (6 December 2017) by the Minister of Health of the Republic of Lithuania on the Amendment of the Order No 49 (28 January 2000) "Regarding the Approval of List of Reimbursed Medicinal Products"*; Nr. V-1389; Ministry of Health: Vilnius, Lithuania, 6 December 2017.

14. ORFARIN 3 mg Tabletės/ORFARIN 5 mg Tabletės. Summary of Product Characteristics. Available online: https://vapris.vvkt.lt/vvkt-web/public/medications (accessed on 4 May 2018).
15. Dragūnas, G.; Ražukas, P.; Urbonas, G.; Zutkis, M. Lėtiniu prieširdžių virpėjimu sergančių pacientų gydymas varfarinu. Ar pasiekiame tikslą? *Lietuvos Bendrosios Praktikos Gydytojas* **2015**, *19*, 297–301.
16. Račkauskas, G.; Zabiela, V.; Marinskis, G.; Baranauskas, A.; Balkute, D.; Alunderyte, J.; Puodžiukynas, A.; Kazakevičius, T.; Kviesulaitis, V.; Aidietis, A. Evaluation of atrial fibrillation management and cardiovascular risk profile in atrial fibrillation patients: A cross-sectional survey. *Medicina (Kaunas)* **2017**, *53*, 19–25. [CrossRef] [PubMed]
17. Boulanger, L.; Kim, J.; Friedman, M.; Hauch, O.; Foster, T.; Menzin, J. Patterns of use of antithrombotic therapy and quality of anticoagulation among patients with non-valvular atrial fibrillation in clinical practice. *Int. J. Clin. Pract.* **2006**, *60*, 258–264. [CrossRef] [PubMed]
18. Wittkowsky, A.K.; Devine, E.B. Frequency and causes of overanticoagulation and underanticoagulation in patients treated with warfarin. *Pharmacotherapy* **2004**, *24*, 1311–1316. [CrossRef] [PubMed]
19. White, H.D.; Gruber, M.; Feyzi, J.; Kaatz, S.; Tse, H.F.; Husted, S.; Albers, G.W. Comparison of outcomes among patients randomized to warfarin therapy according to anticoagulant control: Results from SPORTIF III and V. *Arch. Intern Med.* **2007**, *167*, 239–245. [CrossRef] [PubMed]
20. Connolly, S.J.; Pogue, J.; Eikelboom, J.; Flaker, G.; Commerford, P.; Franzosi, M.G.; Healey, J.S.; Yusuf, S.; Active, W. Investigators. Benefit of oral anticoagulant over antiplatelet therapy in atrial fibrillation depends on the quality of international normalized ratio control achieved by centers and countries as measured by time in therapeutic range. *Circulation* **2008**, *118*, 2029–2037. [CrossRef]
21. Wallentin, L.; Yusuf, S.; Ezekowitz, M.D.; Alings, M.; Flather, M.; Franzosi, M.G.; Pais, P.; Dans, A.; Eikelboom, J.; Oldgren, J.; et al. Efficacy and safety of dabigatran compared with warfarin at different levels of international normalised ratio control for stroke prevention in atrial fibrillation: An analysis of the RE-LY trial. *Lancet* **2010**, *376*, 975–983. [CrossRef]
22. Van Spall, H.G.; Wallentin, L.; Yusuf, S.; Eikelboom, J.W.; Nieuwlaat, R.; Yang, S.; Kabali, C.; Reilly, P.A.; Ezekowitz, M.D.; Connolly, S.J. Variation in warfarin dose adjustment practice is responsible for differences in the quality of anticoagulation control between centers and countries: An analysis of patients receiving warfarin in the randomized evaluation of long-term anticoagulation therapy (RE-LY) trial. *Circulation* **2012**, *26*, 2309–2316. [CrossRef]
23. Pokorney, S.D.; Simon, D.N.; Thomas, L.; Fonarow, G.C.; Kowey, P.R.; Chang, P.; Singer, D.E.; Ansell, J.; Blanco, R.G.; Gersh, B.; et al. Patients' time in therapeutic range on warfarin among US patients with atrial fibrillation: Results from ORBIT-AF registry. *Am. Heart J.* **2015**, *170*, 141–148. [CrossRef] [PubMed]
24. Dolan, G.; Smith, L.A.; Collins, S.; Plumb, J.M. Effect of setting, monitoring intensity and patient experience on anticoagulation control: A systematic review and meta-analysis of the literature. *Curr. Med. Res. Opin.* **2008**, *24*, 1459–1472. [CrossRef]
25. Baker, W.L.; Cios, D.A.; Sander, S.D.; Coleman, C.I. Meta-analysis to assess the quality of warfarin control in atrial fibrillation patients in the United States. *J. Manag. Care Pharm.* **2009**, *15*, 244–252. [CrossRef] [PubMed]
26. Gallagher, A.M.; Setakis, E.; Plumb, J.M.; Clemens, A.; van Staa, T.P. Risks of stroke and mortality associated with suboptimal anticoagulation in atrial fibrillation patients. *Thromb. Haemost.* **2011**, *106*, 968–977. [CrossRef] [PubMed]
27. Björck, F.; Renlund, H.; Lip, G.Y.; Wester, P.; Svensson, P.J.; Själander, A. Outcomes in a warfarin-treated population with atrial fibrillation. *JAMA Cardiol.* **2016**, *1*, 172–180. [CrossRef]
28. Lehto, M.; Niiranen, J.; Korhonen, P.; Mehtälä, J.; Khanfir, H.; Hoti, F.; Lassila, R.; Raatikainen, P. Quality of warfarin therapy and risk of stroke, bleeding, and mortality among patients with atrial fibrillation: Results from the nationwide FinWAF Registry. *Pharmacoepidemiol. Drug Saf.* **2017**, *26*, 657–665. [CrossRef]
29. NICE. Atrial Fibrillation: Management. 18 June 2014. Available online: http://www.nice.org.uk/guidance/cg180/resources/guidance-atrial-fibrillation-the-management-of-atrial-fibrillation-pdf (accessed on 16 May 2018).
30. JCS Joint Working Group. Guidelines for Pharmacotherapy of Atrial Fibrillation (JCS 2013). *Circ. J.* **2014**, *78*, 1997–2021. [CrossRef]
31. Ogawa, S.; Aonuma, K.; Tse, H.-F.; Huang, D.; Huang, J.-L.; Kalman, J.; Kamakura, S.; Nair, M.; Shin, D.-G.; Stiles, M.; et al. The APHRS's 2013 statement on antithrombotic therapy of patients with nonvalvular atrial fibrillation. *J. Arrhythm.* **2013**, *29*, 190–200. [CrossRef]

32. Rose, A.J.; Hylek, E.M.; Ozonoff, A.; Ash, A.S.; Reisman, J.I.; Berlowitz, D.R. Patient characteristics associated with oral anticoagulation control: Results of the Veterans AffaiRs Study to Improve Anticoagulation (VARIA). *J. Thromb. Haemost.* **2010**, *8*, 2182–2191. [CrossRef]
33. Apostolakis, S.; Sullivan, R.M.; Olshansky, B.; Lip, G.Y.H. Factors affecting quality of anticoagulation control among patients with atrial fibrillation on warfarin: The SAMe-TT_2R_2 score. *Chest* **2013**, *144*, 1555–1563. [CrossRef]
34. McAlister, F.A.; Wiebe, N.; Hemmelgarn, B.R. Time in therapeutic range and stability over time for warfarin users in clinical practice: A retrospective cohort study using linked routinely collected health data in Alberta, Canada. *BMJ Open* **2018**, *8*, e016980:1–e016980:8. [CrossRef] [PubMed]
35. Macedo, A.F.; Bell, J.; McCarron, C.; Conroy, R.; Richardson, J.; Scowcroft, A.; Sunderland, T.; Rotheram, N. Determinants of oral anticoagulation control in new warfarin patients: Analysis using data from Clinical Practice Research Datalink. *Thromb. Res.* **2015**, *136*, 250–260. [CrossRef] [PubMed]
36. Dallalzadeh, L.O.; Go, A.S.; Chang, Y.; Borowsky, L.H.; Fang, M.C.; Singer, D.E. Stability of high-quality warfarin anticoagulation in a community-based atrial fibrillation cohort: The Anticoagulation and Risk Factors in Atrial Fibrillation (ATRIA) study. *J. Am. Heart Assoc.* **2016**, *5*, e003482:1–e003482:15. [CrossRef] [PubMed]
37. Çelik, A.; İzci, S.; Kobat, M.A.; Ateş, A.H.; Çakmak, A.; Çakıllı, Y.; Yılmaz, M.B.; Zoghi, M.; WARFARIN-TR Study Collaborates. The awareness, efficacy, safety, and time in therapeutic range of warfarin in the Turkish population: WARFARIN-TR. *Anatol. J. Cardiol.* **2016**, *16*, 595–600. [CrossRef]
38. Palareti, G.; Legnani, C.; Guazzaloca, G.; Lelia, V.; Cosmi, B.; Lunghi, B.; Marchetti, G.; Poli, D.; Pengo, V.; ad hoc Study Group of the Italian Federation of Anticoagulation Clinics. Risks factors for highly unstable response to oral anticoagulation: A case-control study. *Br. J. Haematol* **2005**, *129*, 72–78. [CrossRef] [PubMed]
39. Holbrook, A.; Schulman, S.; Witt, D.M.; Vandvik, P.O.; Fish, J.; Kovacs, M.J.; Svensson, P.J.; Veenstra, D.L.; Crowther, M.; Guyatt, G.H. Evidence-based management of anticoagulant therapy: Antithrombotic Therapy and Prevention of Thrombosis, 9th ed: American College of Chest Physicians Evidence-Based Clinical Practice Guidelines. *Chest* **2012**, *141*, e152S–e184S. [CrossRef] [PubMed]
40. Hellyer, J.A.; Azarbal, F.; Than, C.T.; Fan, J.; Schmitt, S.K.; Yang, F.; Frayne, S.M.; Phibbs, C.S.; Yong, C.; Heidenreich, P.A.; et al. Impact of baseline stroke risk and bleeding risk on warfarin international normalized ratio control in atrial fibrillation (from the TREAT-AF Study). *Am. J. Cardiol.* **2017**, *119*, 268–274. [CrossRef] [PubMed]
41. Schmitt, L.; Speckman, J.; Ansell, J. Quality assessment of anticoagulation dose management: Comparative evaluation of measures of time-in-therapeutic range. *J. Thromb. Thrombolysis* **2003**, *15*, 213–216. [CrossRef] [PubMed]

6

Management of Direct Oral Anticoagulants in Patients with Atrial Fibrillation Undergoing Cardioversion

Giuseppe Coppola, Girolamo Manno, Antonino Mignano *, Mirko Luparelli, Antonino Zarcone, Giuseppina Novo and Egle Corrado

Division of Cardiology, University Hospital "P. Giaccone", University of Palermo, Via del Vespro 129, p.c. 90127 Palermo, Italy; giuseppe.coppola@policlinico.pa.it (G.C.); girolamomanno@hotmail.it (G.M.); mirkolupini@gmail.com (M.L.); zarconeantonino.91@gmail.com (A.Z.); giuseppina.novo@unipa.it (G.N.); eglecorrado@gmail.com (E.C.)

* Correspondence: tonimignano@gmail.com

Abstract: Atrial fibrillation the most common cardiac arrhythmia. Its incidence rises steadily with each decade, becoming a real "epidemic phenomenon". Cardioversion is defined as a rhythm control strategy which, if successful, restores normal sinus rhythm. This, whether obtained with synchronized shock or with drugs, involves a periprocedural risk of stroke and systemic embolism which is reduced by adequate anticoagulant therapy in the weeks before or by the exclusion of left atrial thrombi. Direct oral anticoagulants are safe, manageable, and provide rapid onset of oral anticoagulation; they are an important alternative to heparin/warfarin from all points of view, with a considerable reduction in bleedings and increase in the safety and quality of life of patients.

Keywords: direct oral anticoagulants (DOACs); atrial fibrillation (AF); electrical cardioversion (EC)

1. Introduction

Atrial fibrillation (AF) is the most common cardiac arrhythmia worldwide. It is nowadays a real "epidemic phenomenon" considering an incidence of approximately 25% in patients aged >40 years with high prevalence in elderly patients [1–6]. The worldwide prevalence of atrial fibrillation in the near future will necessitate mandatory, safe, and effective management [5,6].

Cardioversion is defined as a rhythm-control strategy that, if successful, restores normal sinus rhythm. There are two types of cardioversion: pharmacological (the preferred strategy in patients presenting with recent-onset AF; within 48 h) and electrical (the preferred strategy when AF is prolonged). Cardioversion is very important in the management of AF [7,8]; indeed, delays in cardioversion promote atrial remodeling and difficult sinus rhythm restoration, increasing the likelihood of postcardioversion AF recurrence and adding further thromboembolic risk [8–10]. In fact, sinus rhythm restoration, either obtained with electrical cardioversion or with drugs, carries a periprocedural risk of stroke and systemic embolism which is decreased by adequate anticoagulation in the weeks before cardioversion or excluding left atrial thrombi before the procedure [1,9–14] (see Figure 1). For these reasons, prophylactic anticoagulation represents a cornerstone of peri-cardioversion management in patients with AF [1–12], even if, in patients with datable AF (less than 48 h), it is usual to perform cardioversion without transesophageal echocardiogram (TEE) or antecedent oral anticoagulant therapy (OAT) [12–14]. Randomized controlled trials (RCTs) comparing direct oral anticoagulant (DOAC) therapies in patients with AF duration of <48 h are not available. The same applies to patients with hemodynamic instability and AF that can undergo cardioversion immediately [12]. Long-term OAT after cardioversion should be based on the long-term risk of stroke using the CHA2DS2-VASc

(Congestive Heart failure, hypertension, Age ≥75 – doubled-, Diabetes, Stroke –doubled-, Vascular disease, Age 65–74, and Sex female) risk score. If the duration of AF lasted more than 48 h, or its onset is not evaluable, the periprocedural risk of thromboembolism can be as high as 5–7% without anticoagulant therapy [12,14]. In this clinical situation, current guidelines recommend therapeutic anticoagulation for at least 3 weeks before and at least 4 weeks after cardioversion [12–14] (see Figure 1). It is important to underline that the highest risk of thromboembolism is within the first 7 days after cardioversion (>80% of events) with the greatest risk within the first 72 h [15]. An embolic event after cardioversion can be due both to the fact of left atrial thrombi migration or to the subsequent formation and migration of de novo thrombi caused by postcardioversion atrial stunning [8]. The single biggest risk factor for thrombus formation is inadequate anticoagulation [1,12–16]. In the current European Society of Cardiology (ESC) Guidelines for the management of AF [12], the recommendation for anticoagulation with warfarin before cardioversion is in first class for a time ≥3 weeks and must be continued for ≥4 weeks after the procedure, based on pathophysiological and observational data [12]. Compared to vitamin K antagonist (VKA) therapy, the use of DOACs offers potential advantages in the setting of cardioversion, although their use is recommended in Class IIa in the last ESC Guidelines [12]. These advantages include a faster onset of therapeutic anticoagulant effects, avoidance of heparin bridging, and improved quality of life avoiding the mandatory blood sample to control international normalized ratio (INR) range when vitamin K antagonist are used [14].

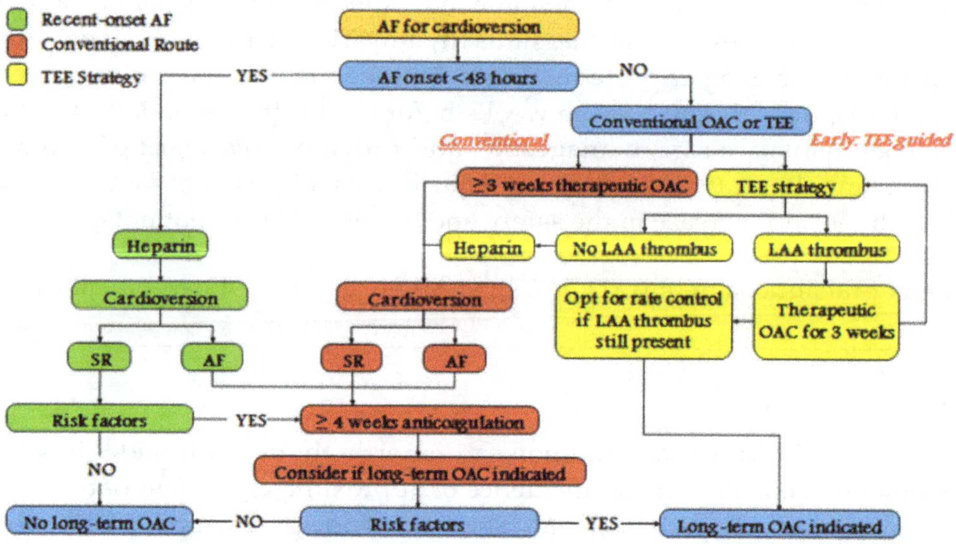

Figure 1. Suggested flow chart for atrial fibrillation (AF) cardioversion on the basis of the current European Society of Cardiology (ESC) Guidelines. Transesophageal echocardiogram (TEE), anticoagulant therapy (OAT), left atrial appendage (LAA), sinus rhythm (SR).

The use of DOACs in this setting of patients is based on subgroup analyses of Randomized Evaluation of Long-Term Anticoagulation Therapy trial (RE-LY) for dabigatran [16], from Rivaroxaban Once Daily Oral Direct Factor Xa Inhibition Compared with Vitamin K Antagonism for Prevention of Stroke and Embolism Trial in Atrial Fibrillation trial (ROCKET AF) for rivaroxaban [17], and from Apixaban for Reduction in Stroke and Other Thromboembolic Events in Atrial Fibrillation trial (ARISTOTLE) for apixaban [18]. Moreover, recent important studies on DOACs suggest new possibilities in cardioversion and deserve to be examined [13,14,19]. These important pieces of evidence have been considered by the American Heart Association (AHA), American College of Cardiology (ACC), and the Heart Rhythm Society (HRS) in the recent 2019 Focused Update of the 2014 AF Guideline [13]. Thus, the aim of this review was to summarize the state-of-the-art methods regarding the use of DOACs in relation to cardioversion.

2. DOACs for Cardioversion in Atrial Fibrillation

From a purely academic and explanatory point of view, we consider four different scenarios regarding cardioversion, which we examine point by point:

- Cardioversion of AF patient treated for >3 weeks with DOACs: we consider the subgroup analyses from RE-LY (dabigatran), ROCKET-AF (rivaroxaban), and ARISTOTLE (apixaban), including important news from the "eXplore the efficacy and safety of once-daily oral riVaroxaban for the prevention of caRdiovascular events in patients with nonvalvular aTrial fibrillation scheduled for cardioversion trial" (X-VeRT study) [20].
- Cardioversion of AF of >48 h in a patient not on DOACs: we consider the X-VeRT study [20] and "Edoxaban versus enoxaparin–warfarin in patients undergoing cardioversion of atrial fi brillation trial" (ENSURE AF) [21].
- Cardioversion of recent onset AF in an anticoagulation-naive patient: in this scenario, the results of the "Eliquis evaluated in acute cardioversion coMpared to usuAl treatmeNts for AnticoagulaTion in subjects with atrial fibrillation trial" (EMANATE trial) are very important [22].
- Patients with evidence of left atrial appendage (LAA) thrombus: we consider the few studies available in the literature on this scenario.

2.1. Cardioversion of AF Patient Treated for >3 Weeks with DOACs

The initial data on the use of DOACs in a clinical setting for cardioversion came from the post-hoc subgroup analysis of randomized control trials (RCTs) RE-LY [16], ROCKET AF [17], and ARISTOTLE [18].

In the RE-LY trial [16,23,24], from a total of 1983 cardioversions, patients received dabigatran 110 mg BID, dabigatran 150 mg BID, and warfarin. It was recommended that patients assigned to dabigatran receive at least 3 weeks of therapy before cardioversion. Stroke and systemic embolism rates at 30 days were 0.77 for dabigatran 110 mg BID, 0.60 for warfarin, 0.30 for dabigatran 150 mg BID, without significant differences among the treatment groups (dabigatran 110 mg versus warfarin, $p = 0.71$; dabigatran 150 mg versus warfarin, $p = 0.40$). Stroke and systemic embolism rates were similar in patients undergoing TEE before cardioversion (25% of patients assigned to dabigatran and 13% of patients assigned to warfarin) and in patients not performing TEE. Major bleeding rates were 1.7% for dabigatran 110 mg group, 0.6% for dabigatran 150 mg, and 0.6% for warfarin (dabigatran 110 mg versus warfarin, $p = 0.06$; dabigatran 150 mg versus warfarin, $p = 0.99$).

The ROCKET AF post-hoc analysis [25] investigated patient outcomes with both cardioversion and catheter ablation procedures; 143 patients underwent electrical cardioversion, 142 underwent pharmacological cardioversion, and 79 underwent catheter ablation. The incidence of stroke or systemic embolism (1.88% versus 1.86%) and death (1.88% versus 3.73%) were similar in the rivaroxaban-treated and warfarin-treated groups. No data were available regarding the use of TEE pre-cardioversion. Major bleeding rates were 18.75% in the rivaroxaban group and 13.04% in the warfarin group. It is important to consider and remember that elective cardioversions were excluded by the enrolling protocol in ROCKET AF, i.e., patients who underwent cardioversion or ablation due to the fact of hemodynamic instability, progressive heart failure, or refractory symptoms despite optimal medical therapy [25].

In the ARISTOTLE trial [18,26], we found 540 cardioversions, and 265 patients received apixaban and 275 received warfarin. A TEE pre-procedural was performed in about 27% of cases. In the first 30 days after cardioversion, no patients experienced a thromboembolic event; one myocardial infarction (MI) and one major bleeding (MB) event occurred in each group, with two deaths in each group. In most cases, cardioversion occurred after months of treatment, with a mean time from enrolment to cardioversion of 243 ± 231 days for patients assigned to warfarin and of 251 ± 248 days for patients assigned to apixaban, far longer than the 3 weeks recommended by international guidelines [27].

Subgroup analyses from RE-LY, ROCKET-AF, and ARISTOTLE underline that electric cardioversion in patients treated with DOACs had a low and similar thromboembolic risk than patients treated with warfarin. According to these data, cardioversion without TEE seems reasonably safe under regular and continued DOAC intake.

2.2. Cardioversion of AF of >48 h in a Patient Not on DOACs Therapy

The X-VeRT, ENSURE-AF, and EMANATE studies [20–22] were evaluated in the context of DOAC-naïve patients, respectively, with rivaroxaban (57% of patients), edoxaban (47%), and apixaban (61%) (see Figure 2).

		ENSURE-AF	X-VeRT	EMANATE	Tot
# of patients	DOAC	1095	978	753	2826
	VKA	1104	492	747	2343
All Strokes	DOAC	2	2	0	4
	VKA	3	2	6	11
Major Bleed	DOAC	3	6	3	12
	VKA	5	4	6	15

Figure 2. Summary of X-VeRT, ENSURE-AF, and EMANATE trials results.

The X-VeRT study [20] is the first prospective randomized trial of DOACs in patients with atrial fibrillation undergoing elective cardioversion. Rivaroxaban was compared with dose adjusted VKA in the prevention of cardiovascular events in 1504 patients with non valvular atrial fibrillation (NVAF) scheduled for early or delayed cardioversion at the discretion of the local cardiologist investigator. In the early approach, oral anticoagulant therapy was given 1–5 days before cardioversion and, in the rivaroxaban arm, a cardioversion was performed at least 4 h after the first dose. In the delayed cardioversion approach, patients were anticoagulated for a range of 3–8 weeks before the procedure. Prophylaxis with rivaroxaban was considered adequate if the pill count was ≥80% in the three weeks preceding the cardioversion. The procedure was TEE guided in 65% of patients treated with an early strategy, whereas a TEE-guided cardioversion was performed in 10% of patients using a delayed strategy, with no significant difference in the rate of TEE employment among the two treatment groups. Primary efficacy endpoints were a composite of stroke and transient ischemic attack (TIA), non- systemic embolism, MI, CV death, while primary safety endpoints were MB. The primary efficacy endpoint occurred in 0.51% of patients in the rivaroxaban arm and 1.02% of patients in the VKAs arm (risk ratio 0.50; 95% CI 0.15–1.73). Majour bleeding (MB) occurred in 0.6% of patients in the rivaroxaban group and in 0.8% of patients in the VKAs group (risk ratio 0.76; 95% CI 0.21–2.67). Rivaroxaban was associated with low rates of adverse outcomes similar to those of VKAs even when data from the early and delayed strategies were analyzed separately. An important difference was found among the two strategies in terms of median time to cardioversion. This data were similar in the early strategy but significantly shorter in the delayed strategy using rivaroxaban versus warfarin (22 days rivaroxaban arm versus 30 days in VKA arm). Only 36% of patients anticoagulated with VKA were cardioverted as scheduled as the INR was not in range, in comparison with 77% in the rivaroxaban arm. According to data from X-VeRT, rivaroxaban can be considered as an effective and safe alternative to VKAs in patients with AF addressed to cardioversion, irrespective of the timing of the procedure. Moreover, X-VeRT showed that rivaroxaban may overcome critical limitations of VKA treatment in the setting of cardioversion, including a significant reduction in time to cardioversion and a considerable reduction of economic expenditure.

In the ENGAGE AF-TIMI 48 trial [28] few patients underwent electrical cardioversion and, therefore, we have limited data about edoxaban in the setting of procedures. Further data about anticoagulation with edoxaban in patients undergoing cardioversion are provided by the ENSURE-AF [21] which is the largest prospective randomized clinical trial of anticoagulation for cardioversion of patients with non-valvular atrial fibrillation. In this trial, 2199 patients scheduled for cardioversion were randomized (1:1) to edoxaban or enoxaparin/warfarin. As in the X-VeRT trial, patients were stratified in two different approaches. In the TEE-guided group, the TEE and cardioversion had to be executed within 3 days of randomization and patients randomly addressed to the edoxaban group had to begin treatment at least 2 h before electrical cardioversion. In the non-TEE-guided group, electrical cardioversion was executed at a minimum of 21 days following the start of anticoagulation. The primary endpoint (PE) was a composite of stroke, systemic embolic event (SEE), MI, and cardiovascular (CV) mortality, while the primary safety endpoint was a composite of major and non-major but clinically relevant bleeding (CRNM). The primary endpoint was similar with edoxaban compared to enoxaparin/warfarin in patients undergoing electrical cardioversion of NVAF (<1% edoxaban arm versus 1% enoxaparin/warfarin, odds ratio (OR) 0·46, 95% CI 0·12–1·43) and was independent of TE or previous anticoagulant therapy. The composite of the PE was numerically lower for edoxaban versus enoxaparin/warfarin and the main difference was due to the cardiovascular mortality, (0.1% in the edoxaban group versus 0.5% in the enoxaparin–warfarin). The primary safety endpoint occurred in 1.5% and 1.0% of patients in the edoxaban versus the enoxaparin/warfarin arm, respectively, and the results were statistically non-significant. There were numerically more major bleedings in the enoxaparin/warfarin arm, while more CRNM bleedings were found in the edoxaban arm. The net clinical outcome (composite of stroke/systemic embolism/myocardial infarction/cardiovascular death/major bleeding) was numerically lower in the edoxaban arm versus the enoxaparin/warfarin arm, but the result was statistically non-significant. In contrast with the X-VeRT study, there was no difference in time to delayed cardioversion among the two treatment groups. This probably means that the ENSURE-AF trial compared edoxaban with the optimized standard care of enoxaparin, bridging the pending therapeutic warfarin. The results suggest that edoxaban may be an effective and safe alternative to enoxaparin/VKA strategy and may allow prompt cardioversion to be performed when following a TEE-guided approach (edoxaban almost 2 h before ECV).

2.3. *Cardioversion of Recent Onset AF, in an Anticoagulation-Naive Patient*

In this very important scenario, a key role is represented by EMANATE study [22]; this was the first study in anticoagulation-naive patients scheduled for cardioversion. All patients received <48 h anticoagulation and 61% were not anticoagulated prior to randomization. One thousand and thirty-eight patients underwent cardioversion, whereas 300 spontaneously restored sinus rhythm; 162 patients were not cardioverted; and in only 855 patients was imaging test (TEE or CT) performed. In some patients randomized to apixaban, according to the investigator, before the cardioversion, a single 10 mg loading dose of apixaban could be administered to achieve exposure at 2 h similar to steady state. Instead the maintenance dose was down titrated to 5 mg. Cardioversion could be performed 2 h after administration of the loading dose; 342 of patients received a loading dose of apixaban. The result of apixaban versus heparin/VKA group showed in EMANATE trial was: 0 versus 6 strokes ($p = 0.0164$), 3 versus 6 major bleeds, 2 versus 1 deaths, and no systemic embolic events in both groups. Among 342 patients receiving the loading dose of apixaban, there were 0 strokes, 1 major bleed, and 1 death. Finally, imaging identified left atrial appendage thrombi in 61 patients; all continued anticoagulation. Among those who underwent second imaging examination (37 ± 11 days after the initial imaging) thrombi resolved in 52% versus 56% in the apixaban and heparin/VKA groups. The EMANATE study supports the use of apixaban in patients with AF undergoing cardioversion. The novelty of this trial was the exclusive enrolment of anticoagulant-naïve patients (62% not receiving, 38% < 48 h) with recently detected AF (new onset or first diagnosed) with a focus on enrolling those amenable to early cardioversion. Also unique to the study, if an immediate cardioversion was planned, there was administration of a loading dose (10 mg) of apixaban at least 2 h before cardioversion. For this reason, potential participants were actively identified in hospital emergency departments which encouraged but did not mandate imaging (TEE or CT).

2.4. *Management of a Patient with Documented Left Atrial Appendage Thrombus*

The left atrial appendage is the site with the highest blood stasis which causes thrombus formation during atrial fibrillation [29]. In fact, about 90% of intracardiac thrombi in patients with cardioembolic events originally develop in the LAA. In patients with evidence of LAA thrombus cardioversion should not be performed. In patients with AF VKA, current guidelines recommend therapy for 3 weeks after diagnosis of an LA/LAA thrombus and long-term therapy for those with a documented residual thrombus [12,30]. Although relevant studies showing differences between DOAC and VKA (small data, although very interesting and encouraging, can be derived from the EMANATE study) do not yet exist, in the past few years, there some evidence has emerged supporting the use of DOACs for LA/LAA thrombus resolution, even if the data are limited to case studies or small case series [31]. The X-TRA study was the first prospective, multicenter study examining thrombus resolution with rivaroxaban in VKA-naïve patients or patients receiving suboptimal or ineffective VKA therapy [31]. This study showed that resolution or reduction of thrombus after rivaroxaban treatment was comparable to the results obtained with VKA therapy according to prior retrospective observational case series and the retrospective CLOT-AF registry [31]. The results suggest that rivaroxaban seems to be a potential option for the treatment of TEE-detected LA/LAA thrombi in patients with AF [31]. Even dabigatran has generated encouraging data regarding its use for LA/LAA thrombus resolution [32]. In a small study with a total of 58 AF patients with LAA thrombus, Xiao et al. [32] demonstrated that dabigatran was effective in the dissolution of LAA thrombus in patients with AF. Ongoing trial RE-LATED-AF will make further clarifications about the use of DOACs in this complex and poorly studied scenario [33].

3. Conclusions

For several years, warfarin has been the primary oral anticoagulant used for patients with AF [34], affirming its superiority over acetylsalicylic acid in reducing thromboembolic risk [1,11–13]. Since 2009 until 2013, the four DOAC registered RCTs have paved the way for a more optimal prevention of thromboembolic risk in patient with AF, reducing hemorrhagic risk; in particular, all DOACs significantly reduced the risk of intracranial hemorrhage (ICH), principally in more complex categories of patients such as in the elderly, frail, and patients with comorbidities (Figure 2) [5,6,35].

Direct oral anticoagulants (DOACs) offer several potential advantages over warfarin therapy in the setting of cardioversion, including removing the need for routine laboratory monitoring and heparin bridging therapy (the latter of which is very important, especially in the case of surgical interventions), as well as having predictable pharmacokinetic and security pharmacodynamic profiles.

Finally, DOACs demonstrated good predictable onset of anticoagulation (since 1 to maximum 4 h) compared with 48 to 72 h for warfarin and up to 5 to 7 days to reach steady state [36,37]. In a very interesting random-effects meta-analysis performed by Brunetti et al. [38], a total of 8564 patients undergoing both electrical and pharmacologic cardioversions for NVAF were included observing, one more time, the effectiveness and safety of DOACs in patients undergoing NVAF.

Unfortunately, today, head-to-head studies do not exist and direct comparisons between DOACs are not possible. Even though other studies concerning DOACs in the context of AF are ongoing (for example, the RE-LATED AF-AFNET 7 trial [33]) and further real-life data are needed, DOACs therapy is an effective and safe strategy in the context of atrial fibrillation patients scheduled for cardioversion.

Author Contributions: First (G.C.) and last (E.C.) author contributed in equal measure, coordinating the drafting of the article and writing the discussion (Sections 2.1–2.4), conclusion and references. G.M. contributed to Sections 2.1–2.4 and references; M.L. contributed to Sections 2.1–2.4 and conclusion, A.M. contributed to introduction, conclusion and references, A.Z. contributed to Section 2.3, Section 2.4, G.N. contributed to Section 2.3, Section 2.4 and conclusion.

References

1. Steffel, J.; Verhamme, P.; Potpara, T.S.; Albaladejo, P.; Antz, M.; Desteghe, L.; Georg Haeusler, K.; Oldgren, J.; Reinecke, H.; Roldan-Schilling, V.; et al. ESC Scientific Document Group. The 2018 European Heart Rhythm Association. Practical Guide on the use of non-vitamin K antagonist oral anticoagulants in patients with atrial fibrillation. *Eur. Heart J.* **2018**, *39*, 1330–1393. [CrossRef] [PubMed]
2. Rietbrock, S.; Heeley, E.; Plumb, J.; van Sta, T. Chronic atrial fibrillation: Incidence, prevalence, and prediction of stroke using the Congestive heart failure, Hypertension, Age >75, Diabetes mellitus, and prior Stroke or transient ischemic attack (CHADS2) risk stratification scheme. *Am. Heart J.* **2008**, *156*, 57–64. [CrossRef] [PubMed]
3. Kulbertus, H.; Lancellotti, P. Fibrillation, an epidemic in the elderly? *Rev. Med. Liege* **2014**, *69*, 301–308. [PubMed]
4. Puccio, D.; Novo, G.; Baiamonte, V.; Nuccio, A.; Fazio, G.; Corrado, E.; Coppola, G.; Muratori, I.; Vernuccio, L.; Novo, S. Atrial fibrillation and mild cognitive impairment: What correlation? *Minerva Cardioangiol.* **2009**, *57*, 143–150.
5. Manno, G.; Novo, G.; Corrado, E.; Coppola, G.; Novo, S. Use of direct oral anticoagulants in very elderly patients: A case report of apixaban in an ultracentenary patient. *J. Cardiovasc. Med. (Hagerstown)* **2019**, *20*, 403–405. [CrossRef] [PubMed]
6. Russo, V.; Carbone, A.; Rago, A.; Golino, P.; Nigro, G. Direct Oral Anticoagulants in octogenarians with atrial fibrillation: it's never too late. *J. Cardiovasc. Pharmacol.* **2019**, *73*, 207–214. [CrossRef]
7. McNamara, R.L.; Tamariz, L.J.; Segal, J.B.; Bass, E.B. Management of atrial fibrillation: Review of the evidence for the role of pharmacologic therapy, electrical cardioversion, and echocardiography. *Ann. Intern. Med.* **2003**, *139*, 1018–1033. [CrossRef]
8. Naccarelli, G.V.; Dell'Orfano, J.T.; Wolbrette, D.L.; Patel, H.M.; Luck, J.C. Cost-effective management of acute atrial fibrillation: Role of rate control, spontaneous conversion, medical and direct current cardioversion, transesophageal echocardiography, and antiembolic therapy. *Am. J. Cardiol.* **2000**, *85*, 36D–45D. [CrossRef]
9. Di Fusco, S.A.; Colivicchi, F.; Aspromonte, N.; Tubaro, M.; Aiello, A.; Santini, M. Direct oral anticoagulants in patients undergoing cardioversion: Insight from randomized clinical trials. *Monaldi Arch. Chest Dis.* **2017**, *87*, 805. [CrossRef]
10. Russo, V; Bottino, R.; Rago, A.; Micco, P.D.; D'Onofrio, A.; Liccardo, B.; Golino, P.; Nigro, G. Atrial Fibrillation and Malignancy: The Clinical Performance of Non-Vitamin K Oral Anticoagulants-A Systematic Review. *Semin. Thromb. Hemost.* **2019**, *45*, 205–214.
11. Andò, G.; Trio, O. New oral anticoagulants versus Warfarin in patients undergoing cardioversion of atrial fibrillation. *Int. J. Cardiol.* **2016**, *225*, 244–246. [CrossRef] [PubMed]
12. Andò, G.; Trio, O.; Carerj, S. New oral anticoagulants versus vitamin K antagonists before cardioversion of atrial fibrillation: A meta-analysis of data from 4 randomized trials. *Expert Rev. Cardiovasc. Ther.* **2015**, *13*, 577–583. [CrossRef] [PubMed]
13. Kirchhof, P.; Benussi, S.; Kotecha, D.; Ahlsson, A.; Atar, D.; Casadei, B.; Castella, M.; Diener, H.C.; Heidbuchel, H.; Hendriks, J.; et al. ESC Scientific Document Group. 2016 ESC Guidelines for the management of atrial fibrillation developed in collaboration with EACTS. *Eur. Heart J.* **2016**, *37*, 2893–2962. [CrossRef] [PubMed]
14. January, C.T.; Wann, L.S.; Calkins, H.; Chen, L.Y.; Cigarroa, J.E.; Cleveland, J.C., Jr.; Ellinor, P.T.; Ezekowitz, M.D.; Field, M.E.; Furie, K.L.; et al. 2019 AHA/ACC/HRS Focused Update of the 2014 AHA/ACC/HRS Guideline for the Management of Patients With Atrial Fibrillation: A Report of the American College of Cardiology/American Heart Association Task Force on Clinical Practice Guidelines and the Heart Rhythm Society. *J. Am. Coll. Cardiol.* **2019**, *74*, 104–132. [PubMed]
15. Trujillo, T.C.; Dobesh, P.P.; Crossley, G.H.; Finks, S.W. Contemporary Management of Direct Oral Anticoagulants During Cardioversion and Ablation for Nonvalvular Atrial Fibrillation. *Pharmacotherapy* **2019**, *39*, 94–108. [CrossRef] [PubMed]

16. Connolly, S.J.; Ezekowitz, M.D.; Yusuf, S.; Eikelboom, J.; Oldgren, J.; Parekh, A.; Pogue, J.; Reilly, P.A.; Themeles, E.; Varrone, J.; et al. for the RE-LY Steering Committee and Investigators. Dabigatran versus warfarin in patients with atrial fibrillation. *N. Engl. J. Med.* **2009**, *361*, 1139–1151. [CrossRef]
17. Patel, M.R.; Mahaffey, K.W.; Garg, J.; Pan, G.; Singer, D.E.; Hacke, W.; Breithardt, G.; Halperin, J.L.; Hankey, G.J.; Piccini, J.P.; et al. ROCKET AF Investigators. Rivaroxaban versus warfarin in nonvalvular atrial fibrillation. *N. Engl. J. Med.* **2011**, *365*, 883–891. [CrossRef]
18. Granger, C.B.; Alexander, J.H.; McMurray, J.J.; Lopes, R.D.; Hylek, E.M.; Hanna, M.; Al-Khalidi, H.R.; Ansell, J.; Atar, D.; Avezum, A.; et al. Apixaban versus warfarin in patients with atrial fibrillation. *N. Engl. J. Med.* **2011**, *0365*, 981–992. [CrossRef] [PubMed]
19. Reilly, P.A.; Lehr, T.; Haertter, S.; Connolly, S.J.; Yusuf, S.; Eikelboom, J.W.; Ezekowitz, M.D.; Nehmiz, G.; Wang, S.; Wallentin, L.; et al. The effect of dabigatran plasma concentrations and patient characteristics on the frequency of ischemic stroke and major bleeding in atrial fibrillation patients: The RE-LY Trial (Randomized Evaluation of Long-Term Anticoagulation Therapy). *J. Am. Coll. Cardiol.* **2014**, *63*, 321–328. [CrossRef]
20. Cappato, R.; Ezekowitz, M.D.; Klein, A.L.; Camm, A.J.; Ma, C.S.; Le Heuzey, J.Y.; Talajic, M.; Scanavacca, M.; Vardas, P.E.; Kirchhof, P.; et al. X-VeRT Investigators. Rivaroxaban vs. vitamin K antagonists for cardioversion in atrial fibrillation. *Eur. Heart J.* **2014**, *35*, 3346–3355. [CrossRef]
21. Goette, A.; Merino, J.L.; Ezekowitz, M.D.; Zamoryakhin, D.; Melino, M.; Jin, J.; Mercuri, M.F.; Grosso, M.A.; Fernandez, V.; Al-Saady, N.; et al. ENSURE-A investigators. Edoxaban versus enoxaparin-warfarin in patients undergoing cardioversion of atrial fibrillation (ENSURE-AF): A randomised, open-label, phase 3b trial. *Lancet* **2016**, *388*, 1995–2003. [CrossRef]
22. Ezekowitz, M.D.; Pollack, C.V., Jr.; Halperin, J.L.; England, R.D.; VanPelt Nguyen, S.; Spahr, J.; Sudworth, M.; Cater, N.B.; Breazna, A.; Oldgren, J.; et al. Apixaban compared to heparin/vitamin K antagonist in patients with atrial fibrillation scheduled for cardioversion: The EMANATE trial. *Eur. Heart J.* **2018**, *39*, 2959–2971. [CrossRef] [PubMed]
23. Lin, H.D.; Lai, C.L.; Dong, Y.H.; Tu, Y.K.; Chan, K.A.; Suissa, S. Re-evaluating Safety and Effectiveness of Dabigatran Versus Warfarin in a Nationwide Data Environment: A Prevalent New-User Design Study. *Drugs Real World Outcomes* **2019**, *6*, 93–104. [CrossRef] [PubMed]
24. Nagarakanti, R.; Ezekowitz, M.D.; Oldgren, J.; Yang, S.; Chernick, M.; Aikens, T.H.; Flaker, G.; Brugada, J.; Kamensky, G.; Parekh, A.; et al. Dabigatran versus warfarin in patients with an analysis of patients undergoing cardioversion. *Circulation* **2011**, *123*, 131–136. [CrossRef] [PubMed]
25. Piccini, J.P.; Stevens, S.R.; Lokhnygina, Y.; Patel, M.R.; Halperin, J.L.; Singer, D.E.; Hankey, G.J.; Hacke, W.; Becker, R.C.; Nessel, C.C.; et al. Outcomes after cardioversion and atrial fibrillation ablation in patients treated with rivaroxaban and warfarin in the ROCKET AF trial. *J. Am. Coll. Cardiol.* **2013**, *61*, 1998–2006. [CrossRef] [PubMed]
26. Lip, G.Y.H.; Khan, A.A.; Olshansky, B. Short-Term Outcomes of Apixaban Versus Warfarin in Patients With Atrial Fibrillation. *Circulation* **2019**, *139*, 2301–2303. [CrossRef] [PubMed]
27. Flaker, G.; Lopes, R.D.; Al-Khatib, S.M.; Hermosillo, A.G.; Hohnloser, S.H.; Tinga, B.; Zhu, J.; Mohan, P.; Garcia, D.; Bartunek, J.; et al. Efficacy and safety of apixaban in patients after cardioversion for atrial fibrillation. *J. Am. Coll. Cardiol.* **2014**, *63*, 1082–1087. [CrossRef]
28. Ruff, C.T.; Giugliano, R.P.; Braunwald, E.; Morrow, D.A.; Murphy, S.A.; Kuder, J.F.; Deenadayalu, N.; Jarolim, P.; Betcher, J.; Shi, M.; et al. Association between edoxaban dose, concentration, anti-Factor Xa activity, and outcomes: An analysis of data from the randomised, double-blind ENGAGE AF-TIMI 48 trial. *Lancet* **2015**, *385*, 2288–2295. [CrossRef]
29. Masci, A.; Barone, L.; Dedè, L.; Fedele, M.; Tomasi, C.; Quarteroni, A.; Corsi, C. The Impact of Left Atrium Appendage Morphology on Stroke Risk Assessment in AtrialFibrillation: A Computational Fluid Dynamics Study. *Front. Physiol.* **2019**, *9*, 1938. [CrossRef]
30. Stabile, G.; Russo, V.; Rapacciuolo, A.; De Divitiis, M.; De Simone, A.; Solimene, F.; D'Onofrio, A.; Iuliano, A.; Maresca, G.; Esposito, F.; et al. Transesophageal echocardiograpy in patients with persistent atrial fibrillation undergoing electrical cardioversion on new oral anticoagulants: A multi center registry. *Int. J. Cardiol.* **2015**, *184*, 283–284. [CrossRef]
31. Lip, G.Y.; Hammerstingl, C.; Marin, F.; Cappato, R.; Meng, I.L.; Kirsch, B.; van Eickels, M.; Cohen, A. X-TRA study and CLOT-AF registry investigators. Left atrial thrombus resolution in atrial fibrillation or flutter:

Results of a prospective study with rivaroxaban (X-TRA) and a retrospective observational registry providing baseline data (CLOT-AF). *Am. Heart J.* **2016**, *178*, 126–134. [CrossRef] [PubMed]

32. Xing, X.F.; Liu, N.N.; Han, Y.L.; Zhou, W.W.; Liang, M.; Wang, Z.L. Anticoagulation efficacy of dabigatran etexilate for left atrial appendage thrombus in patients with atrial fibrillation by transthoracic and transesophageal echocardiography. *Medicine (Baltimore)* **2018**, *97*, e11117. [CrossRef] [PubMed]
33. Ferner, M.; Wachtlin, D.; Konrad, T.; Deuster, O.; Meinertz, T.; von Bardeleben, S.; Münzel, T.; Seibert-Grafe, M.; Breithardt, G.; Rostock, T. Rationale and design of the RE-LATED AF-AFNET 7 trial: Resolution of Left atrial-Appendage Thrombus-Effects of Dabigatran in patients with Atrial Fibrillation. *Clin. Res. Cardiol.* **2016**, *105*, 29–36. [CrossRef] [PubMed]
34. European Atrial Fibrillation Trial Study. Optimal oral anticoagulant therapy in patients with non rheumatic atrial fibrillation and recent cerebral ischemia. *N. Engl. J. Med.* **1995**, *333*, 5–10. [CrossRef] [PubMed]
35. Rago, A.; Papa, A.A.; Cassese, A.; Arena, G.; Magliocca, M.C.G.; D'Onofrio, A.; Golino, P.; Nigro, G.; Russo, V. Clinical Performance of Apixaban vs. Vitamin K Antagonists in Patients with Atrial Fibrillation Undergoing Direct Electrical Current Cardioversion: A Prospective Propensity Score-Matched Cohort Study. *Am. J. Cardiovasc. Drugs* **2019**, *19*, 421–427. [CrossRef] [PubMed]
36. Russo, V.; Rago, A.; Proietti, R.; Di Meo, F.; Papa, A.; Calabrò, P.; D'Onofrio, A.; Nigro, G.; AlTurki, A. Efficacy and safety of the target specific oral anticoagulants for stroke prevention in atrial fibrillation: The real-life evidence. *Ther. Adv. Drug Saf.* **2017**, *8*, 67–75. [CrossRef] [PubMed]
37. Gibson, C.M.; Basto, A.N.; Howard, M.L. Direct Oral Anticoagulants in Cardioversion: A Review of Current Evidence. *Ann. Pharmacother.* **2018**, *52*, 277–284. [CrossRef]
38. Brunetti, N.D.; Tarantino, N.; De Gennaro, L.; Correale, M.; Santoro, F.; Di Biase, M. Direct oral anti-coagulants compared to vitamin-K antagonists in cardioversion of atrial fibrillation: An updated meta-analysis. *J. Thromb. Thromb.* **2018**, *45*, 550–556. [CrossRef] [PubMed]

7

"*A Tale of Two Cities*": Anticoagulation Management in Patients with Atrial Fibrillation and Prosthetic Valves in the Era of Direct Oral Anticoagulants

Giuseppe Palmiero [1,*], Enrico Melillo [1] and Antonino Salvatore Rubino [2]

1 Department of Cardiology, AORN Ospedali dei Colli-Monaldi Hospital, 80131 Naples, Italy
2 Department of Translational Medical Sciences, University of Campania "Luigi Vanvitelli", 80131 Naples, Italy
* Correspondence: g.palmiero@hotmail.it

Abstract: Valvular heart disease and atrial fibrillation often coexist. Oral vitamin K antagonists have represented the main anticoagulation management for antithrombotic prevention in this setting for decades. Novel direct oral anticoagulants (DOACs) are a new class of drugs and currently, due to their well-established efficacy and security, they represent the main therapeutic option in non-valvular atrial fibrillation. Some new evidences are exploring the role of DOACs in patients with valvular atrial fibrillation (mechanical and biological prosthetic valves). In this review we explore the data available in the medical literature to establish the actual role of DOACs in patients with valvular heart disease and atrial fibrillation.

Keywords: novel oral anticoagulants; prosthetic valve replacement; atrial fibrillation

1. Prologue

In 1859 Charles Dickens wrote "*A tale of two cities*", a historical novel set in London and Paris during the French Revolution, a transition period from the monarchical ancient regime to a new form of government. In medicine, now as then, with the introduction into the clinical practice of new therapeutic options for anticoagulation management, a new era is rising, but contrasts are still present. Even in fields of application in which new anticoagulants have proved to be superior to the old molecules (thrombosis prevention in atrial fibrillation and systemic thromboembolism), a sense of comfortability, given by decades of clinical experience of historical anticoagulant drugs, is still contrasting the potential widespread use of new therapeutic option, encouraged by their favorable outcome in terms of efficacy and security.

Moreover, the ancient regime of oral vitamin K antagonists (VKAs) is still dominating the anticoagulation management in prosthetic valve replacement. However, some new evidence seems able to promote a possible revolution in this setting.

2. Introduction

Prosthetic valve replacement represents a historical and effective therapeutic approach for symptoms and outcome improvement in patients with valvular heart disease (VHD) [1]. However, its effectiveness is counterbalanced by complications, whose frequency and severity depend upon valve type and position, as well as other patient-specific risk factors. Thromboembolic events are among those potential prosthesis-related complications, especially early after valve implantation [2].

Biological prosthetic valves, mechanical prosthetic valves, and more recently transcatheter biological prosthetic valve represent the options available in case of natively diseased or damaged heart valves. The decision about the use of one of these prosthetic valves depends upon patient's age, a punctual balance between thromboembolic and bleeding factors, and patient's decision [3].

Long-term anticoagulation therapy has been based historically on oral VKAs [4]. Those agents have been used for some time, accumulating through these decades robust data and clinical experience. For these reasons, despite numerous important limitations, physicians are still confident with their use. Novel direct oral anticoagulants are target-selective agents, including direct thrombin, or factor IIa (dabigatran), and factor Xa inhibitors (apixaban, rivaroxaban, edoxaban). In meta-analysis, including patients across all registration trials, those agents have shown superiority to warfarin (the main VKA agent) for the prevention of stroke and systemic embolism in non-valvular atrial fibrillation [5,6]. DOACs have several pharmacokinetic advantages compared to VKAs: A fixed dose, which avoids the necessity for drug monitoring, rapid onset of action and a short-half life, which limits their action during a short time, few interactions with food and drugs, which makes their use easier and safer. Those characteristics make the DOACs an attractive to VKAs in long-term anticoagulation management of patients with prosthetic valves. However, currently, data showing a net benefit of DOACs in anticoagulation management of prosthetic valve are still lacking.

Recently, in a European Heart Rhythm Association (EHRA) position paper [7] about antithrombotic therapy in atrial fibrillation (AF), a new categorization of VHD in relation to the type of oral anticoagulation use has been proposed. Considering the terms "valvular" and "non-valvular" AF as outdated, the functional EHRA (evaluated heart valves rheumatic or artificial) categorization proposes a distinction in type 1 form, which refers to AF patients with VHD needing therapy with VKAs (moderate-to-severe mitral stenosis of rheumatic origin), and type 2 form, which refers to AF patients with VHD needing therapy with VKAs or DOACs (heart valve regurgitation, aortic stenosis, tricuspid stenosis, pulmonic stenosis, mild mitral stenosis, mitral valve repair, transaortic valve intervention, and bioprosthetic valve replacement). However, this categorization is in contrast with the purpose of the review, namely exploring the possible use of DOACs even in the EHRA type 1 forms, in which these agents are currently contraindicated.

DOACs in AF have showed to but safe and effective in different scenarios: in the elderly [8], in cancer patients [9,10], and in real-life experiences [11,12]. Moreover, DOACs have showed to be well tolerated, with low rates of discontinuation, in real-life [13] as in pivotal trials. Periprocedural and long-time anticoagulation therapy management in patients with AF undergoing interventional procedures represents one of the great chapters related to the use of anticoagulants. Numerous clinical trials have investigated the use of individual drugs in various scenarios and have been translated in recent joint consensus documents among various scientific societies (antithrombotic management in transcatheter valve replacement or repairment [14], percutaneous coronary interventions [15,16], electrophysiological procedures [17], and AF cardioversion [18]). Recent data, analyzing the clinical performance of DOACs in real-world patients who underwent interventional procedures, are emerging. DOACs have shown to be, also in real-world data, both effective and safe in many scenarios (for example, in electrical AF cardioversion [19], also in a population at a high thromboembolic and hemorrhagic risk [20]), confirming the data emerged from dedicated trials. Conversely, real-world data about anticoagulation therapy management in patients undergoing surgical or percutaneous valvular interventions are still missing.

3. Discussion

3.1. Anticoagulation Therapy in Prosthetic Valves

3.1.1. Anticoagulation Therapy in Mechanical Prosthetic Valves

Mechanical prosthetic valves (MPV) are often chosen in younger patients for their intrinsic high durability and low incidence of valve failure. However, these advantages are counterbalanced by a significant increase in thromboembolic events, especially shortly after valve implantation. Multiple thrombotic risk factors are concomitantly present in the vast majority of patients (older age, hypercoagulable state, a history of congestive heart failure, chronic kidney disease or atrial fibrillation, etc.) and for these reasons, long-term anticoagulation is mandatory for MPV and the VKAs are the current standard of care in these patients [3,21].

3.1.2. Anticoagulation Therapy in Biological Prosthetic Valves

Biological prosthetic valves (BPV) are considered less thrombogenic than MPV. However, valve thrombosis in the absence of anticoagulation therapy should not be underestimated, especially in the presence of known risk factors, such as low cardiac output state and structural valve deterioration [2]. Therefore, in patients in sinus rhythm with BPV, following current ACC/AHA guidelines recommendation [22], short-term anticoagulation and antithrombotic management with VKA and low-dose aspirin should be co-administrated for the three to six months after valve implantation. On the other side, ESC/EACTS 2017 guidelines recommend only a short-term (three months) anticoagulation management with VKA after mitral bioprosthetic implantation or surgical valvuloplasty. However, as bioprosthetic aortic valves are considered less thrombogenic than mitral ones [14], short-term antithrombotic management with low-dose aspirin is preferred to anticoagulation therapy. On the other hand, in patients with AF and BPV, long-term anticoagulation with VKA is mandatory, and the general increase in life expectancy is leading to a more frequent association between these two. The thromboembolic risk, in this setting, may be related to both BPV and to AF. However, the incidence of thromboembolic events is similar to those of age-matched patients with chronic AF only [23].

3.1.3. Anticoagulation Therapy After Transcatheter Aortic Valve Implantation

Transcatheter bioprosthetic aortic implantation (TAVI) represents a new therapeutic option for patients with symptomatic severe aortic valve stenosis considered at moderate-to-high risk of surgical replacement. The ESC/EACTS guidelines [3] suggest a dual antiplatelet therapy for the first three to six months after TAVI, followed by lifelong single antiplatelet therapy. In case of high bleeding risk, the dual antiplatelet therapy should be avoided, and the lifelong antithrombotic management should be based on a single antiplatelet therapy. However, new evidence has shown that those valves determine a higher risk of subclinical leaflet thrombosis than surgical prostheses, without significant differences in terms of incidence of stroke [24]. Considering this, current ACC/AHA guidelines [21] have suggested anticoagulation management (non-fractioned heparin for the time interval needed to achieve a 2.5 target INR with VKA) for at least three-months after TAVI, in the absence of a high bleeding risk.

3.2. Role of Direct Oral Anticoagulants in Prosthetic Valves

3.2.1. DOACs in Patients with Atrial Fibrillation and Biological Prosthetic Valves

In AF alone, DOACs represent an effective and safe alternative to VKA. Due to their attractive pharmacokinetic profile, their use has been recently extended to patients with MPV and AF despite the lack of prospective controlled data. Indeed, DOACs have only been restricted for cases with "non-valvular" AF in the currently available trials, and only very few patients with mitral bioprosthesis have been enrolled on the ARISTOTLE [25] and ENGAGE-AF-TIMI48 trials [26].

Guimaraes at al. [27] have recently explored the efficacy and safety of apixaban versus warfarin in patients with AF and prior BPV replacement or valve repair, analyzing the data obtained from patients enrolled in the apixaban pivotal trial (ARISTOTLE). Of more than 18,000 patients enrolled, only 0.6% (104 patients, n = 76 aortic, n = 23 mitral and n = 5 aortic and mitral) had a history of BPV replacement: 55 were randomized to apixaban and 49 to warfarin. Moreover, about 0.3% had a history of valve repair (52 pts, n = 50 mitral and n = 2 aortic): 32 were randomized to apixaban and 20 to warfarin. Efficacy outcomes included stroke or systemic embolism, all-cause stroke, ischemic stroke, myocardial infarction, all-cause death, and cardiovascular death. Safety outcomes included major bleeding, major or clinically evident non-major bleeding, intracranial hemorrhage, gastrointestinal bleeding, and any bleeding. In this subgroup analysis, no significant differences were found between the groups for any of the characteristics analyzed, showing that apixaban is safe and effective also in patients with AF and prior BPV replacement or valve repair. Those results were consistent with results shown in the main ARISTOTLE pivotal trial.

In the edoxaban pivotal ENGAGE AF-TIMI 48 trial patients with left-sided valvular heart disease were enrolled, including those with a history of aortic or mitral valve surgical or transcatheter implantation more than 30 days before randomization [28]. Of more than 21,000 patients enrolled, 0.9% had a previous BPV replacement (191 pts, n = 131 mitral, n = 60 aortic), and among them, 70 patients were randomized to warfarin, 63 patients to high-dose of edoxaban (60 mg daily) and 58 to low-dose of edoxaban (30 mg daily). Primary endpoints included stroke and systemic embolic events, major bleeding, and the primary net clinical outcome. Secondary composite endpoints included ischemic stroke, major adverse cardiac events (myocardial infarction, stroke, or cardiovascular death), and the composite of stroke, all-cause mortality, and life-threatening bleeding. In a subgroup analysis, patients with BPV treated with higher dose edoxaban had similar rates of stroke and major bleeding and lower rates of cardiovascular events (myocardial infarction, cardiovascular death) and primary net clinical outcome compared with warfarin. Patients treated with lower dose edoxaban had similar rates of stroke but lower rates of major bleeding and of the primary net clinical outcome compared with warfarin. In this analysis, edoxaban appears to be a reasonable alternative to warfarin in patients with AF and previous BPV implantation.

However, both the sub-analyses of DOAC pivotal trials have important limitations, including a small sample size and low number of events. Then, to definitively establish the role for alterative anticoagulation to VKA in this setting, larger dedicated controlled trials are needed to definitively assess the safety and efficacy of DOACs.

Russo et al. [29] have proposed in 2018 a multicenter observational study to investigate the efficacy and safety of DOACs in AF patients with BPV or prior surgical valve repair. A total of 122 patients were enrolled. In 92% of cases, warfarin was replaced due to lack of compliance and subtherapeutic INR range. The study population included 24 patients (19.6%) with mitral BPV, 52 patients (43%) with aortic BPV, 41 patients (33.6%) with previous surgical mitral repair, and 5 patients (4%) with a previous surgical aortic repair. Of the total study population, 28.6% were taking apixaban 5 mg twice daily, 24.5% apixaban 2.5 mg twice daily, 18% dabigatran 150 mg twice daily, 13% dabigatran 110 mg twice daily, 9.8% rivaroxaban 20 mg daily, and 5.7% rivaroxaban 15 mg daily. All patients were evaluated for thromboembolic events (ischemic stroke, transient ischemic attack, systemic embolism) as well as major bleeding events during the follow-up period and showed a low mean annual incidence of thromboembolism (0.8%) and major bleeding (1.3%). According to this data, DOAC therapy seems to be an effective and safe treatment alternative for AF patients with BPV or prior surgical valve repair. However, this study is limited by small sample size, a retrospective design, heterogeneous anticoagulation management and lack of VKA control group.

At present, the use of DOACs for the management of concomitant AF following BPV replacement may be considered a valid therapeutic option, with the exception of biological mitral prosthesis implanted in the setting of rheumatic mitral stenosis [30]. However, dedicated double-blinded trials confronting DOACs to VKA in this setting are necessary to evaluate the actual efficacy and safety of recommending the DOACs in patients with bioprosthetic valves.

3.2.2. DOACs in Patients with Atrial Fibrillation and Mechanical Prosthetic Valves

The only published trial investigating the use of a DOACs in mechanical prosthetic valves is the RE-ALIGN Trial [31]. The study made a comparison between dabigatran and warfarin in patients with aortic valve replacement with a mechanical prosthesis for the prophylaxis of thromboembolic events. The study was stopped early after enrollment of only 252 patients due to a significant increase in both thromboembolic (5% in dabigatran group vs. 0% in warfarin group) and bleeding (4% in dabigatran group vs. 2% in warfarin group) events in patients treated with dabigatran compared to conventional therapy with warfarin. Therefore, the use of DOACs in this particular subset of patients appeared of no benefit and excessively harmful, so that the trial was prematurely discontinued. Different mechanisms of action of dabigatran and warfarin can partially explain these findings. In patients with mechanical prosthesis, thrombus formation can derive from contact pathway of coagulation, triggered by exposure of blood to the artificial elements of the valve (ring, struts, leaflets) and from direct release of prothrombotic tissue factor from damaged tissues during surgery. Therefore, VKAs are more effective than dabigatran in this setting by stopping both tissue factor and contact pathway induced coagulation [32].

Despite discouraging results from the RE-ALIGN Trial, Durães and coworkers [33] designed a pilot study to investigate the potential role of rivaroxaban as an alternative to VKA in patients with mechanical prosthetic valves. Their rationale [34,35] was that clotting on the mechanical valves is triggered by the contact and that dabigatran administered in the RE-ALIGN Trial was insufficient to inhibit thrombus formation in this scenario. On the other hand, rivaroxaban is a direct inhibitor of Factor Xa with potential to reduce significantly the generation of thrombin on mechanical prostheses. Accordingly, seven patients with mechanical mitral prosthesis received rivaroxaban 15 mg twice daily and were followed-up for 90 days. At the end of the study, no patients experienced neither thromboembolic nor bleeding adverse events. These findings opened the way to a subsequent randomized controlled trial, whose enrolling phase is expected to end in December 2019.

3.2.3. DOACs After Transcatheter Aortic Valve Implantation in Atrial Fibrillation Patients

The use of DOACs after TAVI has been investigated in the GALILEO trial [36]. In the study, rivaroxaban (10 mg once daily) plus short-term (three months) antiplatelet therapy with low dose aspirin (75 to 100 mg once daily) has been compared to short-term dual antiplatelet therapy management (clopidogrel 75 mg plus aspirin 75 to 100 mg once daily for three months), followed by long-term single antiplatelet management with aspirin alone for thromboembolic prevention after TAVI. The primary efficacy endpoint of the trial is a composite of all-cause death, stroke, systemic embolism, MI, pulmonary embolism, deep vein thrombosis, or symptomatic valve thrombosis. The primary safety endpoint is a composite of life-threatening or disabling bleeding or major bleeding. The trial has been halted precociously: From preliminary data released by Bayer, the rivaroxaban-based antithrombotic strategy has shown an increase in the rates of death or first thromboembolic event (11.4% vs. 8.8%), all-cause death (6.8% vs. 3.3%), and primary bleeding (4.2% vs. 2.4%) compared to antiplatelet-based therapy. Therefore, this confirmed that the use of DOACs is contraindicated after TAVI.

A summary of the main clinical trials and subgroup analysis is reported in Table 1.

Table 1. Summary of the main clinical trials and subgroup analysis assessing the clinical performance of novel oral anticoagulants in patients with bioprosthetic or mechanical heart valve.

Clinical Trial	Prosthetic Valve	N. Patients	Anticoagulant Regimen	Primary Efficacy Endpoint	Safety Endpoint
ARISTOTLE	Biological	104 bioprosthetic valve	Apixaban (n = 55) Warfarin (n = 49)	No significant difference	No significant difference
ENGAGE AF-TIMI 48	Biological	191 bioprosthetic valve	Edoxaban 60 mg (n = 63) Edoxaban 30 mg (n = 58) Warfarin (n = 70)	No significant difference for stroke/systemic embolic events for edoxaban 60 mg (P = 0.15) and edoxaban 30 mg (P = 0.31) vs. warfarin. Lower rates of primary net clinical outcome with edoxaban 60 mg (P = 0.03) and edoxaban 30 mg (P = 0.03)	No significant difference between high dose edoxaban and warfarin (P = 0.26) Lower major bleeding events with edoxaban 30 mg (P = 0.045) vs. warfarin
RE-ALIGN	Mechanical	252 (trial was prematurely stopped)	Dabigatran (150–220–300 mg based on kidney function) Warfarin	9 stroke events (5%) in the dabigatran group No stroke event in the warfarin group	7 major bleeding events (4%) in the dabigatran group 2 major bleeding events (%) in the warfarin group

Table 1. *Cont.*

Clinical Trial	Prosthetic Valve	N. Patients	Anticoagulant Regimen	Primary Efficacy Endpoint	Safety Endpoint
GALILEO	Transcatheter aortic valve replacement	1644 (trial was prematurely stopped)	Rivaroxaban 10 mg + Aspirin 100 for 90 days after TAVR Clopidogrel 75 mg + Aspirin 100 mg for 90 days after TAVR	Death and first thromboembolic events: 11.4% rivaroxaban group vs. 8.8% in antiplatelet group. All-cause death: 6.6% in rivaroxaban group vs. 3.3% in antiplatelet group.	Primary bleeding: 4.2% in rivaroxaban group vs. 2.4% in antiplatelet group.

4. Conclusions

As for all huge transformations occurring in the human history, there always exists a contrast between the forces of changes, which promise to revolutionize the previous status quo, and the forces of reaction, which react against them with the certainties accumulated over the years.

The revolution promised by the novel direct oral anticoagulants in the management of anticoagulant therapy in patients undergoing valve replacement is likely to remain inconclusive: The few clinical trials comparing DOACs to warfarin have been shown to increase the risk of all-cause of mortality, thromboembolic events, and bleeding in patients with MPV. Moreover, a single clinical trial with a single DOAC does not represent robust and clear evidence for dismissing a therapeutic strategy. Furthermore, we should consider that not all DOACs are equal in terms of effectiveness for different indications. Therefore, long-term anticoagulation therapy with VKAs is still mandatory in the setting of mechanical valve replacement.

Even after transcatheter aortic valve replacement, DOACs did not show an advantage over warfarin in terms of thromboembolic bleeding risk reduction. However, the concomitant presence of both thromboembolic and hemorrhagic risk factors, and the lack of robust data, make it difficult to establish the best antithrombotic strategy in this setting.

In patients with BPV, some observations obtained by sub-analysis of pivotal trials data are encouraging. However, in the absence of dedicated double-blinded trials confronting DOACs to VKA in terms of efficacy and safety, there is little evidence of treatment with DOACs in clinical practice in patients with bioprosthetic valves.

Author Contributions: Conceptualization, G.P. and A.S.R.; Resources, G.P and E.M.; Writing—Original Draft Preparation, G.P.; Writing—Review & Editing, E.M. and A.S.R.; Supervision, G.P.

References

1. Reineke, D.; Gisler, F.; Englberger, L.; Carrel, T. Mechanical versus biological aortic valve replacement strategies. *Expert Rev. Cardiovasc. Ther.* **2016**, *14*, 423–430. [CrossRef] [PubMed]
2. Misawa, Y. Valve-related complications after mechanical heart valve implantation. *Surg. Today* **2015**, *45*, 1205–1209. [CrossRef] [PubMed]
3. Baumgartner, H.; Falk, V.; Bax, J.J.; De Bonis, M.; Hamm, C.; Holm, P.J.; Iung, B.; Lancellotti, P.; Lansac, E.; Rodriguez Muñoz, D.; et al. 2017 ESC/EACTS Guidelines for the management of valvular heart disease. *Eur. Heart J.* **2017**, *38*, 2739–2791. [CrossRef] [PubMed]
4. Carnicelli, A.P.; O'Gara, P.T.; Giugliano, R.P. Anticoagulation after heart valve replacement or transcatheter valve implantation. *Am. J. Cardiol.* **2016**, *118*, 1219–1426. [CrossRef] [PubMed]
5. Cohen, A.T.; Hamilton, M.; Mitchell, S.A.; Phatak, H.; Liu, X.; Bird, A.; Tushabe, D.; Batson, S. Comparison of the Novel Oral Anticoagulants Apixaban, Dabigatran, Edoxaban, and Rivaroxaban in the initial and long-term treatment and prevention of venous thromboembolism: Systematic review and network meta-analysis. *PLoS ONE* **2015**, *10*, e0144856. [CrossRef] [PubMed]

6. Lip, G.Y.H.; Collet, J.P.; de Caterina, R.; Fauchier, L.; Lane, D.A.; Larsen, T.B.; Marin, F.; Morais, J.; Narasimhan, C.; Olshansky, B.; et al. Antithrombotic therapy in atrial fibrillation associated with valvular heart disease: Exclusive summary of a joint consensus document from the European Heart Rhythm Association (EHRA) and European Society of Cardiology Working Group on Thrombosis, endorsed by the ESC Working Group on Valvular Heart Disease, Cardiac Arrhythmia Society of Southern Africa (CASSA), Hearth Rhythm Society (HRS), Asia Pacific Herat Rhythm Society (APHRS), South African Heart (SA Heart) Association and Sociedad Latinoamericana de Estimulacion Cardiaca y Electrofisiologia (SOLACE). *Thromb. Haemost.* **2017**, *117*, 2215–2236. [PubMed]
7. Hicks, T.; Stewart, F.; Eising, A. NOACs versus warfarin for stroke prevention in patients with AF: A systematic review and meta-analysis. *Open Heart* **2016**, *3*, e000279. [CrossRef]
8. Russo, V.; Carbone, A.; Rago, A.; Golino, P.; Nigro, G. Direct Oral Anticoagulants in octogenarians with atrial fibrillation: it's never too late. *J. Cardiovasc. Pharmacol.* **2019**, *73*, 207–214. [CrossRef]
9. Russo, V.; Rago, A.; Papa, A.A.; Di Meo, F.; Attena, E.; Golino, P.; D'Onofrio, A.; Nigro, G. Use of Non-Vitamin K Antagonist Oral Anticoagulants in Atrial Fibrillation Patients with Malignancy: Clinical Practice Experience in a Single Institution and Literature Review. *Semin. Thromb. Hemost.* **2018**, *44*, 370–376.
10. Russo, V.; Bottino, R.; Rago, A.; Micco, P.D.; D' Onofrio, A.; Liccardo, B.; Golino, P.; Nigro, G. Atrial Fibrillation and Malignancy: The Clinical Performance of Non-Vitamin K Oral Anticoagulants-A Systematic Review. *Semin. Thromb. Hemost.* **2019**, *45*, 205–214.
11. Russo, V.; Rago, A.; Proietti, R.; Di Meo, F.; Papa, A.A.; Calabrò, P.; D'Onofrio, A.; Nigro, G.; Al Turki, A. Efficacy and safety of the target-specific oral anticoagulants for stroke prevention in atrial fibrillation: the real-life evidence. *Ther. Adv. Drug. Saf.* **2017**, *8*, 67–75. [CrossRef]
12. Russo, V.; Rago, A.; D'Onofrio, A.; Nigro, G. The clinical performance of dabigatran in the Italian real-life experience. *J. Cardiovasc. Med. (Hagerstown).* **2017**, *18*, 922–923. [CrossRef]
13. Verdecchia, P.; D'Onofrio, A.; Russo, V.; Fedele, F.; Adamo, F.; Benedetti, G.; Ferrante, F.; Lodigiani, C.; Paciullo, F.; Aita, A.; et al. Persistence on apixaban in atrial fibrillation patients: A retrospective multicentre study. *J. Cardiovasc. Med. (Hagerstown).* **2019**, *20*, 66–73. [CrossRef]
14. Lip, G.Y.H.; Collet, J.P.; de Caterina, R.; Fauchier, L.; Lane, D.A.; Larsen, T.B.; Marin, F.; Morais, J.; Narasimhan, C.; Olshansky, B.; et al. Antithrombotic therapy in atrial fibrillation associated with valvular heart disease: A joint consensus document from the European Heart Rhythm Association (EHRA) and European Society of Cardiology Working Group on Thrombosis, endorsed by the ESC Working Group on Valvular Heart Disease, Cardiac Arrhythmia Society of Southern Africa (CASSA), Heart Rhythm Society (HRS), Asia Pacific Heart Rhythm Society (APHRS), South African Heart (SA Heart) Association and Sociedad Latinoamericana de Estimulación Cardíaca y Electrofisiología (SOLEACE). *EP Eur.* **2017**, *19*, 1757–1758.
15. Lyp, G.Y.H.; Collet, J.P.; Haude, M.; Byrne, R.; Chung, E.H.; Fauchier, L.; Halvorsen, S.; Lau, D.; Lopez-Cabanillas, N.; Lettino, M.; et al. 2018 Joint European consensus document on the management of antithrombotic therapy in atrial fibrillation patients presenting with acute coronary syndrome and/or undergoing percutaneous cardiovascular interventions: A joint consensus document of the European Heart Rhythm Association (EHRA), European Society of Cardiology Working Group on Thrombosis, European Association of Percutaneous Cardiovascular Interventions (EAPCI), and European Association of Acute Cardiac Care (ACCA) endorsed by the Heart Rhythm Society (HRS), Asia-Pacific Heart Rhythm Society (APHRS), Latin America Heart Rhythm Society (LAHRS), and Cardiac Arrhythmia Society of Southern Africa (CASSA). *EP Eur.* **2019**, *21*, 192–193.
16. Russo, V.; Rago, A.; Proietti, R.; Attena, E.; Rainone, C.; Crisci, M.; Papa, A.A.; Calabrò, P.; D'Onofrio, A.; Golino, P.; et al. Safety and Efficacy of Triple Antithrombotic Therapy with Dabigatran versus Vitamin K Antagonist in Atrial Fibrillation Patients: A Pilot Study. *Biomed Res. Int.* **2019**, 5473240. [CrossRef]
17. Sticherling, C.; Marin, F.; Birnie, D.; Boriani, G.; Calkins, H.; Dan, G.A.; Gulizia, M.; Halvorsen, S.; Hindricks, G.; Kuck, K.H.; et al. Antithrombotic management in patients undergoing electrophysiological procedures: A European Heart Rhythm Association (EHRA) position document endorsed by the ESC Working Group Thrombosis, Heart Rhythm Society (HRS), and Asia Pacific Heart Rhythm Society (APHRS). *Europace* **2015**, *17*, 1197–1214.
18. Russo, V.; Di Napoli, L.; Bianchi, V.; Tavoletta, V.; De Vivo, S.; Cavallaro, C.; Vecchione, F.; Rago, A.; Sarubbi, B.; Calabrò, P.; et al. A new integrated strategy for direct current cardioversion in non-valvular atrial fibrillation patients using short term rivaroxaban administration: The MonaldiVert real life experience. *Int. J. Cardiol.* **2016**, *224*, 454–455. [CrossRef]

19. Russo, V.; Rago, A.; Papa, A.A.; D'Onofrio, A.; Golino, P.; Nigro, G. Efficacy and safety of dabigatran in patients with atrial fibrillation scheduled for transoesophageal echocardiogram-guided direct electrical current cardioversion: A prospective propensity score-matched cohort study. *J. Thromb. Thrombol.* **2018**, *45*, 206–212. [CrossRef]
20. Russo, V.; Bianchi, V.; Cavallaro, C.; Vecchione, F.; De Vivo, S.; Santangelo, L.; Sarubbi, B.; Calabrò, P.; Nigro, G.; D'Onofrio, A. Efficacy and safety of dabigatran in a "real-life" population at high thromboembolic and hemorrhagic risk: Data from MonaldiCare registry. *Eur. Rev. Med. Pharmacol. Sci.* **2015**, *19*, 3961–3967.
21. Nishimura, R.A.; Otto, C.M.; Bonow, R.O.; Carabello, B.A.; Erwin, J.P., 3rd.; Fleisher, L.A.; Jneid, H.; Mack, M.J.; McLeod, C.J.; O'Gara, P.T.; et al. 2017 AHA/ACC focused update of the 2014 AHA/ACC guideline for the management of patients with valvular heart disease: A report of the American College of Cardiology/American Heart Association Task Force on Clinical Practice Guidelines. *Circulation* **2017**, *135*, e1159–e119.
22. Stein, P.D.; Alpert, J.S.; Bussey, H.I.; Dalen, J.E.; Turpie, A.G. Antithrombotic therapy in patients with mechanical and biological prosthetic heart valve. *Chest* **2001**, *119* (Suppl. 1), 220S–227S. [CrossRef]
23. You, J.J.; Singer, D.E.; Howard, P.A.; Lane, D.A.; Eckman, M.H.; Fang, M.C.; Hylek, E.M.; Schulman, S.; Go, A.S.; Hughes, M.; et al. Antithrombotic therapy for atrial fibrillation: Antithrombotic therapy and prevention of thrombosis, 9th ed: American College of Chest Physician Evidence-Based Clinical Practice Guidelines. *Chest* **2012**, *141*, e531S–e575S. [CrossRef]
24. Chakravarty, T.; Sondergaard, L.; Friedman, J.; De Backer, O.; Berman, D.; Kofoed, K.F.; Jilaihawi, H.; Shiota, T.; Abramowitz, Y.; Jørgensen, T.H.; et al. Sublinical leaflet thrombosis in surgical and transcatheter bioprosthetic aortic valves: an observational study. *Lancet* **2017**, *389*, 2383–2392. [CrossRef]
25. Granger, C.B.; Alexander, J.H.; McMurray, J.J.; Lopes, R.D.; Hylek, E.M.; Hanna, M.; Al-Khalidi, H.R.; Ansell, J.; Atar, D.; Avezum, A.; et al. Apixaban versus warfarin in patients with atrial fibrillation. *N. Engl. J. Med.* **2011**, *365*, 981–992. [CrossRef]
26. Giugliano, R.P.; Ruff, C.T.; Braunwald, E.; Murphy, S.A.; Wiviott, S.D.; Halperin, J.L.; Waldo, A.L.; Ezekowitz, M.D.; Weitz, J.I.; Špinar, J.; et al. Edoxaban versus warfarin in patients with atrial fibrillation. *N. Engl. J. Med.* **2013**, *369*, 2093–2104. [CrossRef]
27. Guimaraes, P.O.; Pokorney, S.D.; Lopes, R.D.; Wojdyla, D.M.; Gersh, B.J.; Giczewska, A.; Carnicelli, A.; Lewis, B.S.; Hanna, M.; Wallentin, L.; et al. Efficacy and safety of apixaban vs warfarin in patients with atrial fibrillation and prior bioprosthetic valve replacement of valve repair: Insights from the ARISTOTLE trial. *Clin. Cardiol.* **2019**, *42*, 568–571. [CrossRef]
28. Carnicelli, A.P.; De Caterina, R.; Halperin, J.L.; Renda, G.; Ruff, C.T.; Trevisan, M.; Nordio, F.; Mercuri, M.F.; Antman, E.; Giugliano, R.P.; et al. Edoxaban for the prevention of thromboembolism in patients with atrial fibrillation and bioprosthetic valves. *Circulation* **2017**, *135*, 1273–1275. [CrossRef]
29. Russo, V.; Attena, E.; Mazzone, C.; Esposito, F.; Parisi, V.; Bancone, C.; Rago, A.; Nigro, G.; Sangiuolo, R.; D'Onofrio, A. Non-vitamin K antagonist oral anticoagulants use in patients with atrial fibrillation and bioprosthetic heart valves/prior surgical valve repair: A multicentre clinical practice experience. *Semin. Thromb. Hemost.* **2018**, *44*, 364–369.
30. Steffel, J.; Verhamme, P.; Potpara, T.S.; Albaladejo, P.; Antz, M.; Desteghe, L.; Georg Haeusler, K.; Oldgren, J.; Reinecke, H.; Roldan-Schilling, V.; et al. The 2018 European Heart Rhythm Association Practical Guide on the use of non-vitamin K antagonist oral anticoagulants in patients with atrial fibrillation: Executive summary. *EP Eur.* **2018**, *20*, 1231–1242. [CrossRef]
31. Eikelboom, J.W.; Connolly, S.J.; Brueckmann, M.; Granger, C.B.; Kappetein, A.P.; Mack, M.J.; Blatchford, J.; Devenny, K.; Friedman, J.; Guiver, K.; et al. RE-ALIGN Investigators. Dabigatran versus warfarin in patients with mechanical heart valves. *N. Engl. J. Med.* **2013**, *369*, 1206–1214. [CrossRef]
32. De Caterina, R.; Camm, A.J. What is 'valvular' atrial fibrillation? A reappraisal. *Eur. Heart J.* **2014**, *14*, 3328–3335. [CrossRef]
33. Durães, A.R.; Bitar, Y.S.L.; Lima, M.L.G.; Santos, C.C.; Schonhofen, I.S.; Filho, J.A.L.; Roever, L. Usefulness and Safety of Rivaroxaban in Patients Following Isolated Mitral Valve Replacement with a Mechanical Prosthesis. *Am. J. Cardiol.* **2018**, *122*, 1047–1050. [CrossRef]
34. Durães, A.R.; de Souza Lima Bitar, Y.; Filho, J.A.L.; Schonhofen, I.S.; Camara, E.J.N.; Roever, L.; Cardoso, H.E.D.P.; Akrami, K.M. Rivaroxaban versus Warfarin in Patients with Mechanical Heart Valve: Rationale and Design of the RIWA Study. *Drugs R. D.* **2018**, *18*, 303–308. [CrossRef]

35. Chan, N.C.; Weitz, J.I.; Eikelboom, J.W. Anticoagulation for mechanical heart valves: Will Oral Factor Xa inhibitors be effective. *Arterioscler. Thromb. Vasc. Biol.* **2017**, *37*, 743–745. [CrossRef]
36. Windecker, S.; Tijssen, J.; Giustino, G.; Guimarães, A.H.; Mehran, R.; Valgimigli, M.; Vranckx, P.; Welsh, R.C.; Baber, U.; van Es, G.A.; et al. Trial design: Rivaroxaban for the prevention of major cardiovascular events after transcatheter aortic valve replacement: Rationale and design of the GALILEO study. *Am. Heart J.* **2017**, *184*, 81–87. [CrossRef]

8

Polymorphism of Interleukin 1B may Modulate the Risk of Ischemic Stroke in Polish Patients

Iwona Gorący [1,*], Mariusz Kaczmarczyk [1], Andrzej Ciechanowicz [1], Klaudyna Lewandowska [1], Paweł Jakubiszyn [1], Oksana Bodnar [2], Bartosz Kopijek [3], Andrzej Brodkiewicz [3] and Lech Cyryłowski [4]

1 Department of Clinical and Molecular Biochemistry, Pomeranian Medical University, 70-111 Szczecin, Poland
2 Department of General and Dental Radiology, Pomeranian Medical University, 70-111 Szczecin, Poland
3 Department of Pediatrics, Child Nephrology, Dialysotherapy and Management of Acute Poisoning, Pomeranian Medical University, 71-899 Szczecin, Poland
4 Department of Intervention Radiology, Pomeranian Medical University, 70-111 Szczecin, Poland
* Correspondence: igor@pum.edu.pl

Abstract: *Background and Objectives*: Inflammation plays a crucial role in the pathophysiology of ischemic stroke (IS). Interleukin-1B and interleukin-1 receptor antagonists are key factors in inflammatory processes. Aims: The aims of our study were to evaluate the relationship between genetic variation in interleukin-1B (*IL1B*) rs1143627 and interleukin-1 receptor antagonist (*IL1RN*) variable-number-tandem-repeats (VNTR), and overall IS and subtype prevalence rates. *Materials and Methods:* The analysis included 147 hospitalized Polish patients with IS diagnosed using conventional criteria. The control group consisted of 119 healthy subjects. Genotypes were determined by polymerase chain reaction. *Results:* A significant association between rs1143627 and stroke was found. The -31C *IL1B* polymorphism showed an association with overall IS, OR = 2.30 (1.36–3.87) $p = 0.020$. An association was also detected for LVI (large vessel infarction) subtypes of stroke. After risk factor adjustment (age, diabetes mellitus, dyslipidemia), the C allele was found to be an independent risk factor for LVI, OR = 1.99 (1.05–3.79) $p = 0.036$. Significant association was not observed between *IL1RN* alleles and IS. *Conclusions:* Our results suggest that the C allele of *IL1B* rs1143627 may be associated with susceptibility to overall IS and LVI subtypes of stroke in the Polish population.

Keywords: *IL1B*; *IL1RN*; polymorphism; stroke; inflammation

---

1. Introduction

Ischemic stroke (IS) is a multifactor disease, resulting from classical and genetic risk factors and their interactions. Accumulating evidence supports a critical role of inflammation in the pathogenesis of IS. Interleukin-1 (IL1) is one of the key pro-inflammatory cytokines which plays a key role in this inflammatory process. The IL1 family consists of IL1A, IL1B and one antagonist cytokine, the IL1 receptor antagonist (IL1RA) [1,2]. IL1A and IL1B are inflammatory factors produced by different cell types in response to various stimuli. They affect the endothelial cells, including the induction of adhesion molecules and prothrombotic effects, while the naturally occurring competitive IL1RA may antagonize the immune response. Disturbed balance in the action of IL1A, IL1B and IL1RA leads to the development and progression of atherosclerosis. In fact, earlier studies have shown that increased levels of inflammatory cytokines are associated with vascular ischemic disease [3–5].

The IL1 gene cluster, with loci on chromosome 2, encompasses the *IL1A*, *IL1B*, and *IL1RN* genes. The polymorphisms in this *IL1* gene cluster, including *IL1B* and *IL1RN* (interleukin-1 receptor antagonist, encoding IL1RA), have been commonly studied and appeared to be associated with plasma levels of IL1B and ILRA [6,7].

In experimental studies, several independent groups have reported an early increase in IL1 expression in response to cerebral ischemia in rodents [8,9]. It has also been demonstrated in wild-type (WT) and knock-out IL1RI (IL1RI KO) mice that IL1 may exacerbate ischemic brain injury independently of IL1RI, which suggests the existence of an additional IL1 receptor or receptors in the brain [10]. Currently, IL1 polymorphism is considered to be an independent risk factor for IS development, although some studies have not confirmed this relationship.

The polymorphism in intron 2 of the interleukin receptor antagonist gene (*IL1RN*) is caused by the variable copy number of an 86-bp sequence. The most common allele, allele 1 (*IL1RN*1*), contains two repeats. The alleles 2, 3, 4, and 5 have two, five, three, and six repeats, respectively [11]. The *IL1RN*2* allele of the variable number tandem repeat (VNTR) of *IL1RN* has been reported to be associated with increased ILRA production, which naturally downregulates the immune response [12]. However, some studies have shown that *IL1RN*2* is associated with decreased IL1RA production. IL1B influences the endothelium, including the induction of adhesion molecules and procoagulant activity. Thus, the IL1/IL1RA balance may modulate inflammation processes which may contribute to the pathogenesis of ischemic stroke. A pro-inflammatory profile comprising SNPs in gene encoding regions of *IL1B* and *IL1RN* was further reported to confer an increased risk of atherosclerosis development [13–15] and some studies have reported that *IL1B* and *IL1RN* polymorphisms are associated with genetic risk of IS [16]. However, other studies on different populations did not confirm this and the association remains controversial [17,18].

Ischemic stroke is a disease with devastating consequences, which is why we are still looking for markers enabling early diagnosis. Currently, many risk factors are known for the development of stroke. However, our knowledge concerning the genes which promote the development of stroke is still limited. Our study attempts to explain the role of the genetic variants of *IL1B* (C(-31)T)and *IL1RN*, considered to be key factors regulating inflammatory processes in the development of ischemic stroke. Therefore, we have investigated the possible association between genetic variation in *IL1B* rs1143627 and *IL1RN* VNTR with overall IS and subtypes of IS classified by TOAST (see Materials and Methods) in the Polish population.

2. Materials and Methods

2.1. The Study Group

A total of 147 unrelated patients (80 males and 67 females) were admitted to hospital because of acute brain ischemic stroke (IS): Diagnosed using conventional criteria, including rapidly developed focal or global disturbance of cerebral function lasting more than 24 h, without CT signs of a hemorrhagic lesion in the brain. The study group was from a homogeneous Polish population. All 147 patients underwent clinical scrutiny, investigation of medical history and family anamnesis, evaluation of vascular risk factors, general physical and neurological examinations, routine biochemical analyses, ECG (electrocardiography), and computed tomography (CT) of the brain, within two days of onset.

Data from risk factors were recorded, including arterial hypertension (HT, defined as systolic blood pressure exceeding 140 mmHg or diastolic blood pressure greater than 90 mmHg or previous diagnosis), body mass index (BMI, calculated as weight/height^2), and diabetes (DM, previously diagnosed or a fasting plasma glucose concentration > 7.8 mL/L). Patients were classified as "current smokers" if they reported smoking more than five cigarettes per day. Routine biochemical analyses were done including fasting blood glucose, total cholesterol, HDL cholesterol and triglycerides, liver, and kidney function tests.

The study population was divided according to the TOAST classification [19], which identified five causes of ischemic cerebral infarction: (1) Large artery atherosclerosis (LVI—large-vessel infarction) in 71 patients (46.7%), (2) small-vessel occlusion (SVI—small vessel infarction) in 40 patients (26.3%), (3) cardioembolism (CEI—cardioembolic infarction) in 24 patients (15.8%), (4) stroke of other determined etiology (e.g., non-atherosclerotic artery disease) in no patients, and (5) stroke of unknown etiology in 17 patients (11.2%).

The control group consisted of 119 subjects (65 men, 52 women) who reported non-specific chest complaints and were diagnosed in regard to CAD. They underwent coronary angiography which detected no lesions in coronary arteries. A medical examination ruled out IS and other atherosclerotic diseases as well as a history of ischemic, hemorrhagic, and other brain diseases. The protocol of the study was approved by the Pomeranian Medical University Ethics Committee (nr BN-001/119/03/16.03.2003), with formal informed consent signed by all participants.

2.2. Genotyping

Genomic DNA was isolated from peripheral blood leukocytes using a commercial kit (QIAamp DNA Mini Kit; Qiagen, Hilden, Germany).

For the analysis of C(-31)T *IL1B* gene polymorphism (rs1143627) a polymerase chain reaction/restriction fragments length polymorphism (PCR/RFLP) method was applied with the following primer pair: Forward: 5′ AgA AgC TTC CAC CAA TAC TC, and reverse: 5′ AgC ACC TAg TTg TAA ggA Ag (TIB MOL BIOL, Poznań, Poland). Amplification was performed in volumes of 10 μL containing 40 ng genomic DNA, 0.1 μL of each primer, 5 μL 2xPCR Master Mix (Fermentas, Vilnius, Lithuania). The reactions were run under the following conditions: Denaturation (94 °C, 5 min), annealing (56 °C, 40 s), and extension (72 °C, 8 min). Thirty-five cycles were performed using a Mastercycler gradient machine (Eppendorf, Hamburg, Germany). The resulting product (234 bp) was digested with the Alu I restriction enzyme (MBI Fermentas, Vilnius, Lithuania), and the digestion products were separated in 4% agarose gels. The polymorphic region within intron 2 of the *IL1RN* gene was amplified using polymerase chain reaction (PCR). Genomic DNA (20 ng) served as a template in the 10 μL PCR reaction. This reaction contained the following components: 0.1 μL of each forward primer: 5′ CCC CTC AgC AAC ACT CC, and reverse primer: 5′ ggT CAg AAg ggC AgA gA (TIB MOL BIOL, Berlin, Germany); 5 μL 2xPCR Master Mix (Fermentas, Vilnius, Lithuania) the reaction was performed using standard settings: Denaturation (94 °C, 5 min), annealing (58 °C, 1 min) and extension (72 °C, 8 min), 36 cycles performed using a Mastercycler gradient machine (Eppendorf, Germany). The sizes of amplified products were determined by electrophoresis on 3% agarose gels.

2.3. Statistical Analysis

Statistical analysis was conducted with the R statistical platform (http://cran.r-project.org) using the package SNPassoc (SNPs-based whole-genome association studies. R package version 1.9-2. https://CRAN.R-project.org/package=SNPassoc). In the analysis of single SNPs, multiple inheritance models were used: Co-dominant, dominant, and recessive. Analysis of gene–gene interactions was carried out for the dominant and recessive models. Inheritance models were created with respect to minor alleles. The significance of interactions was calculated by comparing two models with and without the interaction term, using likelihood ratio tests. $p < 0.05$ was considered statistically significant.

3. Results

Demographic characteristics of the IS and control groups, risk factors and TOAST classifications in stroke cases are shown in Table 1. All characteristics did not differ between the two groups except for age (66.9 ± 12.1 vs. 56.8 ± 9.8, $p < 0.0001$) and the frequencies of diabetes mellitus (27% vs. 13%, $p = 0.004$) and dyslipidemia (16%/84% vs. 76%/24%, $p < 0.0001$).

Table 1. Demographic and risk factors of stroke characteristics.

Characteristic	Cases (n = 147)	Control (n = 117)	p
Age (years)	66.9 ± 12.1	56.8 ± 9.8	<0.0001
BMI (kg/m^2)	27.6 ± 4.8	26.9 ± 4.2	0.286
Sex (Males)	54% (80)	56% (65)	0.854
Smoking	32% (47)	24% (28)	0.150
Diabetes mellitus	27% (40)	13% (15)	0.004
Hypertension	60% (88)	51% (60)	0.163
Dyslipidemia	16% (23)	76% (89)	<0.0001
TOAST			
Large-vessel atherosclerosis	46% (68)		
Cardioembolism	17% (25)		
Small-vessel	26% (38)		
Others	11% (16)		

3.1. *Association between Overall IS and Genetic Variation in IL1B and IL1RN*

The genotype distributions were in Hardy–Weinberg equilibrium for *IL1B* (all individuals $p = 0.081$, cases $p = 0.741$, control group $p = 0.073$) and *IL1RN* (all individuals $p = 0.794$, cases $p = 0.867$, control group $p = 0.675$). Observed genotype frequencies for the *IL-1B*:C(-31)T polymorphism (rs1143627) were: 33.3% T/T (n = 88), 43.9% C/T (n = 116), 22.7% C/C (n = 60) and for alleles: 55.3% T and 44.7% C. The genotype frequencies for the *IL1RN* were 39.0% 1/1 (n = 103), 46.2% 1/2 (n = 122), 14.8% 2/2 (n = 39) and for alleles: 62.1% 1 and 37.9% 2. The *IL1RN* alleles 3 and 4 were rare and their frequencies did not significantly differ between the IS patients and the control group (1.9% vs. 1.6%, $p = 0.765$ for allele 3 and 0.3% vs. 1.2%, $p = 0.122$ for allele 4). Baseline characteristics of the study group are shown in Table 1. The results of tests of association of the *IL1RN* and *IL1B* polymorphisms with stroke are summarized in Tables 2 and 3.

Table 2. An association of the *IL1RN* polymorphism with stroke under codominant, dominant, and recessive model.

Model	Control (n = 117)	%	Cases (n = 147)	%	OR	95% CI		p
Codominant								
1/1	54	46.2	49	33.3	1.00			
1/2	49	41.9	73	49.7	1.64	0.97	2.79	0.647 *
2/2	14	12.0	25	17.0	1.97	0.92	4.21	
Dominant								
1/1	54	46.2	49	33.3	1.00			0.358 *
1/2–2/2	63	53.8	98	66.7	1.71	1.04	2.83	
Recessive								
1/1–1/2	103	88.0	122	83.0	1.00			0.650 *
2/2	14	12.0	25	17.0	1.51	0.75	3.05	

* Adjusted by: age, diabetes mellitus, dyslipidemia.

The results of tests for association of the *IL1RN* and *IL1B* polymorphisms with stroke are summarized in Tables 2 and 3. In multivariable modeling, including covariates (age, diabetes mellitus, dyslipidemia), the association of the *ILRN* with stroke was insignificant (Table 2). For the *IL1B* polymorphism, the association under codominant and recessive models was insignificant after adjustment for covariates (age, diabetes mellitus, dyslipidemia), however with the dominant model, the risk of stroke with CT-CC was 2.3 higher than for TT homozygotes (2.30 (1.36–3.87); $p = 0.020$) (Table 3).

Table 3. An association of the *IL-1B* polymorphism with stroke under codominant, dominant, and recessive model.

Model	Control (n = 117)	%	Cases (n = 147)	%	OR	95% CI		p *
Codominant								
T/T	51	43.6	37	25.2	1.00			
C/T	45	38.5	71	48.3	2.17	1.24	3.82	0.065 *
C/C	21	17.9	39	26.5	2.56	1.30	5.05	
Dominant								
T/T	51	43.6	37	25.2	1.00			0.020 *
C/T-C/C	66	56.4	110	74.8	2.30	1.36	3.87	
Recessive								
T/T-C/T	96	82.1	108	73.5	1.00			0.322 *
C/C	21	17.9	39	26.5	1.65	0.91	3.00	

* Adjusted by: Age, diabetes mellitus, dyslipidemia.

In addition to single-locus analyses, we investigated whether the two genes interacted with respect to the modification of stroke risk (Figures 1 and 2). The analysis was conducted with the assumption of dominant or recessive models for each polymorphism and no evidence was found of gene–gene interaction with respect to IS risk. Although the raw p value for the dominant x dominant model was 0.046, it turned out to be non-significant after adjustment for covariates.

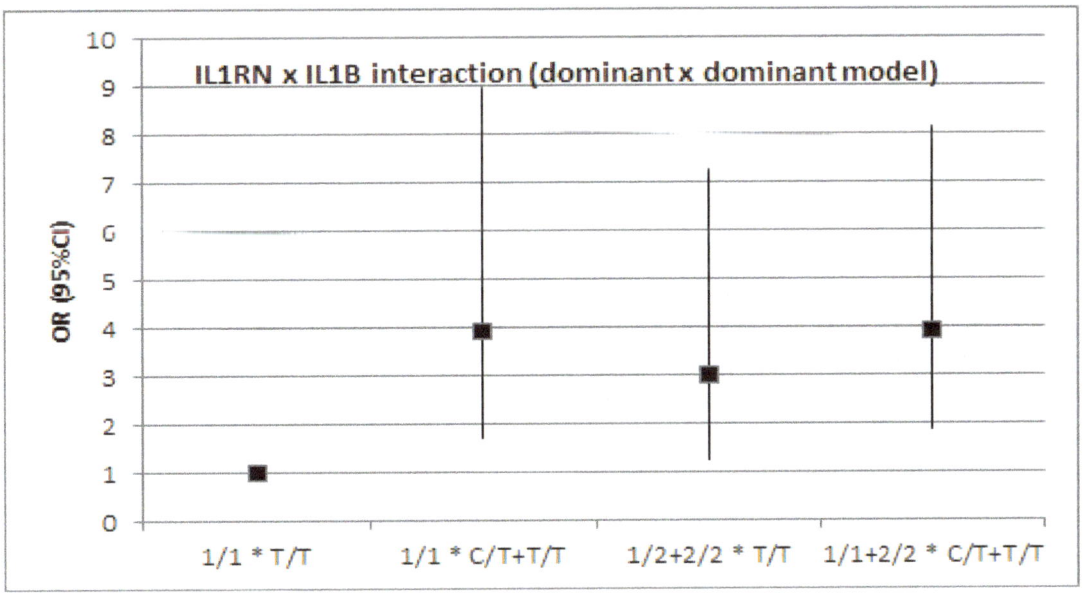

Figure 1. *IL1RN* × *IL1B* interaction (dominant × dominant model). Raw p = 0.046, adjusted p = 0.232 (age, diabetes mellitus, dyslipidemia status).

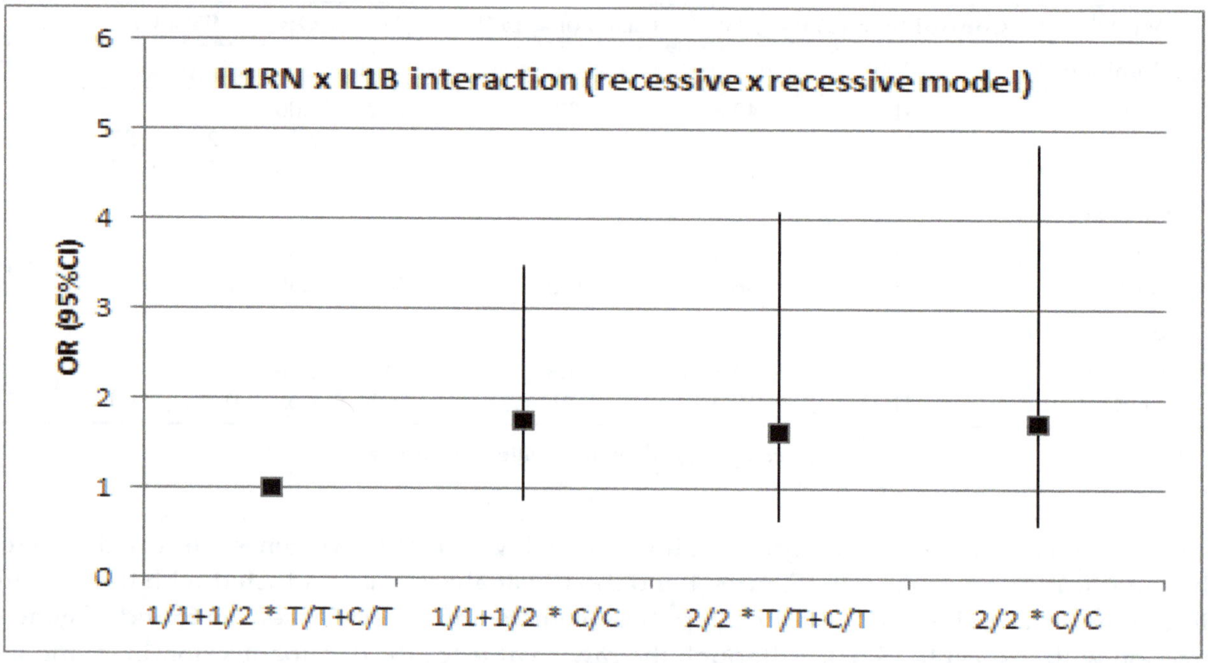

Figure 2. *IL1RN* × *IL1B* interaction (recessive × recessive model). Raw $p = 0.502$, adjusted $p = 0.910$ (age, diabetes mellitus, dyslipidemia status).

3.2. Association between IS and Genetic Variation in IL1B and IL1RN by Stroke Subtype (TOAST)

Each stroke subtype, i.e., CEI, SVI, LVI of the TOAST classification, was compared with control subjects (Tables 4 and 5). No significant associations were found between *IL1RN* and stroke under codominant, dominant, and recessive models by stroke subtype according to TOAST classification (Table 4). For the *IL1B* gene, the carriers of the C allele were significantly overrepresented in LVI subtypes compared with controls with (1.99 (1.05–3.79), $p = 0.036$) (Table 5). For the other subtypes, we did not find any significant correlations (Table 5).

Table 4. An association of the *IL1RN* polymorphism with stroke under codominant, dominant, and recessive models by stroke subtype (TOAST classification).

Model	Control (n = 117)	CEI (n = 25)	OR (95% CI)	p *	SVI (n = 38)	OR (95% CI)	p *	LVI (n = 68)	OR (95% CI)	p *
Codominant										
1/1	54 (46.2)	6 (24.0)	1.00		13 (34.2)	1.00		25 (36.8)	1.00	
1/2	49 (41.9)	14 (56.0)	2.57 (0.92–7.21)		19 (50.0)	1.61 (0.72–3.60)		34 (50.0)	1.50 (0.79–2.86)	
2/2	14 (12.0)	5 (20.0)	3.21 (0.85–12.09)	0.388	6 (15.8)	1.78 (0.57–5.52)	0.947	9 (13.2)	1.39 (0.53–3.63)	0.974
Dominant										
1/1	54 (46.2)	6 (24.0)	1.00		13 (34.2)	1.00		25 (36.8)	1.00	
1/2–2/2	63 (53.8)	19 (76.0)	2.71 (1.01–7.28)	0.261	25 (65.8)	1.65 (0.77–3.53)	0.854	43 (63.2)	1.47 (0.80–2.72)	0.982
Recessive										
1/1–1/2	103 (88.0)	20 (80.0)	1.00		32 (84.2)	1.00		59 (86.8)	1.00	
2/2	14 (12.0)	5 (20.0)	1.84 (0.60–5.68)	0.695	6 (15.8)	1.38 (0.49–3.88)	0.752	9 (13.2)	1.12 (0.46–2.75)	0.823

* Adjusted by: Age, diabetes mellitus, dyslipidemia.

Table 5. An association of the *IL1B* polymorphism with stroke under codominant, dominant, and recessive models by stroke subtype (TOAST classification).

Model	Control (n = 117)	CEI (n = 25)	OR (95% CI)	p *	SVI (n = 38)	OR (95% CI)	p *	LVI (n = 68)	OR (95% CI)	p *
Codominant										
T/T	51 (43.6)	5 (20.0)	1.00		8 (21.1)	1.00		19 (27.9)	1.00	
C/T	45 (38.5)	14 (56.0)	3.17 (1.06–9.50)		19 (50.0)	2.69 (1.07–6.74)		33 (48.5)	1.97 (0.99–3.93)	
C/C	21 (17.9)	6 (24.0)	2.91 (0.80–10.60)	0.074	11 (28.9)	3.34 (1.18–9.48)	0.236	16 (23.5)	2.05 (0.89–4.72)	0.069
Dominant										
T/T	51 (43.6)	5 (20.0)	1.00		8 (21.1)	1.00		19 (27.9)	1.00	
C/T-C/C	66 (56.4)	20 (80.0)	3.09 (1.09–8.80)	0.305	30 (78.9)	2.90 (1.22–6.86)	0.106	49 (72.1)	1.99 (1.05–3.79)	0.036
Recessive										
T/T-C/T	96 (82.1)	19 (76.0)	1.00		27 (71.1)	1.00		52 (76.5)	1.00	
C/C	21 (17.9)	6 (24.0)	1.44 (0.51–4.05)	0.225	11 (28.9)	1.86 (0.80–4.34)	0.874	16 (23.5)	1.41 (0.68–2.93)	0.993

* Adjusted by: Age, diabetes mellitus, dyslipidemia.

4. Discussion

Ischemic stroke is a disease of complex etiology, and it is generally accepted that both environmental and genetic factors play a crucial role in the development of the disease. Although there are many studies which have indicated that inflammatory cytokines and their genetic polymorphisms play an important role in the pathogenesis of IS, the results are still controversial. In this study, two important polymorphisms of the IL1 cluster were investigated for their association with stroke. We have not shown any connection between genetic variants of *ILRN* VNTR with overall stroke or subtypes. This is in line with previous studies on IS [20]. In contrast some studies, have reported an association of the *IL1RN* with stroke [21]. This inconsistency could be explained with the rather relatively small size of study groups than differences between populations. However, we have shown that the *IL1B*:T(-31)C polymorphism is independently associated with overall IS and subtype of IS in the homogeneous Polish population.

For the *IL1B*:C(-31)T polymorphism, we found that carriers of the C allele were associated with a higher risk of overall stroke. Moreover, we found that CT/CC genotypes can increase the risk of subtypes of IS. The relationship of *IL1B* polymorphism and stroke has been examined in several previous studies and our results remain in line with those presented so far. Extensive studies on the *IL1B* polymorphism at position -511 have indicated that *IL1B:*-511T carriers had higher levels of IL1B than *IL1B*:-511C and were associated with increased risk of IS [22]. It is also worth mentioning the study by Iacoviello et al. [23] which is the main source of research heterogeneity because this study reported that TT homozygotes of *IL1B*:-511 are associated with a decreased risk of IS. However, patients in this study were relatively young. Thus, the association between *IL1B* polymorphism and IL1B production still remains controversial. A recent study has documented that IL1B mRNA was increased in the TT genotype [24] whereas Hall et al. [25] showed a 2–3-fold increase in IL1B protein secretion in subjects with the T allele at -511 and the C allele at -31.

We found no interaction between *IL1RN* and *IL1B* concerning IS risk assuming the dominant x dominant and recessive x recessive models. The gene–gene interaction was analyzed using a linear model in which only two (and the same) inheritance patterns for each locus were considered. This approach could possibly have less power as compared with a non-parametric and model-free multifactor dimensionality reduction method that has been shown to have reasonable power to detect epistasis [26].

The polymorphism of *IL1B* at -31 is tightly linked with the polymorphism at -511. However, it is unclear whether the C or T allele of *IL1B* -31 is associated with high expression. We have not measured the plasma IL1B and IL1RA levels and this can be considered as a limitation of our study. It is worth emphasizing that genetic variations of *IL1B* -31 and von Willebrand factor are associated with the recanalization rate of fibrinolysis with tissue-type plasminogen activator, and thus with treatment efficacy [27]. As the authors report, the mechanisms by which these SNPs modulate recanalization could be related to homeostasis modulation by modification of coagulation factor activities. Manso et al. [28] also tested the inflammatory genes *IL1B*, interleukin 6 (*IL6*), myeloperoxidase (*MPO*), and *TNF* with stroke susceptibility, and demonstrated that only two SNPs of *IL6* and one *MPO* single-nucleotide polymorphism were significantly associated with stroke risk in their sample. Probably, an observed lesser genetic influence is related to widespread classical risk factors, or lifestyle. Some studies have reported that *IL1B*:C(-31)T and *IL1RN*:VNTR polymorphisms are significantly correlated with the development of CAD, and thus atherosclerosis process [3,29]. However, other studies conducted in different populations have not confirmed this and these associations still remain controversial. In our previous study we showed no association between polymorphisms of *IL1B*:C(-31)T/*IL1RN* (VNTR) or their haplotypes and CAD in the Polish population [30], which may suggest lesser importance of genetic factors in the development of atherosclerotic diseases in our population.

Nevertheless, IL1B is a potent pro-inflammatory cytokine and plays a major role in the development of both inflammation processes and thrombosis. It is hypothesized that in IS development, IL1B is involved in thrombus formation rather than in atherosclerosis progression because IL1 induces tissue factor and plasminogen activator inhibitor type 1 gene expression [31]. However, this cytokine can induce complex biological effects by the regulation of gene expression of multiple cell types [32]. Therefore, more mechanisms should be considered in the development of IS, although both inflammatory and prothrombotic mechanisms seem to play a fundamental role. The formation of a thrombus leading to occlusion of a vessel is the endpoint which is influenced by many factors (genes, hypertension, hyperlipidemia, diabetes mellitus, etc.), and the gene–environment interaction can be of great importance. Thus, the *IL1B* C allele may not be associated directly with IS per se, but could be modulating cytokines in the inflammatory processes that affect the development of atherosclerosis resulting in IS. It has been shown that genetic variants of *IL1B* that predict higher inflammatory phenotypes modify the risk of Lp(a) in mediating long-term cardiovascular events [33]. These results indicate that *IL1B* can modify many pathways involved in the development of atherosclerosis and thus, cardiovascular events. Additionally, some studies have also reported that the risk of stroke increases with the number of high-risk genotypes in proinflammatory gene polymorphisms carried by an individual, thus suggesting that such polymorphisms may act synergistically [34]. We have evaluated genetic variants of only two genes which are crucial in inflammation. IS is a very complicated and extremely complex disease and its pathomechanism is still not fully explained. It is not yet known how many risk factors in the development of atherosclerosis could be modulated by the genetic variants of *IL1B*, which acts as a key regulator in inflammatory processes.

In different populations with varying intensity of classical risk factors, the impact of genetics may be found to have a variable extent. Previous studies have reported that ethnicity or regional locations are very important in the determination of environmental risk factors [35]. One of advantages of the present study is that it included a well-characterized and homogeneous patients' group (from the northwest region of Poland), but it should be emphasized that our society has strongly expressed classical risk factors for IS. It should be noted that observed differences between the study group and the controls could interfere with the assessment of the role for the *IL1RN* polymorphism in the development of IS. Diabetes, which is a widely recognized risk factor for the development of atherosclerosis, has been more frequent in IS patients, while dyslipidemia has been less frequent. However, the IS patients had been already treated (b-blocker, statin, etc.) which could have downregulated to some extent the inflammatory process agents, while the control group comprised subjects without treatment for this. Moreover, the control group was slightly younger than the IS group, which may have had some impact on the obtained results, and could be considered another limitation of our study. The population included in the study was homogeneous (monoethnic, Polish) and, therefore, our data need to be confirmed in different ethnic groups.

5. Conclusions

The complex interplay between genetic backgrounds, clinical and lifestyle factors, and the environment may ultimately lead to the development of stroke. In the present study, we present supporting evidence for a role of the *IL1B* inflammatory gene in stroke susceptibility. Our findings confirm previous genetic observations, highlighting the need for further functional studies, particularly in view of the possible utility of *IL1B* as a diagnostic biomarker for stroke.

Author Contributions: Conceptualization, I.G. and L.C.; data curation, M.K. and B.K.; formal analysis, L.C.; funding acquisition, A.C.; investigation, K.L. and O.B.; methodology, K.L. and P.J.; project administration, A.C. and A.B.; resources, P.J. and O.B.; software, M.K. and A.B.; supervision, I.G. and A.C.; validation, M.K.; visualization, M.K. and B.K.; writing—original draft, I.G.; writing—review & editing, I.G. and L.C.

References

1. Bochner, B.S.; Luscinskas, F.W.; Gimbrone, M.A., Jr.; Newman, W.; Sterbinsky, S.A.; Derse-Anthony, C.P.; Klunk, D.; Schleimer, R.P. Adhesion of human basophils, eosinophils, and neutrophils to interleukin-1 activated endothelial cells: Contributions of endothelial adhesion molecules. *J. Exp. Med.* **1991**, *173*, 1553–1557. [CrossRef] [PubMed]

2. Dinarello, C.A. Biologic basis for interleukin-1 in disease. *Blood* **1996**, *87*, 2095–2147. [PubMed]
3. Marculescu, R.; Endler, G.; Schillinger, M.; Iordanova, N.; Exner, M.; Hayden, E.; Huber, K.; Wagner, O.; Mannhalter, C. Interleukin-1 receptor antagonist genotype is associated with coronary atherosclerosis in patients with type 2 diabetes. *Diabetes* **2002**, *51*, 3582–3585. [CrossRef] [PubMed]
4. Rios, D.L.; Cerqueira, C.C.; Bonfim-Silva, R.; Araújo, L.J.; Pereira, J.F.; Gadelha, S.R.; Barbosa, A.A. Interleukin-1 beta and interleukin-6 polymorphism associations with angiographically assessed coronary artery disease in Brazilians. *Cytokine* **2010**, *50*, 292–296. [CrossRef] [PubMed]
5. Zhang, Y.M.; Zhong, L.J.; He, B.X.; Li, W.C.; Nie, J.; Wang, X.; Chen, X.T. The correlation between polymorphism at position—511 C/T in the promoter region of interleukin 1B and the severity of coronary heart disease. *Zhonhua Yi Xue Yi Chuan Xue Za Zhi* **2006**, *3*, 86–88.
6. Santilla, S.; Savinainen, K.; Hurme, M. Presence of the IL-1RA allele2(IL1RN*2) is associated with enhanced IL-1beta production in vitro. *Scan. J. Immunol.* **1998**, *47*, 195–198. [CrossRef]
7. Blakemore, A.I.; Tarlow, J.K.; Cork, M.J.; Gordon, C.; Emery, P.; Duff, G.W. Interleukin-1 receptor antagonist gene polymorphism as a disease severity factor in systemic lupus erythematosus. *Artritis Rheum.* **1994**, *37*, 1380–1385. [CrossRef] [PubMed]
8. Davies, C.A.; Loddick, S.A.; Toulmond, S.; Stroemer, R.P.; Hunt, J.; Rothwell, N.J. The progression and topographic distribution of interleukin-1beta expression after permanent middle cerebral artery occlusion in the rat. *J. Cereb. Blood Flow Metab.* **1999**, *19*, 87–98. [CrossRef]
9. Touzani, O.; Boutin, H.; Chuquet, J.; Rothwell, N. Potential mechanisms of interleukin-1 involvement in cerebral ischaemia. *J. Neuroimmunol.* **1999**, *100*, 203–215. [CrossRef]
10. Touzani, O.; Boutin, H.; LeFeuvre, R.; Parker, L.; Miller, A.; Luheshi, G.; Rothwell, N. Interleukin-1 influences ischemic brain damage in the mouse independently of the interleukin-1 receptor. *J. Neurosc.* **2002**, *22*, 38–43. [CrossRef]
11. Tarlow, J.K.; Blakemore, A.I.; Lennard, A.; Solari, R.; Hughes, H.N.; Steinkasserer, A.; Duff, G.W. Polymorphism in human IL-1 receptor antagonist gene intron 2 is caused by variable numbers of an 86-bp tandem repeat. *Hum. Genet.* **1993**, *91*, 403–404. [CrossRef] [PubMed]
12. Hurme, M.; Santila, S. IL-1 receptor antagonist (IL-Ra) plasma levels are co-ordinately regulated by both IL-Ra and IL-1beta genes. *Eur. J. Immunol.* **1998**, *47*, 195–198.
13. Worrall, B.B.; Azhar, S.; Nyquist, P.A.; Ackerman, R.H.; Hamm, T.L.; DeGraba, T.J. Interleukin-1 receptor antagonist gene polymorphisms in carotid atherosclerosis. *Stroke* **2003**, *34*, 790–793. [CrossRef] [PubMed]
14. Fragoso, J.M.; Delgadillo, H.; Llorente, L.; Chuquiure, E.; Juárez-Cedillo, T.; Vallejo, M.; Lima, G.; Furuzawa-Carballeda, J.; Peña-Duque, M.A.; Martínez-Ríos, M.A.; et al. Interleukin 1 receptor antagonist polymorphisms are associated with the risk of developing acute coronary syndrome in Mexicans. *Immunol. Lett.* **2010**, *133*, 106–111. [CrossRef] [PubMed]
15. Francis, S.E.; Camp, N.J.; Dewberry, R.M.; Gunn, J.; Syrris, P.; Carter, N.D.; Jeffery, S.; Kaski, J.C.; Cumberland, D.C.; Duff, G.W.; et al. Interleukin-1 receptor antagonist gene polymorphism and coronary artery disease. *Circulation* **1999**, *99*, 861–866. [CrossRef] [PubMed]
16. Olofsson, P.S.; Sheikine, Y.; Jatta, K.; Ghaderi, M.; Samnegård, A.; Eriksson, P.; Sirsjö, A. A functional interleukin-1 receptor antagonist polymorphism influences atherosclerosis development. The interleukin-1 beta: Interleukin-1 receptor antagonist balance in atherosclerosis. *Circ. J.* **2009**, *73*, 1531–1536. [CrossRef] [PubMed]
17. Yan, W.; Chen, Z.Y.; Chen, J.Q.; Chen, H.M. Association between the interleukin-1B gene—511C/T polymorphism and ischemic stroke: An update meta-analysis. *Genet. Mol. Res.* **2016**, *15*. [CrossRef]
18. Li, N.; He, Z.; Xu, J.; Liu, F.; Deng, S.; Zhang, H. Association of PDE4D and IL-1 gene polymorphism with ischemic stroke in a Han Chinese population. *Brain Res. Bull.* **2010**, *81*, 38–42. [CrossRef]
19. Adams, H.P., Jr.; Bendixen, B.H.; Kappelle, L.J.; Biller, J.; Love, B.B.; Gordon, D.L.; Marsh, E.E., 3rd. Classification of subtype of acute ischemic stroke: Definitions for use in a multicenter clinical trial. *Stroke* **1993**, *24*, 35–41. [CrossRef]
20. Yang, Y.; Wu, W.; Wang, L.; Ding, Y. Lack of association between interleukin-1β receptor antagonist gene 86-bp VNTR polymorphism and ischemic stroke: A meta-analysis. *Medicine* **2018**, *97*, e11750. [CrossRef]
21. Noha, A.R.; Hanan, S.M. Influence of interleukin-1 gene cluster polymorphism on the susceptibility and outcomes of acute stroke in Egyptian patients. *Cell Biochem. Biophys.* **2015**, *71*, 637–647.
22. Nemetz, A.; Nosti-Escanilla, M.P.; Molnár, T.; Köpe, A.; Kovács, A.; Fehér, J.; Tulassay, Z.; Nagy, F.; García-González, M.A.; Peña, A.S. IL-1B gene polymorphism influence the course and severity of

inflammatory bowel disease. *Immunogenetics* **1999**, *49*, 527–531. [CrossRef] [PubMed]

23. Iacoviello, L.; Di Castelnuovo, A.; Gattone, M.; Pezzini, A.; Assanelli, D.; Lorenzet, R.; Del Zotto, E.; Colombo, M.; Napoleone, E.; Amore, C.; et al. Polymorphisms of the interleukin-1beta gene affect the risk of myocardial infarction and ischemic stroke at young age and the response of mononuclear cells to stimulation in vitro. *Arterioscler. Thromb. Vasc. Biol.* **2005**, *25*, 222–227. [CrossRef] [PubMed]
24. Kimura, R.; Nishioka, T.; Soemantri, A.; Ishida, T. Cis-acting effect of the IL-1B C-31T polymorphism on IL-1beta mRNA expression. *Genes Immun.* **2005**, *5*, 571–575.
25. Hall, S.K.; Perregaux, D.G.; Gabel, C.A.; Woodworth, T.; Durham, L.K.; Huizinga, T.W.; Breedveld, F.C.; Seymour, A.B. Correction of polymorphic variation in the promoter region of the interleukin-1β gene with secretion of interleukin 1β protein. *Arthritis Reum.* **2004**, *50*, 1976–1983. [CrossRef] [PubMed]
26. Wei, L.K.; Menon, S.; Griffiths, L.R.; Gan, S.H. Signaling pathway genes for blood pressure, folate and cholesterol levels among hypertensives: An epistasis analysis. *J. Hum. Hypertens.* **2015**, *29*, 99–104. [CrossRef] [PubMed]
27. Fernández-Cadenas, I.; Del Río-Espínola, A.; Giralt, D.; Domingues-Montanari, S.; Quiroga, A.; Mendióroz, M.; Ruíz, A.; Ribó, M.; Serena, J.; Obach, V.; et al. IL1B and VWF variants are associated with fibrynolitic early recanalization in patients with ischemic stroke. *Stroke* **2012**, *43*, 2659–2665. [CrossRef] [PubMed]
28. Manso, H.; Krug, T.; Sobral, J.; Albergaria, I.; Gaspar, G.; Ferro, J.M.; Oliveira, S.A.; Vicente, A.M. Variants in the inflammatory IL6 and MPO genes modulate stroke susceptibility through main effects and gene–gene interactions. *J. Cereb. Blood Flow Metab.* **2011**, *31*, 1751–1759. [CrossRef] [PubMed]
29. Rechciński, T.; Grebowska, A.; Kurpesa, M.; Sztybrych, M.; Peruga, J.Z.; Trzos, E.; Rudnicka, W.; Krzemińska-Pakuła, M.; Chmiela, M. Interleukin-1b and interleukin-1 receptor inhibitor gene cluster polymorphisms in patients with coronary artery disease after percutaneous angioplasty or coronary artery bypass grafting. *Kardiol. Pol.* **2009**, *67*, 601–610.
30. Gorący, J.; Gorący, I.; Safranow, K.; Taryma, O.; Adler, G.; Ciechanowicz, A. Lack of association of interleukin-1 gene cluster polymorphisms with angiographically documented coronary artery disease: Demonstration of association with hypertension in the Polish population. *Arch. Med. Res.* **2011**, *42*, 426–432. [CrossRef] [PubMed]
31. Larsson, P.; Ulfhammer, E.; Karlsson, L.; Bokarewa, M.; Wåhlander, K.; Jern, S. Effects of IL-1beta and IL-6 on tissue-type plasminogen activator expression in vascular endothelial cells. *Thromb. Res.* **2008**, *123*, 342–351. [CrossRef] [PubMed]
32. Lynch, M.A. Neuroinflammatory changes negatively impact on LTP: A focus on IL-1beta. *Brain Res.* **2015**, *1621*, 197–204. [CrossRef] [PubMed]
33. Naka, K.K.; Bechlioullis, A.; Marini, A.; Sionis, D.; Vakalis, K.; Triantis, G.; Wilkins, L.; Rogus, J.; Kornman, K.S.; Witztum, J.L.; et al. Interleukin-1 genotypes modulate the long-term effect of lipoprotein (a) on cardiovascular events: The Ioannina study. *J. Clin. Lipidol.* **2018**, *12*, 338–347. [CrossRef] [PubMed]
34. Flex, A.; Gaetani, E.; Papaleo, P.; Straface, G.; Proia, A.S.; Pecorini, G.; Tondi, P.; Pola, P.; Pola, R. Proinflammatory genetic profiles in subjects with history of ischemic stroke. *Stroke* **2004**, *35*, 2270–2275. [CrossRef] [PubMed]
35. Koukkou, E.; Watts, G.F.; Mazurkiewicz, J.; Lowy, C. Ethnic differences in lipid and lipoprotein metabolism in pregnant women of African and Caucasian origin. *J. Clin. Pathol.* **1994**, *47*, 1105–1107. [CrossRef] [PubMed]

9

Diagnosis and Management of Left Atrium Appendage Thrombosis in Atrial Fibrillation Patients Undergoing Cardioversion

Enrico Melillo [1,*], Giuseppe Palmiero [1], Adele Ferro [2], Paola Elvira Mocavero [3], Vittorio Monda [1] and Luigi Ascione [1]

[1] Department of Cardiology, AO dei Colli, Monaldi Hospital, 80131 Naples, Italy
[2] Institute of Biostructure and Bioimaging, National Council Research, 80131 Naples, Italy
[3] Anesthesiology and Intensive Care Unit, AO dei Colli, Monaldi Hospital, 80131 Naples, Italy
* Correspondence: doc.emelillo88@gmail.com

Abstract: Atrial fibrillation is the most common cardiac arrhythmia and is associated with an increased risk of stroke and thromboembolic complications. A rhythm control strategy with both electrical and pharmacological cardioversion is recommended for patients with symptomatic atrial fibrillation. Anticoagulant therapy for 3–4 weeks prior to cardioversion is recommended in order to avoid thromboembolic events deriving from restoring sinus rhythm. Transesophageal echocardiography has a pivotal role in this setting, excluding the presence of left atrial appendage thrombus before cardioversion. The aim of this review is to discuss the epidemiology and risk factors for left atrial appendage thrombosis, the role of echocardiography in the decision making before cardioversion, and the efficacy of different anticoagulant regimens on the detection and treatment of left atrial appendage thrombosis.

Keywords: atrial fibrillation; cardioversion; oral anticoagulation therapy; left atrial appendage thrombosis; transesophageal echocardiography

---

1. Introduction

Atrial fibrillation (AF) is the most common sustained arrhythmia, with a prevalence of 0.4% in the general population and 9% in octogenarian patients [1]. Patients with AF have a higher risk of cardiovascular complications, including a 3–5 -old increase of stroke [2]. A 4–5 fold risk of systemic embolism (SE) [3] and a higher risk of heart failure (HF) development [4]. Without prior adequate anticoagulation, cardioversion (CV) (both electric and pharmacological) in patients with AF is associated with a non-negligible risk of thromboembolic events [5]. Consequently, for patients with AF >48 h onset, the current guidelines recommend anticoagulant therapy for at least three weeks before and four weeks after CV [6]. The transesophageal echocardiogram (TOE) is a diagnostic method that allows a detailed evaluation of the anatomy and function of the left atrial appendage (LAA), and is considered the gold standard for identifying or excluding left atrium (LA) and LAA thrombosis [6]. Vitamin K antagonists (VKAs) have traditionally been considered the gold standard for thromboembolic prophylaxis before CV; however, novel oral anticoagulants (NOACs) have also been studied, and are increasingly employed in this setting [7–9]. The aim of this review is to discuss the risk factors and diagnostic modalities of LAA thrombosis in AF patients undergoing CV, and to provide a summary and update of the therapeutic strategies to prevent and resolve LAA thrombosis.

2. Risk Factors of Left Atrial Appendage Thrombosis

LAA is the most prominent site of LA thrombus formation, with more than 90% of thrombi generating within this anatomical structure [10]. Extra-appendage thrombosis is a very rare finding in non-valvular AF and, when present, an LAA thrombus is usually concomitant [11]. The CHA_2DS_2-VASc score incorporates the more common stroke risk factors seen in everyday clinical practice, and is recommended to guide anticoagulant therapy in AF patients. CHA_2DS_2-VASc and older $CHADS_2$ scoring systems are also good predictors of LAA thrombosis. CHA_2DS_2-VASc showed a higher sensibility and specificity for LAA thrombus detection, and severe impairment of left ventricle systolic function is a powerful predictor of LAA thrombosis [12–14]. Moreover, the addition of the AF type (persistent AF) and renal function to the CHA_2DS_2-VASc score may better stratify thromboembolic risk and could identify patients who do not need preprocedural TOE [15]. In AF patients with low thromboembolic risk, the CHA_2DS_2-VASc score seems more able to identify low-risk individuals with a low probability of LAA thrombus, as seen in two retrospective studies totaling 1100 AF patients where no LAA thrombi were identified in individuals with a CHA_2DS_2-VASc score <2 [16,17]. Conversely, a low $CHADS_2$ score is less reliable in predicting the risk of LAA thrombus formation [18].

Moreover, the addition of biomarkers such as brain natriuretic peptide can improve the risk stratification of CHADS2 and CHA_2DS_2-VASc scores for LAA thrombus [19,20].

3. The Role of Echocardiography before Cardioversion

3.1. Transthoracic Echocardiography

Transthoracic echocardiography (TTE) should be performed for the clinical evaluation of every AF patient. TTE provides a comprehensive evaluation of cardiac anatomy and function that can help to define the type of AF and to identify patients with high risk of LAA thrombosis. Firstly, echocardiographic assessment is necessary to diagnose valvular AF, defined by the presence of moderate–severe mitral stenosis or a prosthetic valve, which is necessarily treated with VKAs anticoagulant therapy [6]. TTE provides an overall assessment of left ventricle ejection fraction (LVEF), a risk marker of both stroke and LAA thrombus presence before CV [21]. An LVEF < 40% is considered an equivalent of the congestive HF criterion in the CHA_2DS_2-VASc score, while a normal LVEF has been associated with a low prevalence of LAA thrombosis in AF patients undergoing TOE [22]. Evaluation of LA dimension is fundamental in assessing risk of LAA thrombosis and the probability of successful rhythm control [23]. The measurement of antero-posterior LA diameter has been traditionally considered the gold standard for LA dimension assessment. However, growing evidence suggests that the LA volume index (LAVI) is a more powerful predictor of LAA thrombus. [22]. Furthermore, a combination of LVEF-to-LAVI ratio <1.5 showed a 100% sensitivity in predicting the presence of LAA thrombus, therefore identifying a low-risk population before CV [24].

TTE provides markers to predict the probability of successful rhythm control before CV. LAVI, LVEF, diastolic function, E/è wave ratio, and LV hypertrophy can influence the outcome of rhythm control strategy [25,26]. The HATCH score (which stands for hypertension, age 75 years, thromboembolic event, pulmonary disease, and HF) summarizes the main markers affecting the likelihood of a successful CV [27].

The assessment of LA function with 2D speckle tracking echocardiography (STE) is a promising tool in the clinical evaluation of AF patients. Normal LA strain analysis with STE has three phases: active filling phase (reservoir), passive emptying phase (conduit), and booster pump phase (pump), which corresponds to LA contraction at the end of the ventricular diastole. In AF patients, the booster pump phase is missing, and the most reliable parameter is the peak systolic reservoir strain. STE deformation analysis is highly correlated with the amount of LA interstitial fibrosis and remodeling process occurring in AF patients [28]. A reduced peak positive strain has been associated with lower LAA emptying velocities, with an LA prothrombotic state, and with higher incidence of LAA thrombosis [29,30].

3.2. Transesophageal Echocardiography and Intracardiac Echocardiography

TOE is considered the gold standard modality for diagnosis of LAA thrombi with a sensitivity and specificity of 95%–100% [31]. Current guidelines recommend TOE as an alternative to periprocedural anticoagulation in patients with >48 h AF duration or when the exact duration and onset of AF cannot be determined [6]. Moreover, in patients where thrombosis is identified, a repeat TOE after 3–4 weeks of anticoagulation should be considered before CV [6]. Modern multiplane TOE enables a visual assessment of LAA thrombi (Figure 1) or other potential intracardiac sources of embolism. TOE allows visual diagnosis of spontaneous echo contrast (SEC), also called "smoke" (Figure 2B), and "sludge" (Figure 2A), a dense and marked SEC, which is a precursor of thrombus formation and has a greater prognostic significance than smoke alone [32]. LAA mechanical function can be assessed from TOE with pulsed wave Doppler sample volume placed 1 cm below LAA ostium. LAA emptying velocities <20 cm/s are associated with a higher prevalence of SEC and LAA thrombosis [33] (Figure 2B). A combined use of color and pulsed-wave Doppler with contrast echocardiography can provide incremental information in aiding the diagnosis of LAA thrombosis in patients with doubtful diagnosis [34].

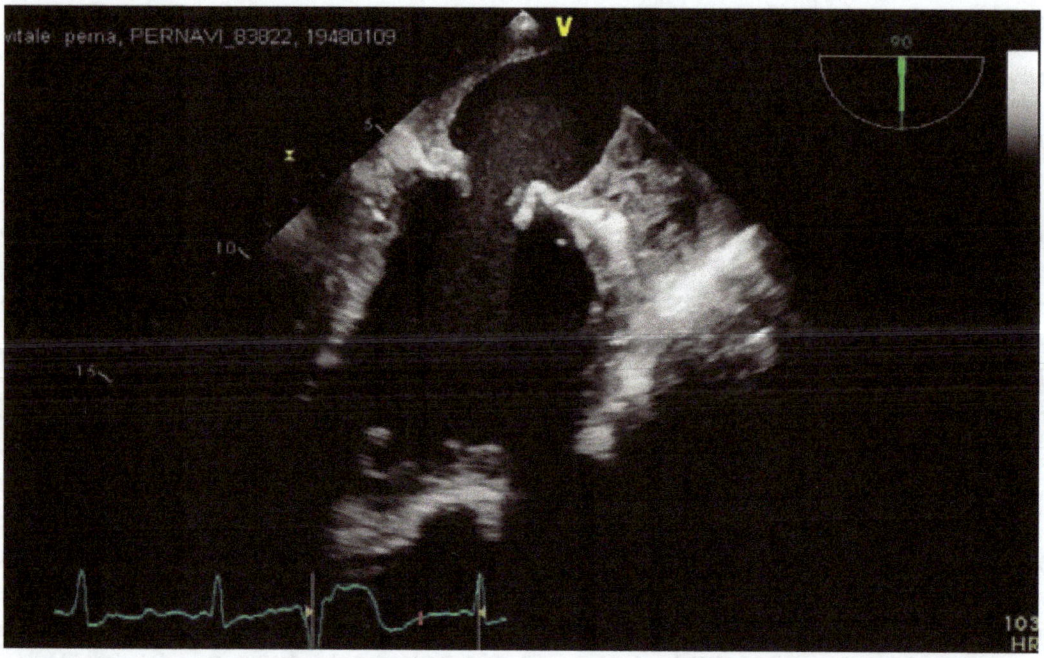

Figure 1. Transesophageal echocardiogram (TOE) intercommissural view showing massive left atrium (LA) and left atrial appendage (LAA) thrombosis.

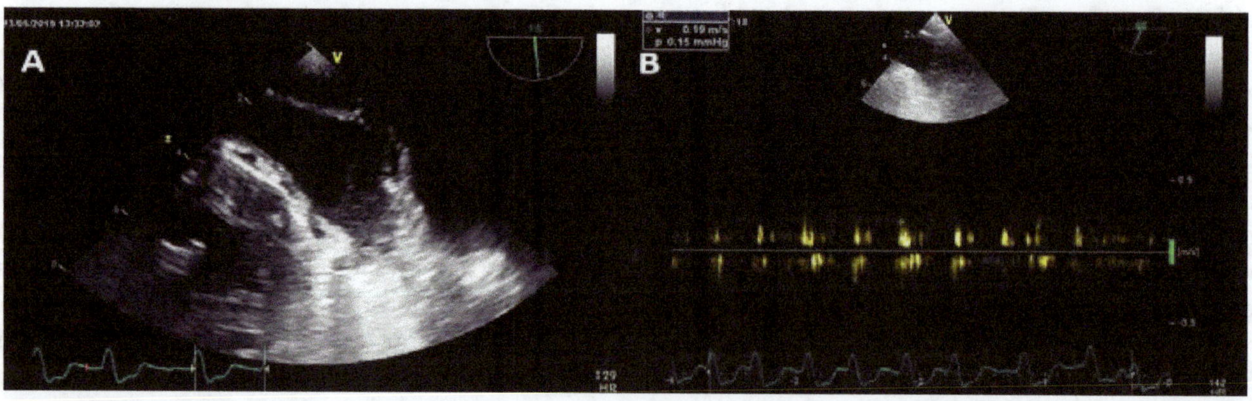

Figure 2. Detection of sludge in LAA with swirling effect (**A**) and associated low LAA emptying velocities (**B**).

However, despite the high sensitivity for thrombus detection, there are some potential limitations of the traditional bidimensional TOE. TOE may misdiagnose thrombi <2 mm, which have high embolic potential, especially in the setting of complex multilobed LAA anatomy [35]. Moreover, the LAA has a complex and highly variable three-dimensional morphology, which can render its assessment difficult using 2D TOE alone. In particular, the presence of pectinate muscles, multilobed appendage morphology, SEC, or acoustic shadowing from the Coumadin ridge might be misinterpreted as thrombi, and could prevent the accurate evaluation of the LAA with traditional 2D imaging [36]. 3D TOE improves the evaluation of LAA anatomy, overcoming some limitations associated with 2D imaging. 3D TOE enables a multiplanar reconstruction that provides a more extensive evaluation of the LAA (especially of complex multilobe morphologies), and a better depiction of the surrounding anatomical landmarks [37] (Figure 3). There is a lack of evidence regarding the sensitivity and specificity of 3D TOE for detecting LAA thrombosis. However, a recent report suggests that 3D TOE should be suggested when the diagnosis of LAA thrombosis remains equivocal after a detailed 2D analysis [36]. Moreover, with the widespread diffusion of LAA percutaneous closure techniques and increasing operator experience in 3D imaging, it is reasonable that 3D TOE will have a growing role in the diagnosis of LAA thrombosis.

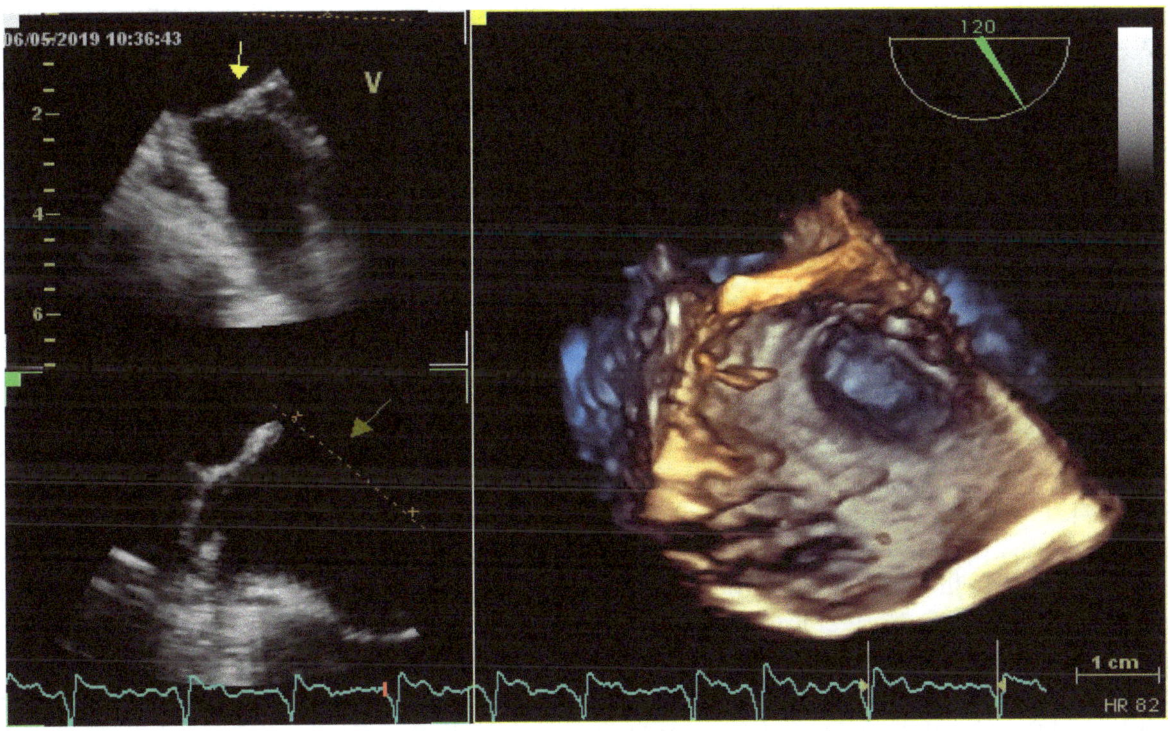

Figure 3. A three-dimensional TOE imaging of LAA.

Finally, intracardiac echocardiography (ICE) is an alternative imaging method of the LAA, usually indicated when TOE is contraindicated or not obtainable. ICE is performed with an 8–10 Fr catheter introduced through femoral venous access and advanced in right heart chambers under fluoroscopic guidance [38]. In the absence of interatrial transseptal crossing, the LAA can be displayed indirectly through the right ventricle outflow tract and the pulmonary artery, considering their close anatomical relationship [39]. Although ICE is less sensitive than TOE for thrombus detection [40], it can serve as a complementary method—especially when equivocal TOE findings require further evaluation. However, considering its invasive nature, in practice ICE is mainly performed in the catheterization laboratory during planned interventional cardiac procedures and when TOE is contraindicated.

4. Prevention and Treatment of Left Atrial Appendage Thrombosis

CV is associated with an increased risk of thromboembolic events and strokes. For patients with AF >48 h onset, current guidelines recommend anticoagulant therapy for at least three weeks before and four weeks after CV [6]. The reason for three weeks of anticoagulation before electrical CV derives from a study suggesting that at least 14 days are needed for fibroblastic infiltration and organization of an LAA thrombus [41]. The four weeks of anticoagulation after CV are due to postprocedural LA stunning, with marked impairment of Doppler-derived indexes of LA contraction that contribute to a higher risk of thromboembolic stroke [5,42].

VKAs are considered the gold standard for thromboembolic prophylaxis before CV, and are the only recommended treatment in patients with valvular AF [6]. Previous studies suggest that the incidence of LA/LAA thrombosis under treatment with VKAs ranges between 0.6% and 7%, depending on population study and sample size [43–45]. The narrow therapeutic interval and difficulties in keeping a target time in therapeutic range are considered the main limitations of VKA therapy.

NOACs are safe and effective alternatives to VKA therapy [46–49], and are currently considered as first-line therapy for long-term stroke prevention in patients with nonvalvular AF [6]. The overall safety and efficacy profile of NOACs have been confirmed in different clinical scenarios [50–58]. The clinical performance of NOACs in the setting of acute and elective CV has been addressed by three prospective randomized trials. In the X-VeRT trial, 1504 patients with AF of either >48 h or unknown duration undergoing CV were randomized to once-daily rivaroxaban or VKA [7]. The composite endpoint of stroke or systemic embolism after CV occurred in 1.02% of patients on VKAs and in 0.51% of patients on rivaroxaban. More recently, the ENSURE-AF trial randomized 2199 patients with AF >48 h and <1 year duration undergoing electrical cardioversion to 60 mg edoxaban once daily or warfarin with enoxaparin bridging [8]. The primary efficacy composite endpoint of stroke, systemic embolic event, myocardial infarction, and cardiovascular mortality at 28 days post CV occurred in 1.0% of patients of both arms. The EMANATE trial randomized 1500 patients with AF of ≤48 h onset to apixaban or heparin/VKA [9]. The trial showed a significant reduction with apixaban in strokes (0% vs. 0.8%) and in major bleeding (0.4% vs. 0.8%) at 30 days compared to warfarin. The favorable clinical profile of NOACs in patients undergoing CV has also been confirmed in a recent metanalysis [59,60] and in real-world studies [61–66].

Probably as a result of this evidence, a recent multicentric European registry addressing NOAC strategies before CV showed a trend towards an increasing use of NOACs and a significant decrease of VKA use [67]. However, in this registry 68.5% of patients received VKA anticoagulant therapy before CV and clinicians appeared to hesitate to embrace NOAC usage before CV [67].

In a real-world clinical scenario, the average time to CV was shorter with NOACs compared to warfarin [62]. Moreover, a budget impact analysis showed that the potential use of an early rivaroxaban strategy before direct-current CV could lead to a significant saving of costs related to procedure [68]. Therefore, considering these positive points and the effective clinical profile versus warfarin, it is reasonable that the use of the NOAC anticoagulation strategy before CV could increase in coming years.

Although randomized trials have addressed the efficacy and clinical profile of NOACs versus warfarin before CV, the prevalence of LA/LAA thrombus after adequate anticoagulation with NOACs remains a relatively unaddressed issue. In the X-VeRT study, a relatively high occurrence of LAA thrombi (18.2%) was observed in the 33 patients enrolled in the trial who underwent TOE before elective CV [7]. However, only about 10% of patients scheduled for elective CV in the X-VeRT trial underwent TOE, and these data could explain the high percentage of LAA thrombosis. In the ENSURE-AF trial, 47 patients (8%) in the edoxaban arm and 42 patients (7.1%) in the enoxaparin-warfarin arm had LAA thrombosis on pre-CV TOE [8]. In the EMANATE trial, LA/LAA thrombus was detected in 61 patients (4%), 30 in the apixaban group, and 31 in the heparin/VKA group, in over 829 patients who underwent TOE before CV [9].

There is a paucity of data on the prevalence of LAA thrombosis on NOAC therapy before CV in a real-life setting. A multicenter real-world study performed in AF patients undergoing TOE 12 h before CV or catheter ablation reported LAA thrombus in 3.6% of patients (15/414) with no significant difference between dabigatran, rivaroxaban, and apixaban [69]. Another recent real-world study showed LAA thrombosis in 7/127 patients (5.5%) and SEC in 24/127 (18.9%) [70].

Therefore, these data firstly suggest that LAA thrombosis is not a negligible event despite adequate anticoagulation, and that—although not universally accepted—a TOE-guided CV strategy is mandatory in order to reduce the burden of thromboembolic periprocedural events and to reduce bleeding events [71].

Once an LAA thrombus is identified, effective anticoagulation is recommended for at least three weeks or until LAA thrombus resolution is detected on follow-up TOE [6]. In this setting, VKA therapy for four weeks with repeat TOE showed resolution of thrombi in 80%–89% patients who were not previously anticoagulated [72,73]. If LAA thrombus occurs despite therapeutic anticoagulation, different strategies can be pursued, including switching to NOACs. Data are lacking on LAA resolution after NOACs therapy, and principally comprise case reports, where NOACs were initiated after failure of VKAs therapy or low time in therapeutic range [74–76]. The X-TRA multicenter prospective trial explored the use of rivaroxaban for the treatment of firstly-diagnosed LAA thrombus in 53 patients with available baseline and follow-up TOE [77]. About 75% of the patients had no prior anticoagulant therapy, while approximately one-quarter were treated with subtherapeutic VKA therapy. After six weeks of treatment, repeat TOE found a resolution of LAA thrombi in 41.5% of patients, 19% had LAA thrombi reduced in size, while 17% were unchanged and 22.5% had an increase in thrombi size [77].

In a recent retrospective study, among the 1485 patients with AF undergoing TOE, LAA thrombus or sludge was detected in 117 patients (7.8%) [78]. Of these, 39 (33%) were prescribed an NOAC, with rivaroxaban being the most frequently prescribed (54%). On repeat TOE, LAA thrombus resolution was seen in 37 patients (58.7%) with higher resolution rates, although not statistically significant, with NOAC therapy. A recent report on TOE showed 4.7% of LA/LAA thrombosis in 864 AF patients [79]. Follow-up TOE was performed in 22 patients, and 19 of them had LA/LAA thrombus resolution. In this real-world study, the preferred anticoagulant strategy was an uptitration of NOAC dosages and keeping higher INR values for warfarin therapy. However, a reduced NOAC dosage was most frequently associated with LA/LAA thrombi detection [79].

In conclusion, there is still a lack of solid evidence on the efficacy and safety of NOACs in LAA thrombus resolution. Current ongoing randomized trials comparing NOACs with VKAs in LA/LAA thrombosis resolution (rivaroxaban NCT03792152; dabigatran NCT02256683) will provide further evidence in this clinical scenario.

5. Conclusions

- The incidence of LAA thrombosis in AF patients undergoing CV is not a negligible event despite adequate anticoagulant therapy.
- A TOE-guided CV is a mandatory strategy in order to reduce the burden of periprocedural thromboembolic events.
- Although VKAs have been historically considered the cornerstone anticoagulant therapy before CV, growing evidence show that NOACs are safe and effective alternatives in this setting.
- Further and extended data are needed to assess the efficacy and safety profile of NOACs for the treatment of LAA thrombosis.

Author Contributions: E.M. and G.P. designed the paper structure; E.M., G.P., A.F., and P.E.M. performed the literature review; E.M. wrote the paper; V.M. and L.A. were responsible for final supervision and approval of the paper.

Acknowledgments: None to declare.

References

1. Feinberg, W.M.; Blackshear, J.L.; Laupacis, A.; Kronmal, R.; Hart, R.G. Prevalence, age distribution, and gender of patients with atrial fibrillation. Analysis and implications. *Arch. Intern. Med.* **1995**, *155*, 469–473. [CrossRef] [PubMed]
2. Wolf, P.A.; Abbott, R.D.; Kannel, W.B. Atrial fibrillation as an independent risk factor for stroke: The Framingham Study. *Stroke* **1991**, *22*, 983–988. [CrossRef] [PubMed]
3. Frost, L.; Engholm, G.; Johnsen, S.; Moller, H.; Henneberg, E.W.; Husted, S. Incident thromboembolism in the aorta and the renal, mesenteric, pelvic, and extremity arteries after discharge from the hospital with a diagnosis of atrial fibrillation. *Arch. Intern. Med.* **2001**, *161*, 272–276. [CrossRef] [PubMed]
4. Wang, T.J.; Larson, M.G.; Levy, D.; Vasan, R.S.; Leip, E.P.; Wolf, P.A.; D'Agostino, R.B.; Murabito, J.M.; Kannel, W.B.; Benjamin, E.J. Temporal relations of atrial fibrillation and congestive heart failure and their joint influe.nce on mortality: The Framingham Heart Study. *Circulation* **2003**, *107*, 2920–2925. [CrossRef] [PubMed]
5. Airaksinen, K.E.; Gronberg, T.; Nuotio, I.; Nikkinen, M.; Ylitalo, A.; Biancari, F.; Hartikainen, J.E. Thromboembolic complications after cardioversion of acute atrial fibrillation: The FinCV (Finnish CardioVersion) study. *J. Am. Coll. Cardiol.* **2013**, *62*, 1187–1192. [CrossRef] [PubMed]
6. Kirchhof, P.; Benussi, S.; Kotecha, D.; Ahlsson, A.; Atar, D.; Casadei, B.; Castella, M.; Diener, H.C.; Heidbuchel, H.; Hendriks, J.; et al. 2016 ESC guidelines for the management of atrial fibrillation developed in collaboration with EACTS. *Europace* **2016**, *18*, 1609–1678. [CrossRef]
7. Cappato, R.; Ezekowitz, M.D.; Klein, A.L.; Camm, A.J.; Ma, C.S.; Le Heuzey, J.Y.; Talajic, M.; Scanavacca, M.; Vardas, P.E.; Kirchhof, P.; et al. Rivaroxaban vs. vitamin K antagonists for cardioversion in atrial fibrillation. *Eur. Heart J.* **2014**, *35*, 3346–3355. [CrossRef]
8. Goette, A.; Merino, J.L.; Ezekowitz, M.D.; Zamoryakhin, D.; Melino, M.; Jin, J.; Mercuri, M.F.; Grosso, M.A.; Fernandez, V.; Al-Saady, N.; et al. Edoxaban versus enoxaparin–warfarin in patients undergoing cardioversion of atrial fibrillation (ENSURE-AF): A randomised, open-label, phase 3b trial. *Lancet* **2016**, *388*, 1995–2003. [CrossRef]
9. Ezekowitz, M.D.; Pollack, C.V., Jr.; Halperin, J.L.; England, R.D.; VanPelt Nguyen, S.; Spahr, J.; Sudworth, M.; Cater, N.B.; Breazna, A.; Oldgren, J.; et al. Apixaban compared to heparin/vitamin K antagonist in patients with atrial fibrillation scheduled for cardioversion: The EMANATE trial. *Eur. Heart J.* **2018**, *39*, 2959–2971. [CrossRef]
10. Schotten, U.; Verheule, S.; Kirchhof, P.; Goette, A. Pathophysiological mechanisms of atrial fibrillation: A translational appraisal. *Physiol. Rev.* **2011**, *91*, 265–325. [CrossRef]
11. Cresti, A.; García-Fernández, M.A.; Sievert, H.; Mazzone, P.; Baratta, P.; Solari, M.; Geyer, A.; De Sensi, F.; Limbruno, U. Prevalence of extra-appendage thrombosis in non-valvular atrial fibrillation and atrial flutter in patients undergoing cardioversion: A large Transeophageal Echo study. *EuroIntervention* **2019**, *15*, e225–e230. [CrossRef]
12. Yarmohammadi, H.; Klosterman, T.; Grewal, G.; Alraies, M.C.; Varr, B.C.; Lindsay, B.; Zurick, A.O.; Shrestha, K.; Tang, W.H.; Bhargava, M.; et al. Efficacy of the $CHADS_2$ scoring system to assess left atrial thrombogenic milieu risk before cardioversion of non-valvular atrial fibrillation. *Am. J. Cardiol.* **2013**, *112*, 678–683. [CrossRef] [PubMed]
13. Zylla, M.; Pohlmeier, M.; Hess, A.; Mereles, D.; Kieser, M.; Bruckner, T.; Scholz, E.; Zitron, E.; Schweizer, P.A.; Katus, H.A.; et al. Prevalence of intracardiac thrombi under phenprocoumon, direct oral anticoagulants (dabigatran and rivaroxaban), and bridging therapy in patients with atrial fibrillation and flutter. *Am. J. Cardiol.* **2015**, *115*, 635–640. [CrossRef]
14. Willens, H.J.; Gomez-Marin, O.; Nelson, K.; DeNicco, A.; Moscucci, M. Correlation of CHADS2 and CHA2DS2-VASc scores with transesophageal echocardiography risk factors for thromboembolism in a multiethnic United States population with nonvalvular atrial fibrillation. *J. Am. Soc. Echocardiogr.* **2013**, *26*, 175–184. [CrossRef]
15. Sikorska, A.; Baran, J.; Pilichowska-Paszkiet, E.; Sikora-Frąc, M.; Kryński, T.; Piotrowski, R.; Stec, S.; Zaborska, B.; Kułakowski, P. Risk of left atrial appendage thrombus in patients scheduled for ablation for atrial fibrillation: Beyond the CHA2DS2VASc score. *Pol. Arch. Med. Wewnętrznej* **2015**, *125*, 921–928. [CrossRef]

16. Uz, O.; Atalay, M.; Dogan, M.; Isilak, Z.; Yalcin, M.; Uzun, M.; Kardesoglu, E.; Cebeci, B.S. The CHA2DS2-VASc score as a predictor of left atrial thrombus in patients with non-valvular atrial fibrillation. *Med. Princ. Pract.* **2014**, *23*, 234–238. [CrossRef] [PubMed]
17. Tang, R.B.; Dong, J.Z.; Liu, X.P.; Long, D.Y.; Yu, R.H.; Du, X.; Liu, X.H.; Ma, C.S. Is CHA2DS2-VASc score a predictor of left atrial thrombus in patients with paroxysmal atrial fibrillation? *Thromb. Haemost.* **2011**, *105*, 1107–1109. [CrossRef] [PubMed]
18. Yarmohammadi, H.; Varr, B.C.; Puwanant, S.; Lieber, E.; Williams, S.J.; Klostermann, T.; Jasper, S.E.; Whitman, C.; Klein, A.L. Role of CHADS2 score in evaluation of thromboembolic risk and mortality in patients with atrial fibrillation undergoing direct current cardioversion (from the ACUTE Trial Substudy). *Am. J. Cardiol.* **2012**, *110*, 222–226. [CrossRef] [PubMed]
19. Ochiumi, Y.; Kagawa, E.; Kato, M.; Sasaki, S.; Nakano, Y.; Itakura, K.; Takiguchi, Y.; Ikeda, S.; Dote, K. Usefulness of brain natriuretic peptide for predicting left atrial appendage thrombus in patients with unanticoagulated nonvalvular persistent atrial fibrillation. *J. Arrhythmia* **2015**, *31*, 307–312. [CrossRef]
20. Habara, S.; Dote, K.; Kato, M.; Sasaki, S.; Goto, K.; Takemoto, H.; Hasegawa, D.; Matsuda, O. Prediction of left atrial appendage thrombi in non-valvular atrial fibrillation. *Eur. Heart J.* **2007**, *28*, 2217–2222. [CrossRef] [PubMed]
21. Lip, G.Y.; Nieuwlaat, R.; Pisters, R.; Lane, D.A.; Crijns, H.J. Refining clinical risk stratification for predicting stroke and thromboembolism in atrial fibrillation using a novel risk factor-based approach: The euro heart survey on atrial fibrillation. *Chest* **2010**, *137*, 263–272. [CrossRef] [PubMed]
22. Ayirala, S.; Kumar, S.; O'Sullivan, D.M.; Silverman, D.I. Echocardiographic predictors of left atrial appendage thrombus formation. *J. Am. Soc. Echocardiogr.* **2011**, *24*, 499–505. [CrossRef] [PubMed]
23. Marchese, P.; Bursi, F.; Delle Donne, G.; Malavasi, V.; Casali, E.; Barbieri, A.; Melandri, F.; Modena, M.G. Indexed left atrial volume predicts the recurrence of non-valvular atrial fibrillation after successful cardioversion. *Eur. J. Echocardiogr.* **2011**, *12*, 214–221. [CrossRef] [PubMed]
24. Doukky, R.; Khandelwal, A.; Garcia Sayan, E.; Gage, H. External validation of a novel transthoracic echocardiographic tool in predicting left atrial appendage thrombus formation in patients with nonvalvular atrial fibrillation. *Eur. Heart J. Cardiovasc. Imaging* **2013**, *14*, 876–881. [CrossRef] [PubMed]
25. Donal, E.; Lip, G.Y.; Galderisi, M.; Goette, A.; Shah, D.; Marwan, M.; Lederlin, M.; Mondillo, S.; Edvardsen, T.; Sitges, M.; et al. EACVI/EHRA Expert Consensus Document on the role of multi-modality imaging for the evaluation of patients with atrial fibrillation. *Eur. Heart J. Cardiovasc. Imaging* **2016**, *17*, 355–383. [CrossRef] [PubMed]
26. Fornengo, C.; Antolini, M.; Frea, S.; Gallo, C.; Grosso Marra, W.; Morello, M.; Gaita, F. Prediction of atrial fibrillation recurrence after cardioversion in patients with left-atrial dilation. *Eur. Heart J. Cardiovasc. Imaging* **2015**, *16*, 335–341. [CrossRef]
27. de Vos, C.B.; Pisters, R.; Nieuwlaat, R.; Prins, M.H.; Tieleman, R.G.; Coelen, R.J.S.; van den Heijkant, A.C.; Allessie, M.A.; Crijns, H.J. Progression from paroxysmal to persistent atrial fibrillation clinical correlates and prognosis. *J. Am. Coll. Cardiol.* **2010**, *55*, 725–731. [CrossRef]
28. Cameli, M.; Mandoli, G.E.; Loiacono, F.; Sparla, S.; Iardino, E.; Mondillo, S. Left atrial strain: A useful index in atrial fibrillation. *Int. J. Card.* **2016**, *220*, 208–213. [CrossRef]
29. Cameli, M.; Lunghetti, S.; Mandoli, G.E.; Righini, F.M.; Lisi, M.; Curci, V.; Di Tommaso, C.; Solari, M.; Nistor, D.; Gismondi, A.; et al. Left Atrial Strain Predicts Pro-Thrombotic State in Patients with non-valvular Atrial Fibrillation. *J. Atr. Fibrillation* **2017**, *10*, 1641. [CrossRef]
30. Costa, C.; Alujas, T.G.; Valente, F.; Aranda, C.; Rodríguez-Palomares, J.; Gutierrez, L.; Maldonado, G.; Galian, L.; Teixidó, G.; Evangelista, A. Left atrial strain: A new predictor of thrombotic risk and successful electrical cardioversion. Echo Research and practice. *Echo Res. Pract.* **2016**, *3*, 45–52. [CrossRef]
31. Manning, W.J.; Weintraub, R.M.; Waksmonski, C.A.; Haering, J.M.; Rooney, P.S.; Maslow, A.D.; Johnson, R.G.; Douglas, P.S. Accuracy of transesophageal echocardiography for identifying left atrial thrombi. A prospective, intraoperative study. *Ann. Intern. Med.* **1995**, *123*, 817–822. [CrossRef] [PubMed]
32. Troughton, R.W.; Asher, C.R.; Klein, A.L. The role of echocardiography in atrial fibrillation and cardioversion. *Heart* **2003**, *89*, 1447–1454. [CrossRef] [PubMed]
33. Black, I.W. Spontaneous echo contrast: Where there's smoke there's fire. *Echocardiography* **2000**, *17*, 373–382. [CrossRef] [PubMed]

34. Ruiz-Arango, A.; Landolfo, C. A novel approach to the diagnosis of left atrial appendage thrombus using contrast echocardiography and power Doppler imaging. *Eur. J. Echocardiogr.* **2008**, *9*, 329–333. [CrossRef] [PubMed]

35. Veinot, J.P.; Harrity, P.J.; Gentile, F.; Khandheria, B.K.; Bailey, K.R.; Eickholt, J.T.; Seward, J.B.; Tajik, A.J.; Edwards, W.D. Anatomy of the normal left atrial appendage: A quantitative study of age-related changes in 500 autopsy hearts—implications for echocardiographic examination. *Circulation* **1997**, *96*, 3112–3115. [CrossRef] [PubMed]

36. Squara, F.; Bres, M.; Baudouy, D.; Schouver, E.D.; Moceri, P.; Ferrari, E. Transesophageal echocardiography for the assessment of left atrial appendage thrombus: Study of the additional value of systematic real time 3D imaging after regular 2D evaluation. *Echocardiography* **2018**, *35*, 474–480. [CrossRef] [PubMed]

37. Nakajima, H.; Seo, Y.; Ishizu, T.; Yamamoto, M.; Machino, T.; Harimura, Y.; Kawamura, R.; Sekiguchi, Y.; Tada, H.; Aonuma, K. Analysis of the left atrial appendage by three-dimensional transesophageal echocardiography. *Am. J. Cardiol.* **2010**, *106*, 885–892. [CrossRef] [PubMed]

38. Basman, C.; Parmar, Y.J.; Kronzon, I. Intracardiac Echocardiography for Structural Heart and Electrophysiological Interventions. *Curr. Cardiol. Rep.* **2017**, *19*, 102. [CrossRef]

39. Baran, J.; Stec, S.; Pilichowska-Paszkiet, E.; Zaborska, B.; Sikora-Frąc, M.; Kryński, T.; Michałowska, I.; Łopatka, R.; Kułakowski, P. Intracardiac Echocardiography for Detection of Thrombus in the Left Atrial Appendage. *Circ. Arrhythmia Electrophysiol.* **2013**, *6*, 1074–1081. [CrossRef] [PubMed]

40. Saksena, S.; Sra, J.; Jordaens, L.; Kusumoto, F.; Knight, B.; Natale, A.; Kocheril, A.; Nanda, N.C.; Nagarakanti, R.; Simon, A.M.; et al. A prospective comparison of cardiac imaging using intracardiac echocardiography with transesophageal echocardiography in patients with atrial fibrillation: The intracardiac echocardiography guided cardioversion helps interventional procedures study. *Circ. Arrhythmia Electrophysiol.* **2010**, *3*, 571–577. [CrossRef] [PubMed]

41. Goldman, M.J. The management of chronic atrial fibrillation. *Prog. Cardiovasc. Dis.* **1960**, *2*, 465–479. [CrossRef]

42. Manning, W.J.; Leeman, D.E.; Gotch, P.J. Pulsed Doppler evaluation of atrial mechanical function after electrical cardioversion of atrial fibrillation. *J. Am. Coll. Cardiol.* **1989**, *13*, 617–623. [CrossRef]

43. Scherr, D.; Dalal, D.; Chilukuri, K.; Dong, J.; Spragg, D.; Henrikson, C.A.; Nazarian, S.; Cheng, A.; Berger, R.D.; Abraham, T.P.; et al. Incidence and predictors of left atrial thrombus prior to catheter ablation of atrial fibrillation. *J. Cardiovasc. Electrophysiol.* **2009**, *20*, 379–384. [CrossRef] [PubMed]

44. Wallace, T.W.; Atwater, B.D.; Daubert, J.P.; Voora, D.; Crowley, A.L.; Bahnson, T.D.; Hranitzky, P.M. Prevalence and clinical characteristics associated with left atrial appendage thrombus in fully anticoagulated patients undergoing catheter-directed ablation of atrial fibrillation. *J. Cardiovasc. Electrophysiol.* **2010**, *21*, 849–852. [CrossRef] [PubMed]

45. Anselmino, M.; Garberoglio, L.; Gili, S.; Bertaglia, E.; Stabile, G.; Marazzi, R.; Themistoclakis, S.; Solimene, F.; Frea, S.; Marra, W.G.; et al. Left atrial appendage thrombi relate to easily accessible clinical parameters in patients undergoing atrial fibrillation transcatheter ablation: A multicentre study. *Int. J. Cardiol.* **2017**, *241*, 218–222. [CrossRef] [PubMed]

46. Connolly, S.J.; Ezekowitz, M.D.; Yusuf, S.; Eikelboom, J.; Oldgren, J.; Parekh, A.; Pogue, J.; Reilly, P.A.; Themeles, E.; Varrone, J.; et al. RELY Steering Committee and Investigators, Dabigatran versus warfarin in patients with atrial fibrillation. *N. Engl. J. Med.* **2009**, *361*, 1139–1151. [CrossRef] [PubMed]

47. Patel, M.R.; Mahaffey, K.W.; Garg, J.; Pan, G.; Singer, D.E.; Hacke, W.; Breithardt, G.; Halperin, J.L.; Hankey, G.J.; Piccini, J.P.; et al. Rivaroxaban versus warfarin in nonvalvular atrial fibrillation. *N. Engl. J. Med.* **2011**, *365*, 883–891. [CrossRef] [PubMed]

48. Granger, C.B.; Alexander, J.H.; McMurray, J.J.; Lopes, R.D.; Hylek, E.M.; Hanna, M.; Al-Khalidi, H.R.; Ansell, J.; Atar, D.; Avezum, A.; et al. Apixaban versus warfarin in patients with atrial fibrillation. *N. Engl. J. Med.* **2011**, *365*, 981–992. [CrossRef]

49. Giugliano, R.P.; Ruff, C.T.; Braunwald, E.; Murphy, S.A.; Wiviott, S.D.; Halperin, J.L.; Waldo, A.L.; Ezekowitz, M.D.; Weitz, J.I.; Špinar, J.; et al. Edoxaban versus warfarin in patients with atrial fibrillation. *N. Engl. J. Med.* **2013**, *369*, 2093–2104. [CrossRef]

50. Russo, V.; Carbone, A.; Rago, A.; Golino, P.; Nigro, G. Direct Oral Anticoagulants in octogenarians with atrial fibrillation: it's never too late. *J. Cardiovasc. Pharmacol.* **2019**, *73*, 207–214. [CrossRef]

51. Russo, V.; Attena, E.; Mazzone, C.; Melillo, E.; Rago, A.; Galasso, G.; Riegler, L.; Parisi, V.; Rotunno, R.; Nigro, G.; et al. Real-life Performance of Edoxaban in Elderly Patients with Atrial Fibrillation: A Multicenter Propensity Score-Matched Cohort Study. *Clin. Ther.* **2019**. [CrossRef] [PubMed]
52. Russo, V.; Rago, A.; Proietti, R.; Attena, E.; Rainone, C.; Crisci, M.; Papa, A.A.; Calabrò, P.; D'Onofrio, A.; Golino, P.; et al. Safety and Efficacy of Triple Antithrombotic Therapy with Dabigatran versus Vitamin K Antagonist in Atrial Fibrillation Patients: A Pilot Study. *BioMed Res. Int.* **2019**, *2019*, 5473240. [CrossRef] [PubMed]
53. Russo, V.; Bottino, R.; Rago, A.; Di Micco, P.; D'Onofrio, A.; Liccardo, B.; Golino, P.; Nigro, G. Atrial Fibrillation and Malignancy: The Clinical Performance of Non-Vitamin K Oral Anticoagulants-A Systematic Review. *Semin. Thromb. Hemost.* **2019**, *45*, 205–214. [PubMed]
54. Russo, V.; Attena, E.; Mazzone, C.; Esposito, F.; Parisi, V.; Bancone, C.; Rago, A.; Nigro, G.; Sangiuolo, R.; D'Onofrio, A. Nonvitamin K Antagonist Oral Anticoagulants Use in Patients with Atrial Fibrillation and Bioprosthetic Heart Valves/Prior Surgical Valve Repair: A Multicenter Clinical Practice Experience. *Semin. Thromb. Hemost.* **2018**, *44*, 364–369. [PubMed]
55. Russo, V.; Rago, A.; Papa, A.A.; Di Meo, F.; Attena, E.; Golino, P.; D'Onofrio, A.; Nigro, G. Use of Non-Vitamin K Antagonist Oral Anticoagulants in Atrial Fibrillation Patients with Malignancy: Clinical Practice Experience in a Single Institution and Literature Review. *Semin. Thromb. Hemost.* **2018**, *44*, 370–376. [PubMed]
56. Russo, V.; Rago, A.; Proietti, R.; Di Meo, F.; Antonio Papa, A.; Calabrò, P.; D'Onofrio, A.; Nigro, G.; AlTurki, A. Efficacy and safety of the target-specific oral anticoagulants for stroke prevention in atrial fibrillation: The real-life evidence. *Ther. Adv. Drug Saf.* **2017**, *8*, 67–75. [CrossRef] [PubMed]
57. Russo, V.; Bianchi, V.; Cavallaro, C.; Vecchione, F.; De Vivo, S.; Santangelo, L.; Sarubbi, B.; Calabro, P.; Nigro, G.; D'Onofrio, A. Efficacy and safety of dabigatran in a "real-life" population at high thromboembolic and hemorrhagic risk: Data from MonaldiCare registry. *Eur. Rev. Med. Pharmacol. Sci.* **2015**, *19*, 3961–3967.
58. Russo, V.; Rago, A.; D'Onofrio, A.; Nigro, G. The clinical performance of dabigatran in the Italian real-life experience. *J. Cardiovasc. Med.* **2017**, *18*, 922–923. [CrossRef]
59. Telles-Garcia, N.; Dahal, K.; Kocherla, C.; Lip, G.Y.H.; Reddy, P.; Dominic, P. Non-vitamin K anticoagulants oral anticoagulants are as safe and effective as warfarin for cardioversion of atrial fibrillation: A systematic review and meta-analysis. *Int. J. Cardiol.* **2018**, *268*, 143–148. [CrossRef]
60. Gibson, C.M.; Basto, A.N.; Howard, M.L. Direct Oral Anticoagulants in Cardioversion: A Review of Current Evidence. *Ann. Pharmacother.* **2018**, *52*, 277–284. [CrossRef]
61. Itäinen, S.; Lehto, M.; Vasankari, T.; Mustonen, P.; Kotamäki, M.; Numminen, A.; Lahtela, H.; Bah, A.; Hartikainen, J.; Hekkala, A.M.; et al. Non-vitamin K antagonist oral anticoagulants in atrial fibrillation patients undergoing elective cardioversion. *Europace* **2018**, *20*, 565–568. [CrossRef] [PubMed]
62. Frederiksen, A.S.; Albertsen, A.E.; Christesen, A.M.S.; Vinter, N.; Frost, L.; Møller, D.S. Cardioversion of atrial fibrillation in a real-world setting: Non-vitamin K antagonist oral anticoagulants ensure a fast and safe strategy compared to warfarin. *Europace* **2018**, *20*, 1078–1085. [CrossRef] [PubMed]
63. Russo, V.; Rago, A.; Papa, A.A.; D'Onofrio, A.; Golino, P.; Nigro, G. Efficacy and safety of dabigatran in patients with atrial fibrillation scheduled for transoesophageal echocardiogram-guided direct electrical current cardioversion: A prospective propensity score-matched cohort study. *J. Thromb. Thrombolysis* **2018**, *45*, 206–212. [CrossRef]
64. Russo, V.; Di Napoli, L.; Bianchi, V.; Tavoletta, V.; De Vivo, S.; Cavallaro, C.; Vecchione, F.; Rago, A.; Sarubbi, B.; Calabrò, P.; et al. A new integrated strategy for direct current cardioversion in non-valvular atrial fibrillation patients using short term rivaroxaban administration: The MonaldiVert real life experience. *Int. J. Cardiol.* **2016**, *224*, 454–455. [CrossRef] [PubMed]
65. Rago, A.; Papa, A.A.; Cassese, A.; Arena, G.; Magliocca, M.C.G.; D'Onofrio, A.; Golino, P.; Nigro, G.; Russo, V. Clinical Performance of Apixaban vs. Vitamin K Antagonists in Patients with Atrial Fibrillation Undergoing Direct Electrical Current Cardioversion: A Prospective Propensity Score-Matched Cohort Study. *Am. J. Cardiovasc. Drugs* **2019**, *19*, 421–427. [CrossRef]
66. Stabile, G.; Russo, V.; Rapacciuolo, A.; De Divitiis, M.; De Simone, A.; Solimene, F.; D'Onofrio, A.; Iuliano, A.; Maresca, G.; Esposito, F.; et al. Transesophageal echocardiograpy in patients with persistent atrial fibrillation undergoing electrical cardioversion on new oral anticoagulants: A multi center registry. *Int. J. Cardiol.* **2015**, *184*, 283–284. [CrossRef] [PubMed]

67. Papp, J.; Zima, E.; Bover, R.; Karaliute, R.; Rossi, A.; Szymanski, C.; Troccoli, R.; Schneider, J.; Fagerland, M.W.; Camm, A.J.; et al. Changes in oral anticoagulation for elective cardioversion: Results from a European cardioversion registry. *Eur. Heart J. Cardiovasc. Pharmacother.* **2017**, *3*, 147–150. [CrossRef]
68. Russo, V.; Rago, A.; Papa, A.A.; Bianchi, V.; Tavoletta, V.; DE, S.V.; Cavallaro, C.; Nigro, G.; D'Onofrio, A. Budget impact analysis of rivaroxaban vs. warfarin anticoagulation strategy for direct current cardioversion in non-valvular atrial fibrillation patients: The MonaldiVert Economic Study. *Minerva Cardioangiol.* **2018**, *66*, 1–5.
69. Bertaglia, E.; Anselmino, M.; Zorzi, A.; Russo, V.; Toso, E.; Peruzza, F.; Rapacciuolo, A.; Migliore, F.; Gaita, F.; Cucchini, U.; et al. NOACs and atrial fibrillation: Incidence and predictors of left atrial thrombus in the real world. *Int. J. Cardiol.* **2017**, *249*, 179–183. [CrossRef]
70. Hwang, J.; Park, H.S.; Jun, S.W.; Choi, S.W.; Lee, C.H.; Kim, I.C.; Cho, Y.K.; Yoon, H.J.; Kim, H.; Nam, C.W.; et al. The incidence of left atrial appendage thrombi on transesophageal echocardiography afterpretreatment with apixaban for cardioversion in the real-world practice. *PLoS ONE* **2018**, *13*, e0208734. [CrossRef]
71. Klein, A.L.; Grimm, R.A.; Murray, R.D.; Apperson-Hansen, C.; Asinger, R.W.; Black, I.W.; Davidoff, R.; Erbel, R.; Halperin, J.L.; Orsinelli, D.A.; et al. Use of Transesophageal Echocardiography to Guide Cardioversion in Patients with Atrial Fibrillation. *N. Engl. J. Med.* **2001**, *344*, 1411–1420. [CrossRef] [PubMed]
72. Corrado, G.; Tadeo, G.; Beretta, S.; Tagliagambe, L.M.; Manzillo, G.F.; Spata, M.; Santarone, M. Atrial thrombi resolution after prolonged anticoagulation in patients with atrial fibrillation. *Chest* **1999**, *115*, 140–143. [CrossRef] [PubMed]
73. Collins, L.J.; Silverman, D.I.; Douglas, P.S.; Manning, W.J. Cardioversion of Nonrheumatic Atrial Fibrillation. Reduced Thromboembolic Complications with 4 Weeks of Precardioversion Anticoagulation Are Related to Atrial Thrombus Resolution. *Circulation* **1995**, *92*, 160–163. [CrossRef] [PubMed]
74. Hammerstingl, C.; Pötzsch, B.; Nickenig, G. Resolution of giant left atrial appendage thrombus with rivaroxaban. *Thromb. Haemost.* **2013**, *109*, 583–584.
75. Takasugi, J.; Yamagami, H.; Okata, T.; Toyoda, K.; Nagatsuka, K. Dissolution of the left atrial appendage thrombus with rivaroxaban therapy. *Cerebrovasc. Dis.* **2013**, *36*, 322–323. [CrossRef]
76. Vidal, A.; Vanerio, G. Dabigatran and left atrial appendage thrombus. *J. Thromb. Thrombolysis* **2012**, *34*, 545–547. [CrossRef] [PubMed]
77. Lip, G.Y.; Hammerstingl, C.; Marin, F.; Cappato, R.; Meng, I.L.; Kirsch, B.; van Eickels, M.; Cohen, A. Left atrial thrombus resolution in atrial fibrillation or flutter: Results of a prospective study with rivaroxaban (X-TRA) and a retrospective observational registry providing baseline data (CLOT-AF). *Am. Heart J.* **2016**, *178*, 126–134. [CrossRef] [PubMed]
78. Niku, A.D.; Shiota, T.; Siegel, R.J.; Rader, F. Prevalence and Resolution of Left Atrial Thrombus in Patients with Nonvalvular Atrial Fibrillationand Flutter with Oral Anticoagulation. *Am. J. Cardiol.* **2019**, *123*, 63–68. [CrossRef] [PubMed]
79. Lee, W.C.; Fang, C.Y.; Chen, Y.L.; Fang, H.Y.; Chen, H.C.; Liu, W.H.; Fu, M.; Chen, M.C. Left Atrial or Left Atrial Appendage Thrombus Resolution After Adjustment of Oral Anticoagulant Treatment. *J. Stroke Cerebrovasc. Dis.* **2019**, *28*, 90–96. [CrossRef] [PubMed]

10

The Role of Cardiovascular and Metabolic Comorbidities in the Link between Atrial Fibrillation and Cognitive Impairment

Ahmed AlTurki [1,*], Jakub B. Maj [1], Mariam Marafi [2], Filippo Donato [3], Giovanni Vescovo [3], Vincenzo Russo [4] and Riccardo Proietti [3]

1 Division of Cardiology, McGill University Health Center, Montreal, QC H3G1A4, Canada; jakub.maj@mail.mcgill.ca
2 Department of Neurology and Neurosurgery, Montreal Neurological Institute, Montreal, QC H3A2B4, Canada; mariamarafie@gmail.com
3 Department of Cardiac, Thoracic, and Vascular Sciences, University of Padua, 35121 Padua, Italy; filippodonato89@gmail.com (F.D.); gm.vescovo@libero.it (G.V.); riccardoproietti6@gmail.com (R.P.)
4 Department of Medical Translational Sciences, University of Campania "Luigi Vanvitelli"-Monaldi Hospital, 80131 Naples, Italy; v.p.russo@libero.it
* Correspondence: ahmedalturkimd@gmail.com

Abstract: Atrial fibrillation (AF) is the most common arrhythmia encountered in clinical practice with implications on long-term outcomes. Metabolic disorders including diabetes mellitus and obesity are independent predictors of atrial fibrillation and present therapeutic targets to reduce both the incidence and duration burden of atrial fibrillation. The presence of pericardial fat in direct contact with cardiac structures, as well the subsequent release of proinflammatory cytokines, may play an important role in this connection. Atrial fibrillation is an independent predictor of cognitive impairment and dementia. While clinical stroke is a major contributor, other factors such as cerebral hypoperfusion and microbleeds play important roles. New evidence suggests that atrial fibrillation and cognitive impairment may be downstream events of atrial cardiomyopathy, which may be caused by several factors including metabolic syndrome, obesity, and obstructive sleep apnea. The mechanisms linking these comorbidities to cognitive impairment are not yet fully elucidated. A clearer understanding of the association of AF with dementia and cognitive impairment is imperative. Future studies should focus on the predictors of cognitive impairment among those with AF and aim to understand the potential mechanisms underlying these associations. This would inform strategies for the management of AF aiming to prevent continued cognitive impairment.

Keywords: atrial fibrillation; metabolic syndrome; obesity; cognitive impairment; dementia

---

1. Introduction

Atrial fibrillation (AF) is the most common significant arrhythmia and is increasingly prevalent [1]. Hospitalization due to AF has increased by 60% in the United States in the last 20 years and is expected to affect 20 million Americans by 2030 [2]. AF may be complicated by thromboembolic events and heart failure, and it is associated with an increase in mortality [3]. Metabolic disorders including hypertension and diabetes have been shown to significantly increase the risk of these complications in those with AF [4]. In addition, obesity and obstructive sleep apnea have also been associated with AF [5].

Cognitive decline and dementia have emerged as associated risks in patients with atrial fibrillation [6]. A significant portion of this risk is attributable to cerebrovascular thromboembolic events that lead to vascular dementia [7]. However, AF has been shown to be a risk factor for cognitive impairment and dementia independent of stroke [8]. In this review, we will examine the association between metabolic disorders and AF as well as the possible role of these cardiovascular and metabolic comorbidities in the pathogenesis of cognitive impairment in patients with AF.

2. Obesity and Metabolic Syndrome

Atrial fibrillation is associated with heart failure, obesity, diabetes, hypertension, and hyperthyroidism [9]. Obesity has been shown to be an independent risk factor for AF [10], and this association has been observed in multiples studies thus far [11–13]. Wang et al. [11], analyzed the data of the Framingham Heart Study, a long-standing, multigenerational, longitudinal study of cardiovascular disease, and found that body mass index (BMI) independently predicted AF when adjusted for other risk factors [11]. Each BMI unit increase was associated with a 4% risk increase of AF. Overall, obese men and women had a 52% and 46% greater risk of AF, respectively, when compared to nonobese participants. One of the largest studies to date was a nationwide, prospective cohort from Denmark of 47,589 individuals, where each increase in BMI per unit increased the risk of AF by 8% and 6% in men and women, respectively [14]. In individuals with a BMI over 30, the adjusted hazard ratio for AF was 2.35 in men and 1.99 in women [14]. The association between obesity and AF is independent of ethnicity. In two large cohort studies of 28,449 Japanese individuals and 14,598 American individuals, a significant association between obesity and AF was shown [15,16]. Umetani et al. [17], reported a three-fold risk of AF in individuals with BMI > 25, after adjusting for age and left atrial (LA) size, and that obesity was the strongest metabolic risk factor for AF [17]. In the Atherosclerosis Risk in Communities (ARIC) study, 20% of incident AF could be attributed to obesity. Wanahita conducted a meta-analysis of 16 studies and found a 49% increase in the risk of AF in individuals with a BMI above 30 [13].

Adipose tissue is known to release multiple compounds, many of which are proinflammatory cytokines [18]. Central obesity is strongly associated with insulin resistance [19]. In addition, obesity is associated with the activation of the sympathetic nervous system and renin-angiotensin system, leading to hypertension [20]. These elements define the metabolic syndrome. Metabolic syndrome can practically be considered as a collection of cardiovascular and metabolic imbalances that are associated with a higher risk of developing cardiovascular atherosclerotic disease. Key features include abdominal obesity, dyslipidemia, hypertension, and insulin resistance [21]. Metabolic syndrome has an estimated prevalence of 20% in North America [22], which underlines the need to identify, manage, and prevent potential complications [21].

Metabolic syndrome has been shown to be associated with atrial remodeling and fibrosis, atrial synchronicity, autonomic abnormalities, mitochondrial dysfunction, and increased LA size [23,24]. An electrophysiological study of patients with AF has shown that left atrial low-voltage zones were identified more commonly in patients with metabolic syndrome (46%) than in patients without metabolic syndrome (8.2%). Metabolic syndrome was an independent predictor of left atrial low voltage with 11 times the odds [20]. Each component of metabolic syndrome has been demonstrated to be associated with an increased risk of AF [23]. It is not only the diagnosis of diabetes mellitus that has an association with AF, but increased fasting glucose also independently predicts the risk of AF. Each increase of 18 mg/dL is linked with a 33% increased risk of AF [25].

One mechanism in which obesity may lead to AF is through the presence of pericardial fat, which is of importance because of its contiguity with the heart and a shared blood supply [26]. Pericardial fat is highly metabolically active and releases proinflammatory cytokines. Critically, pericardial fat is more strongly associated with metabolic risk than BMI. Thus, pericardial fat may play a major role in the risk of AF observed with obesity [26].

3. Obesity as a Therapeutic Target to Decrease Metabolic Comorbidities

From a pharmacological perspective regarding weight loss, there is little evidence of the benefit in reducing the risk of AF with medications used in diabetes that induce significant weight loss and improve insulin sensitivity, such as glucagon-like peptide -1 receptor agonists, sodium-glucose transport protein 2 (SGLT2), and dipeptidyl peptidase-4 (DPP-4) inhibitors [23]. Osteopontin, a proinflammatory adhesion protein that is upregulated in obese individuals with hypertension, may be a pharmacological target to prevent atrial remodeling [27].

Interventions of weight management have been shown to affect atrial remodeling in a proportional manner and to reduce AF burden. The benefits of weight loss were seen from the structural perspective in a study conducted by Abed and colleagues that showed a significant decrease in the left atrial area and interventricular septal thickness in subjects that lost 14.3 kg, compared to the control group that lost 3.6 kg [28]. In addition, patients who lost significant amounts of weight also experienced a reduction in AF, as well as AF symptom-related frequency and severity [28]. However, there appears to be a minimal threshold of weight loss for AF burden to decrease [23]. The Long-Term Effect of Goal-Directed Weight Management in an Atrial Fibrillation Cohort (LEGACY) study aimed to assess the long-term impact of weight loss on AF rhythm control in patients who were obese, as defined by a BMI of 27 kg/m^2 [29]. Similarly, in the LEGACY study, subjects with BMI > 27 that lost >10% of body mass had a six-fold decrease of arrhythmias compared to individuals that lost less than 10% of body mass. Patients that lost >5% of body mass, but did not reach the 10% threshold, actually had a two-fold increase in arrhythmia recurrence [29].

Weight control measures that involve medical interventions, rather than exercise or diet, have also been shown to be effective. Bariatric surgery is able to produce significant weight loss that is more sustainable in comparison to nonsurgical interventions [30]. This has been shown to have dramatic effects on metabolic comorbidities, such as hypertension and diabetes mellitus, and may return the patient to a normotensive and normoglycemic state. Reductions in cholesterol have also been noted. This mirrors the effect of weight loss by nonsurgical interventions [28,29]. Interestingly, bariatric surgery has been shown to decrease incident AF as well as reduce the burden of AF in obese individuals [31]. In the Swedish Obese Subjects study, investigators compared 2000 individuals that underwent bariatric surgery to a matched cohort of 2000 patients that received usual care [31]. After a median 19 years follow-up period, incident AF had occurred in 12.4% of patients that underwent bariatric surgery compared to 16.8% of those that received usual care with a 29% relative risk reduction in incident AF [31]. Lynch and colleagues replicated this finding [32].

4. Fibrotic Atrial Cardiomyopathy

Metabolic syndrome, which results in hypertension, inflammation, endothelial dysfunction, and myocardial steatosis, leads to left atrial fibrosis and dilatation [23]. Inflammation is the main driver of atrial fibrosis; a proposed mechanism in metabolic syndrome is through the accumulation of intracellular triglycerides and free fatty acids. These deposits appear to be toxic to the atrial myocytes, leading to myocardial apoptosis and fibrosis. The resulting atrial fibrosis leads to structural and electrical remodeling of the left atrium. Atrial dilatation leads to the activation of the renin–angiotensin–aldosterone system, which in itself leads to further myocyte fibrosis, apoptosis, and vasoconstriction by angiotensin II and aldosterone [24]. Atrial fibrosis causes the development of electrical remodeling by delaying interatrial conduction with prolongation of atrial activation time and cycle length, and these changes are enhanced by augmented atrial stretch from obesity. Atrial stretch causes prolongation of the action potential and shortens refractory periods which allow physiological rhythm to be overtaken by reentrant wave fronts from the pulmonary veins, which result in atrial fibrillation. Recurrent episodes of AF enhance atrial remodeling that will promote further events in time.

Atrial cardiomyopathy, therefore, is hypothesized to be the result of these multiple metabolic derangements including hypertension, diabetes, and metabolic syndrome [33]. In turn, AF may also independently be associated with strokes and cognitive decline. This notion is supported by findings seen in patients with subclinical AF in whom studies found a significant increase in stroke risk [34]. The classical theory is that AF causes blood to stagnate in the left atrium that leads to a stroke. However, data from patients with subclinical device-detected AF put this theory into question. There was no temporal relationship between AF episodes and stroke events, with the majority of AF episodes occurring >30 days prior to the stroke event [35,36]. This lends credence to the notion that atrial hypocontractility and impaired atrial endothelial function in the context of atrial cardiomyopathy contribute significantly to stroke events and do not require the presence of AF [33]. In a recent consensus document by the European Heart Rhythm Association that examined the current literature on the subject, hypertension, obesity, and diabetes mellitus were noted to lead to atrial cardiomyopathy through the promotion of changes to the cardiac myocyte, fibrosis, and noncollagenous infiltration [37].

5. Atrial Fibrillation (AF) and Cognitive Function

Both atrial fibrillation and dementia are common diseases that share similar risk factors, but the association between them appears to be independent of shared risk factors. Table 1 summarizes the current body of literature demonstrating the association between AF and dementia. An improved understanding of the predictors of cognitive impairment in patients with AF, and the potential underlying mechanisms, is critical for the management of AF with the aim to prevent adverse outcomes in these patients [38].

Several studies have documented the association of AF and cognitive impairment. In 935 participants of the ARIC study with no prior history of strokes, incident AF was associated with a more rapid decline in executive function and verbal fluency [39]. The association was only found in those with subclinical strokes, which suggested a thromboembolic cause of the association. Ott and colleagues assessed data from a cross-sectional study with 6584 participants, of whom 9.6% had cognitive impairment and 4.2% had dementia [40]. The most common causes of dementia were Alzheimer's disease (75%), vascular dementia (15%), and undefined dementia (11%). Participants with AF had twice the odds of having dementia compared to those without AF.

Other studies have shown that the association between AF and cognitive decline goes beyond thromboembolic disease. Marzona and colleagues performed a combined post hoc analysis of two prospective multicenter trials, Telmisartan, Ramipril, or Both in Patients at High Risk for Vascular Events (ONTARGET) and The Telmisartan Randomised Assessment Study in ACE intolerant subjects with cardiovascular Disease (TRANSCEND), which comprised 31,506 patients aged 55 years and older with cardiovascular disease or diabetes [41]. At baseline, 3.3% had AF, while 6.5% developed AF during follow-up (median 56 months). AF was associated with a 14% increased risk of cognitive decline and a 16% increased risk of new-onset dementia; these results were independent of any history of overt stroke [41]. Santangeli published a systematic review of eight prospective studies that included over 77,000 patients. The risk of dementia in AF patients was increased by 40% (hazard ratio (HR) 1.42, 95% confidence interval (CI) 1.17–1.72, $p = 0.002$) [6]. Kim and colleagues analyzed data from a large population-based cohort. The association between incident AF and subsequent incident dementia was assessed in 262,611 participants aged 60 years and older that were free of stroke and dementia in Korea between 2005 and 2012. Incident AF was observed in 10,435 participants over a time frame of 1,629,903 person-years at a rate of 0.64% per year. During that time period, incident dementia occurred at a rate of 4.1 and 2.7 per 100 person-years in those with incident AF and a propensity score-matched AF-free group, respectively. Incident AF increased the risk of dementia by 50% (HR 1.52; 95% CI 1.43–1.63). Incident AF was associated with an increased risk of both Alzheimer's (HR 1.31, 95% CI 1.20–1.43) and vascular dementia (HR 2.11, 95% CI 1.85–2.41). Oral anticoagulation in patients who developed incident AF was associated with a reduced risk of incident dementia (HR 0.61, 95% CI 0.54–0.68), while higher CHA2DS2-VASc scores were associated with an increased risk of dementia [42].

AF is associated with an increased risk of progressive cognitive impairment in patients who have not suffered from a stroke. In a secondary analysis of the Cardiovascular Health Study, patients with AF had a more rapid decline of cognitive function compared to patients with sinus rhythm [43], as assessed by the Mini Mental State Exam. Cognitive impairment risk is greater in AF patients with heart failure, diabetes, and kidney disease [44]. A higher risk of dementia in patients with AF that have not suffered from strokes is found in both men and women. In a large study of 35,608 patients without a history of AF or dementia, of whom 40.4% were women, the five-year rates of AF were higher in men than women (14.0% in men versus 11.9% in women; $p < 0.0001$). However, dementia rates (1.1% in women versus 0.9% in men; $p = 0.09$) were similar in women and men. Among the patients who developed AF, the five-year rate of dementia in women was 2.9%, versus 2.3% in men ($p = 0.180$) [45].

Multiple mechanisms of cognitive dysfunction due to atrial fibrillation have been postulated. The most intuitive mechanism is ischemic stroke causing cognitive decline. The risk of ischemic stroke is four to five times greater in individuals with atrial fibrillation. Subclinical strokes contribute significantly to cognitive decline. AF is significantly associated with subclinical strokes, which has been shown to confer a two- to seven-fold increase in odds [8]. Chronic brain hypoperfusion is believed to be a second mechanism of cognitive decline in AF. Cardiac output can decrease as a result of beat-to-beat variability, leading to hypoperfusion and hypoxia of the brain. Animal models have shown that hypoperfusion of the brain reduces clearance of amyloid beta, which may lead to Alzheimer's dementia [7]. In a modeling analysis performed to assess the hemodynamic effect of AF on brain perfusion, the variance in R-R intervals as well as loss of atrioventricular synchrony led to a reduction in cerebral blood flow that led to repetitive hypoperfusions [46]. Lastly, systemic inflammation is increased in patients with AF, as evidenced by elevated markers such as C-reactive protein and tumor necrosis factor and may lead to cognitive impairment via cerebrovascular dysfunction [7]. Systemic inflammation may cause cerebral microinfarction with subsequent cognitive dysfunction via endothelial dysfunction, tissue factor release, and platelet activation [38]. Intensive lipid-lowering treatment with 40 mg atorvastatin and 10 mg ezetimibe, which has been shown to have anti-inflammatory properties, slows neurocognitive deterioration and cortical volume loss [47].

Table 1. Important studies in the association between atrial fibrillation and dementia.

Study First Author (Year)	Study Details	Outcomes
Bunch et al., [48]	Prospective database 3-year follow-up 16,848 with AF and 16,848 age/gender matched controls without AF.	0.9% of the AF patients and 0.5% of the no AF patients
Dublin et al., [49]	Prospective cohort study. A population-based sample of 3045 community-dwelling adults aged 65 and older without dementia or clinical stroke followed from 1994 to 2008. AF identified using codes	572 participants (18.8%) developed dementia (449 with Alzheimer's disease). The adjusted hazard ratio associated with AF was 1.38 (95% confidence interval (CI) = 1.10–1.73) for all-cause dementia and 1.50 (95% CI = 1.16–1.94) for possible or probable Alzheimer's disease).
De Bruijn et al. [50]	Prospective cohort study 6514 dementia-free participants in the prospective population-based Rotterdam Study 20 years of follow-up Clinical criteria	Incident AF was associated with an increased risk of dementia in younger participants (<67 years: 1.81; 1.11–2.94 vs. ≥67 years: 1.12; 0.85–1.46; $p = 0.02$ for interaction)
Ding et al. [51]	Prospective cohort study 2685 dementia-free participants from the Swedish National Study on Aging and Care who were regularly examined from 2001–2004 to 2010–2013. 9 years of follow-up Clinical criteria	AF was significantly associated with an increased risk of all-cause dementia (HR = 1.40, 95% CI: 1.11–1.77) and vascular and mixed dementia (HR = 1.88, 95% CI: 1.09–3.23)
Marzona et al. [41]	Post-hoc analysis of two randomized controlled trials, TRANSCEND and ONTARGET 31,506 participants 56 months follow up Clinical outcomes	AF was associated with an increased risk of incident dementia (HR 1.30, 95% CI 1.14–1.49)
Rusanen et al. [52]	2000 participants who were randomly selected from four separate, population-based samples originally studied in midlife 25 year follow up Clinical outcomes	AF in late-life was an independent risk factor for dementia (HR 2.61, 95% CI 1.05–6.47; $p = 0.039$) and AD (HR 2.54, 95% CI 1.04–6.16; $p = 0.040$)

6. Future Directions

Given the increased prevalence of AF, metabolic syndrome, and cognitive impairment, it is imperative that our understanding of the associations and interactions of these entities also increases. Prospective studies with well-defined and adjudicated predictors and outcomes are needed. This includes clear criteria for the subdivisions of dementia and prolonged screening for AF prior to the commencement of studies. New technology that allows continuous ambulatory monitoring of AF will significantly increase our ability to screen for AF. The Apple Heart Study, which enrolled 419,093 participants, disclosed the preliminary findings that 2161 participants (0.5%) received a pulse notification for AF. These patients were then invited to wear an electrocardiogram patch, and AF was identified in 34% of participants [53] Studies assessing the efficacy of a variety of treatment modalities for prevention and treatment of cognitive impairment in the context of AF will inform future clinical practice. Ongoing trials such as Blinded Randomized Trial of Anticoagulation to Prevent Ischemic Stroke and Neurocognitive Impairment in AF (BRAIN-AF) (NCT02387229) will assess whether anticoagulation is effective in patients without traditional risk factors for stroke. Ongoing improvement in imaging may allow further characterization of cerebral changes and explain mechanisms of the association between AF and dementia.

7. Conclusions

AF is associated with cognitive impairment and dementia via stroke-dependent and independent mechanisms. Metabolic comorbidities are independent predictors of AF and may be a cause of atrial cardiomyopathy, which would in turn contribute to AF as well as non-stroke-related mechanisms. Further studies are required to elucidate and identify predictors of this association. Such knowledge may inform future management of AF.

Author Contributions: *Concept and design*, A.A., M.M., V.R., and R.P.; *data procurement and literature review*, A.A., J.B.M., M.M., F.D., and G.V.; *drafting of manuscript*, A.A., J.B.M., and M.M.; *critical review of manuscript*: A.A., J.B.M., M.M., F.D., G.V., V.R., and R.P.

References

1. Miyasaka, Y.; Barnes, M.E.; Gersh, B.J.; Cha, S.S.; Bailey, K.R.; Abhayaratna, W.P.; Seward, J.B.; Tsang, T.S. Secular trends in incidence of atrial fibrillation in Olmsted County, Minnesota, 1980 to 2000, and implications on the projections for future prevalence. *Circulation* **2006**, *114*, 119–125. [CrossRef] [PubMed]
2. Homan, E.A.; Reyes, M.V.; Hickey, K.T.; Morrow, J.P. Clinical Overview of Obesity and Diabetes Mellitus as Risk Factors for Atrial Fibrillation and Sudden Cardiac Death. *Front. Physiol.* **2018**, *9*, 1847. [CrossRef] [PubMed]
3. Lin, Y.S.; Chen, T.H.; Chi, C.C.; Lin, M.S.; Tung, T.H.; Liu, C.H.; Chen, Y.L.; Chen, M.C. Different Implications of Heart Failure, Ischemic Stroke, and Mortality Between Nonvalvular Atrial Fibrillation and Atrial Flutter-a View from a National Cohort Study. *J. Am. Heart Assoc.* **2017**, *6*, e006406. [CrossRef] [PubMed]
4. Lip, G.Y.H.; Nieuwlaat, R.; Pisters, R.; Lane, D.A.; Crijns, H.J.G.M. Refining Clinical Risk Stratification for Predicting Stroke and Thromboembolism in Atrial Fibrillation Using a Novel Risk Factor-Based Approach: The Euro Heart Survey on Atrial Fibrillation. *Chest* **2010**, *137*, 263–272. [CrossRef] [PubMed]
5. Gami, A.S.; Hodge, D.O.; Herges, R.M.; Olson, E.J.; Nykodym, J.; Kara, T.; Somers, V.K. Obstructive Sleep Apnea, Obesity, and the Risk of Incident Atrial Fibrillation. *J. Am. Coll. Cardiol.* **2007**, *49*, 565–571. [CrossRef] [PubMed]
6. Santangeli, P.; Di Biase, L.; Bai, R.; Mohanty, S.; Pump, A.; Cereceda Brantes, M.; Horton, R.; Burkhardt, J.D.; Lakkireddy, D.; Reddy, Y.M.; et al. Atrial fibrillation and the risk of incident dementia: A meta-analysis. *Heart Rhythm.* **2012**, *9*, 1761–1768. [CrossRef] [PubMed]
7. Alonso, A.; Arenas de Larriva, A.P. Atrial Fibrillation, Cognitive Decline and Dementia. *Eur. Cardiol.* **2016**, *11*, 49–53. [CrossRef]

8. Dietzel, J.; Haeusler, K.G.; Endres, M. Does atrial fibrillation cause cognitive decline and dementia? *EP Eur.* **2017**, *20*, 408–419. [CrossRef]
9. Patel, N.J.; Deshmukh, A.; Pant, S.; Singh, V.; Patel, N.; Arora, S.; Shah, N.; Chothani, A.; Savani, G.T.; Mehta, K.; et al. Contemporary trends of hospitalization for atrial fibrillation in the United States, 2000 through 2010: Implications for healthcare planning. *Circulation* **2014**, *129*, 2371–2379. [CrossRef]
10. Choe, W.S.; Choi, E.K.; Han, K.D.; Lee, E.J.; Lee, S.R.; Cha, M.J.; Oh, S. Association of metabolic syndrome and chronic kidney disease with atrial fibrillation: A nationwide population-based study in Korea. *Diabetes Res. Clin. Pract.* **2019**, *148*, 14–22. [CrossRef]
11. Wang, T.J.; Parise, H.; Levy, D.; D'Agostino, R.B.; Wolf, P.A.; Vasan, R.S.; Benjamin, E.J. Obesity and the Risk of New-Onset Atrial Fibrillation. *JAMA* **2004**, *292*, 2471–2477. [CrossRef] [PubMed]
12. Asad, Z.; Abbas, M.; Javed, I.; Korantzopoulos, P.; Stavrakis, S. Obesity is associated with incident atrial fibrillation independent of gender: A meta-analysis. *J. Cardiovasc. Electrophysiol.* **2018**, *29*, 725–732. [CrossRef] [PubMed]
13. Wanahita, N.; Messerli, F.H.; Bangalore, S.; Gami, A.S.; Somers, V.K.; Steinberg, J.S. Atrial fibrillation and obesity—results of a meta-analysis. *Am. Heart J.* **2008**, *155*, 310–315. [CrossRef] [PubMed]
14. Frost, L.; Hune, L.J.; Vestergaard, P. Overweight and obesity as risk factors for atrial fibrillation or flutter: The Danish Diet, Cancer, and Health Study. *Am. J. Med.* **2005**, *118*, 489–495. [CrossRef]
15. Huxley, R.R.; Lopez, F.L.; Folsom, A.R.; Agarwal, S.K.; Loehr, L.R.; Soliman, E.Z.; Maclehose, R.; Konety, S.; Alonso, A. Absolute and attributable risks of atrial fibrillation in relation to optimal and borderline risk factors: The Atherosclerosis Risk in Communities (ARIC) study. *Circulation* **2011**, *123*, 1501–1508. [CrossRef]
16. Watanabe, H.; Tanabe, N.; Watanabe, T.; Darbar, D.; Roden, D.M.; Sasaki, S.; Aizawa, Y. Metabolic syndrome and risk of development of atrial fibrillation: The Niigata preventive medicine study. *Circulation* **2008**, *117*, 1255–1260. [CrossRef]
17. Umetani, K.; Kodama, Y.; Nakamura, T.; Mende, A.; Kitta, Y.; Kawabata, K.; Obata, J.E.; Takano, H.; Kugiyama, K. High prevalence of paroxysmal atrial fibrillation and/or atrial flutter in metabolic syndrome. *Circ. J.* **2007**, *71*, 252–255. [CrossRef]
18. Berg, A.H.; Scherer, P.E. Adipose Tissue, Inflammation, and Cardiovascular Disease. *Circ. Res.* **2005**, *96*, 939–949. [CrossRef]
19. Hocking, S.; Samocha-Bonet, D.; Milner, K.L.; Greenfield, J.R.; Chisholm, D.J. Adiposity and insulin resistance in humans: The role of the different tissue and cellular lipid depots. *Endocr. Rev.* **2013**, *34*, 463–500. [CrossRef]
20. Hajhosseiny, R.; Matthews, G.K.; Lip, G.Y. Metabolic syndrome, atrial fibrillation, and stroke: Tackling an emerging epidemic. *Heart Rhythm.* **2015**, *12*, 2332–2343. [CrossRef]
21. Grundy, S.M.; Cleeman, J.I.; Daniels, S.R.; Donato, K.A.; Eckel, R.H.; Franklin, B.A.; Gordon, D.J.; Krauss, R.M.; Savage, P.J.; Smith, S.C.; et al. Diagnosis and Management of the Metabolic Syndrome. *Circulation* **2005**, *112*, 2735–2752. [CrossRef] [PubMed]
22. Park, Y.-W.; Zhu, S.; Palaniappan, L.; Heshka, S.; Carnethon, M.R.; Heymsfield, S.B. The Metabolic Syndrome: Prevalence and Associated Risk Factor Findings in the US Population from the Third National Health and Nutrition Examination Survey, 1988–1994. *JAMA Intern. Med.* **2003**, *163*, 427–436. [CrossRef] [PubMed]
23. Bell, D.S.H.; Goncalves, E. Atrial fibrillation and type 2 diabetes: Prevalence, etiology, pathophysiology and effect of anti-diabetic therapies. *Diabetes Obes. Metab.* **2019**, *21*, 210–217. [CrossRef] [PubMed]
24. Goudis, C.A.; Korantzopoulos, P.; Ntalas, I.V.; Kallergis, E.M.; Ketikoglou, D.G. Obesity and atrial fibrillation: A comprehensive review of the pathophysiological mechanisms and links. *J. Cardiol.* **2015**, *66*, 361–369. [CrossRef]
25. Cho, M.E.; Craven, T.E.; Cheung, A.K.; Glasser, S.P.; Rahman, M.; Soliman, E.Z.; Stafford, R.S.; Johnson, K.C.; Bates, J.T.; Burgner, A.; et al. The association between insulin resistance and atrial fibrillation: A cross-sectional analysis from SPRINT (Systolic Blood Pressure Intervention Trial). *J. Clin. Hypertens. (Greenwich)* **2017**, *19*, 1152–1161. [CrossRef]
26. Al-Rawahi, M.; Proietti, R.; Thanassoulis, G. Pericardial fat and atrial fibrillation: Epidemiology, mechanisms and interventions. *Int. J. Cardiol.* **2015**, *195*, 98–103. [CrossRef]
27. Hohl, M.; Lau, D.H.; Muller, A.; Elliott, A.D.; Linz, B.; Mahajan, R.; Hendriks, J.M.L.; Bohm, M.; Schotten, U.; Sanders, P.; et al. Concomitant Obesity and Metabolic Syndrome Add to the Atrial Arrhythmogenic Phenotype in Male Hypertensive Rats. *J. Am. Heart Assoc.* **2017**, *6*, e006717. [CrossRef]

28. Abed, H.S.; Wittert, G.A.; Leong, D.P.; Shirazi, M.G.; Bahrami, B.; Middeldorp, M.E.; Lorimer, M.F.; Lau, D.H.; Antic, N.A.; Brooks, A.G.; et al. Effect of Weight Reduction and Cardiometabolic Risk Factor Management on Symptom Burden and Severity in Patients with Atrial Fibrillation: A Randomized Clinical Trial. *JAMA* **2013**, *310*, 2050–2060. [CrossRef]
29. Pathak, R.K.; Middeldorp, M.E.; Meredith, M.; Mehta, A.B.; Mahajan, R.; Wong, C.X.; Twomey, D.; Elliott, A.D.; Kalman, J.M.; Abhayaratna, W.P.; et al. Long-Term Effect of Goal-Directed Weight Management in an Atrial Fibrillation Cohort: A Long-Term Follow-Up Study (LEGACY). *J. Am. Coll. Cardiol.* **2015**, *65*, 2159–2169. [CrossRef]
30. Kalman, J.M.; Nalliah, C.J.; Sanders, P. Surgical Weight Loss and Atrial Fibrillation: A Convenient Paradigm to Evaluate a Complex Problem. *J. Am. Coll. Cardiol.* **2016**, *68*, 2505–2507. [CrossRef]
31. Jamaly, S.; Carlsson, L.; Peltonen, M.; Jacobson, P.; Sjöström, L.; Karason, K. Bariatric Surgery and the Risk of New-Onset Atrial Fibrillation in Swedish Obese Subjects. *J. Am. Coll. Cardiol.* **2016**, *68*, 2497–2504. [CrossRef] [PubMed]
32. Lynch, K.T.; Mehaffey, J.H.; Hawkins, R.B.; Hassinger, T.E.; Hallowell, P.T.; Kirby, J.L. Bariatric surgery reduces incidence of atrial fibrillation: A propensity score–matched analysis. *Surg. Obes. Relat. Dis.* **2019**, *15*, 279–285. [CrossRef] [PubMed]
33. Guichard, J.-B.; Nattel, S. Atrial Cardiomyopathy. *J. Am. Coll. Cardiol.* **2017**, *70*, 756. [CrossRef]
34. AlTurki, A.; Marafi, M.; Russo, V.; Proietti, R.; Essebag, V. Subclinical Atrial Fibrillation and Risk of Stroke: Past, Present and Future. *Medicina* **2019**, *55*, 611. [CrossRef] [PubMed]
35. Brambatti, M.; Connolly, S.J.; Gold, M.R.; Morillo, C.A.; Capucci, A.; Muto, C.; Lau, C.P.; Gelder, I.C.V.; Hohnloser, S.H.; Carlson, M.; et al. Temporal Relationship Between Subclinical Atrial Fibrillation and Embolic Events. *Circulation* **2014**, *129*, 2094–2099. [CrossRef] [PubMed]
36. Daoud, E.G.; Glotzer, T.V.; Wyse, D.G.; Ezekowitz, M.D.; Hilker, C.; Koehler, J.; Ziegler, P.D. Temporal relationship of atrial tachyarrhythmias, cerebrovascular events, and systemic emboli based on stored device data: A subgroup analysis of TRENDS. *Heart Rhythm.* **2011**, *8*, 1416–1423. [CrossRef]
37. Goette, A.; Kalman, J.M.; Aguinaga, L.; Akar, J.; Cabrera, J.A.; Chen, S.A.; Chugh, S.S.; Corradi, D.; D'Avila, A.; Dobrev, D.; et al. EHRA/HRS/APHRS/SOLAECE expert consensus on atrial cardiomyopathies: Definition, characterization, and clinical implication. *EP Eur.* **2016**, *18*, 1455–1490. [CrossRef]
38. Gallinoro, E.; D'Elia, S.; Prozzo, D.; Lioncino, M.; Natale, F.; Golino, P.; Cimmino, G. Cognitive Function and Atrial Fibrillation: From the Strength of Relationship to the Dark Side of Prevention. Is There a Contribution from Sinus Rhythm Restoration and Maintenance? *Medicina* **2019**, *55*, 587. [CrossRef]
39. Chen, L.Y.; Lopez, F.L.; Gottesman, R.F.; Huxley, R.R.; Agarwal, S.K.; Loehr, L.; Mosley, T.; Alonso, A. Atrial Fibrillation and Cognitive Decline-The Role of Subclinical Cerebral Infarcts. *Stroke* **2014**, *45*, 2568–2574. [CrossRef]
40. Ott, A.; Breteler, M.M.B.; Bruyne, M.C.d.; Harskamp, F.V.; Grobbee, D.E.; Hofman, A. Atrial Fibrillation and Dementia in a Population-Based Study. *Stroke* **1997**, *28*, 316–321. [CrossRef]
41. Marzona, I.; O'Donnell, M.; Teo, K.; Gao, P.; Anderson, C.; Bosch, J.; Yusuf, S. Increased risk of cognitive and functional decline in patients with atrial fibrillation: Results of the ONTARGET and TRANSCEND studies. *Can. Med. Assoc. J.* **2012**, *184*, E329–E336. [CrossRef] [PubMed]
42. Kim, D.; Yang, P.-S.; Yu, H.T.; Kim, T.-H.; Jang, E.; Sung, J.-H.; Pak, H.-N.; Lee, M.-Y.; Lee, M.-H.; Lip, G.Y.H.; et al. Risk of dementia in stroke-free patients diagnosed with atrial fibrillation: Data from a population-based cohort. *Eur. Heart J.* **2019**, *40*, 2313–2323. [CrossRef] [PubMed]
43. Thacker, E.L.; McKnight, B.; Psaty, B.M.; Longstreth, W.T.; Sitlani, C.M.; Dublin, S.; Arnold, A.M.; Fitzpatrick, A.L.; Gottesman, R.F.; Heckbert, S.R. Atrial fibrillation and cognitive decline. A longitudinal cohort study. *Neurology* **2013**, *81*, 119–125. [CrossRef] [PubMed]
44. Coma, M.; González-Moneo, M.J.; Enjuanes, C.; Velázquez, P.P.; Espargaró, D.B.; Pérez, B.A.; Tajes, M.; Garcia-Elias, A.; Farré, N.; Sánchez-Benavides, G.; et al. Effect of Permanent Atrial Fibrillation on Cognitive Function in Patients with Chronic Heart Failure. *Am. J. Car.* **2016**, *117*, 233–239. [CrossRef]
45. Golive, A.; May, H.T.; Bair, T.L.; Jacobs, V.; Crandall, B.G.; Cutler, M.J.; Day, J.D.; Mallender, C.; Osborn, J.S.; Weiss, J.P. The Impact of Gender on Atrial Fibrillation Incidence and Progression to Dementia. *Am. J. Car.* **2018**, *122*, 1489–1495. [CrossRef]

46. Anselmino, M.; Scarsoglio, S.; Saglietto, A.; Gaita, F.; Ridolfi, L. Transient cerebral hypoperfusion and hypertensive events during atrial fibrillation: A plausible mechanism for cognitive impairment. *Sci. Rep.* **2016**, *6*, 28635. [CrossRef]
47. Lappegård, K.T.; Pop-Purceleanu, M.; van Heerde, W.; Sexton, J.; Tendolkar, I.; Pop, G. Improved neurocognitive functions correlate with reduced inflammatory burden in atrial fibrillation patients treated with intensive cholesterol lowering therapy. *J. Neuroinflamm.* **2013**, *10*, 844. [CrossRef]
48. Bunch, T.J.; Crandall, B.G.; Weiss, J.P.; May, H.T.; Bair, T.L.; Osborn, J.S.; Anderson, J.L.; Muhlestein, J.B.; Horne, B.D.; Lappe, D.L.; et al. Patients treated with catheter ablation for atrial fibrillation have long-term rates of death, stroke, and dementia similar to patients without atrial fibrillation. *J. Cardiovasc. Electrophysiol.* **2011**, *22*, 839–845. [CrossRef]
49. Dublin, S.; Anderson, M.L.; Haneuse, S.J.; Heckbert, S.R.; Crane, P.K.; Breitner, J.C.; McCormick, W.; Bowen, J.D.; Teri, L.; McCurry, S.M.; et al. Atrial fibrillation and risk of dementia: a prospective cohort study. *J. Am. Geriatr. Soc.* **2011**, *59*, 1369–1375. [CrossRef]
50. de Bruijn, R.F.; Heeringa, J.; Wolters, F.J.; Franco, O.H.; Stricker, B.H.; Hofman, A.; Koudstaal, P.J.; Ikram, M.A. Association Between Atrial Fibrillation and Dementia in the General Population. *JAMA Neurol.* **2015**, *72*, 1288–1294. [CrossRef]
51. Ding, M.; Fratiglioni, L.; Johnell, K.; Santoni, G.; Fastbom, J.; Ljungman, P.; Marengoni, A.; Qiu, C. Atrial fibrillation, antithrombotic treatment, and cognitive aging. A population-based study. *Neurology* **2018**, *91*, e1732–e1740. [CrossRef] [PubMed]
52. Rusanen, M.; Kivipelto, M.; Levälahti, E.; Laatikainen, T.; Tuomilehto, J.; Soininen, H.; Ngandu, T. Heart diseases and long-term risk of dementia and Alzheimer's disease: a population-based CAIDE study. *J. Alzheimers Dis.* **2014**, *42*, 183–191. [CrossRef] [PubMed]
53. Turakhia, M.P.; Desai, M.; Hedlin, H.; Rajmane, A.; Talati, N.; Ferris, T.; Desai, S.; Nag, D.; Patel, M.; Kowey, P. Rationale and design of a large-scale, app-based study to identify cardiac arrhythmias using a smartwatch: The Apple Heart Study. *Am. Heart J.* **2019**, *207*, 66–75. [CrossRef] [PubMed]

11

Detrimental Impact of Chronic Obstructive Pulmonary Disease in Atrial Fibrillation: New Insights from Umbria Atrial Fibrillation Registry

Fabio Angeli [1,*], Gianpaolo Reboldi [2], Monica Trapasso [2], Adolfo Aita [3], Giuseppe Ambrosio [1] and Paolo Verdecchia [3]

1 Division of Cardiology and Cardiovascular Pathophysiology, Hospital S. Maria della Misericordia, 06156 Perugia, Italy
2 Department of Medicine, University of Perugia, 06156 Perugia, Italy
3 Fondazione Umbra Cuore e Ipertensione-ONLUS and Division of Cardiology, Hospital S. Maria Della Misericordia, 06156 Perugia, Italy
* Correspondence: angeli.internet@gmail.com

Abstract: *Background and objectives:* Chronic obstructive pulmonary disease (COPD) is a leading cause of morbidity and mortality worldwide. Among extra-pulmonary manifestations of COPD, atrial fibrillation (AF) is commonly observed in clinical practice. The coexistence of COPD and AF significantly affects the risk of cardiovascular morbidity and mortality. Nonetheless, the mechanisms explaining the increased risk of vascular events and death associated to the presence of COPD in AF are complex and not completely understood. We analyzed data from an Italian network database to identify markers and mediators of increased vascular risk among subjects with AF and COPD. *Materials and Methods:* Cross-sectional analysis of the Umbria Atrial Fibrillation (Umbria-FA) Registry, a multicenter, observational, prospective on-going registry of patients with non-valvular AF. Of the 2205 patients actually recruited, 2159 had complete clinical data and were included in the analysis. *Results:* the proportion of patients with COPD was 15.6%. COPD patients had a larger proportion of permanent AF when compared to the control group (49.1% vs. 34.6%, $p < 0.0001$) and were more likely to be obese and current smokers. Other cardiovascular risk factors including chronic kidney disease (CKD), peripheral artery disease and subclinical atherosclerosis were more prevalent in COPD patients (all $p < 0.0001$). COPD was also significantly associated with higher prevalence of previous vascular events and a history of anemia (all $p < 0.0001$). The thromboembolic and bleeding risk, as reflected by the CHA_2DS_2VASc and HAS-BLED scores, were higher in patients with COPD. Patients with COPD were also more likely to have left ventricular (LV) hypertrophy at standard ECG than individuals forming the cohort without COPD ($p = 0.018$). *Conclusions:* AF patients with COPD have a higher risk of vascular complications than AF patients without this lung disease. Our analysis identified markers and mediators of increased risk that can be easily measured in clinical practice, including LV hypertrophy, CKD, anemia, and atherosclerosis of large arteries.

Keywords: chronic obstructive pulmonary disease; atrial fibrillation; cardiovascular risk; outcome; prognosis

---

1. Introduction

Chronic obstructive pulmonary disease (COPD) is a major global public health problem, being a leading cause of morbidity and mortality worldwide [1,2]. It is currently rated the fourth most common cause of death and predicted to be the third in the next ten years [2].

Among extra-pulmonary manifestations of COPD, atrial fibrillation (AF) is commonly observed in clinical practice [3,4]. An accumulating body of evidence suggests that COPD is independently associated with this type of arrhythmia [5] and the presence of COPD in AF patients significantly affects outcomes and risk of all-cause mortality [6–10]. In the modern era of anticoagulation therapy, some post-hoc analyses of clinical trials demonstrated that COPD is strongly associated with cardiovascular and non-cardiovascular mortality in AF: data from the Apixaban for Reduction in Stroke and Other Thromboembolic Events in Atrial Fibrillation (ARISTOTLE) trial [9] demonstrated that, after multivariable adjustment for confounders, COPD was associated with a higher risk of all-cause mortality (adjusted hazard ratio [HR]: 1.60, 95% confidence interval [CI]: 1.36 to 1.88, $p < 0.001$) and both cardiovascular and non-cardiovascular mortality. Similarly, the Rivaroxaban Once Daily Oral Direct Factor Xa Inhibition Compared with Vitamin K Antagonism for Prevention of Stroke and Embolism Trial in Atrial Fibrillation (ROCKET AF) [10] showed that COPD was independently associated with higher mortality, suggesting that optimal prevention and treatment of COPD may improve survival.

Nonetheless, the pathophysiological mechanisms underlying the increased risk of vascular events and death associated to the presence of COPD in AF are complex and not completely understood [7]. There is also a paucity of information on risk factors and mediators of vascular events in patients with COPD and AF in most studies [5].

To this purpose, we performed a cross-sectional analysis on a large cohort of AF patients to investigate the interplays between these two conditions. Specifically, we used the unique features of our Italian network database (see methods) to further elucidate and identify markers and mediators of increased vascular risk among subjects with AF and COPD.

2. Materials and Methods

2.1. Population

We performed a cross-sectional analysis of the Umbria Atrial Fibrillation (Umbria-FA) Registry approved by CEAS-Umbria on date 20 September 2012—Number 1976/12, a multicenter, observational, prospective on-going registry of patients with non-valvular AF (see Appendix A).

Details of this Registry have been reported elsewhere [11]. Enrollment is being performed in 22 Hospitals or out-patient facilities in the setting of the Italian Health System, beginning in January 2013. All patients sign a written informed consent and the study is conducted in accordance with the EU Note for Guidance on Good Clinical Practice CPMP/ECH/135/95 and the Declaration of Helsinki. Each participating centre (see Appendix A) obtained the approval by the Ethics Committees at regional-local levels.

For enrollment, patients must be affected by AF at entry into the Registry or, in case of paroxysmal or persistent AF currently in sinus rhythm, by evidence of AF within one year before entry (standard ECG, ECG-Holter monitoring, or pacemaker diagnostics are also accepted for diagnosis of AF) [11].

Our Italian Network database on AF has the potential to evaluate in detail the key features of AF patients and major gaps in the Guidelines [12,13] implementation in clinical practice, when compared to other registries. Indeed, the initial evaluation of Umbria-FA Registry include a detailed clinical examination, 12-lead electrocardiogram (ECG), laboratory tests and, when feasible, an echocardiographic study.

Based on characteristics of AF episodes, five types of AF are distinguished: first diagnosed, paroxysmal, persistent, long-standing persistent, and permanent AF [12,13]. Standard 12-lead ECG is recorded during brief end-expiratory apnea and left ventricular (LV) hypertrophy at ECG is diagnosed using the BMI-corrected Perugia criterion [14].

The presence of COPD was defined according to documented medical history, as collected by physicians at study site-level. This assessment was performed by any physician during the clinical interview with the patient and by searching through medical records [1]. As for other risk factors, Investigators were asked to follow international guidelines to define COPD [1].

2.2. Statistical Analysis

We used STATA 14 (StataCorp, College Station, TX, USA) and R software version 3 (R Foundation for Statistical Computing, Vienna, Austria). Data are presented as mean ± standard deviation (SD) for continuous variables and proportions for categorical variables. Differences in proportions between groups were analyzed using the χ^2 test. Mean values of variables were compared by independent sample t-test. In 2-tailed tests, p values < 0.05 were considered statistically significant.

3. Results

Of the 2205 patients recruited on 31 October 2018 in the Umbria-AF Registry, 2159 had complete clinical data (Figure 1) and were included in the final analysis. The proportion of patients with COPD was 15.6% with a mean age equal to 79.2 ± 8.4 (median: 77). Figure 1 also summarizes the types of AF in the two groups: as depicted, COPD patients had a larger proportion of permanent AF (49.1% vs. 34.6%, $p < 0.0001$). The main characteristics of recruited patients (including risk factors, comorbid conditions and previous vascular events in the two groups) are shown in Table 1.

Patients with COPD were more likely to be obese and current smokers. While hypertension showed a similar prevalence among the two groups, other cardiovascular risk factors (including diabetes and chronic kidney disease (CKD)) were more prevalent in COPD patients (all $p < 0.0001$). Prevalence of patients with established peripheral artery disease (PAD) was 13.9% in the COPD group and 4.7% in the control group ($p < 0.0001$). Subclinical atherosclerosis of large arteries was present in 15% of patients with COPD and 8% in the control group ($p < 0.0001$).

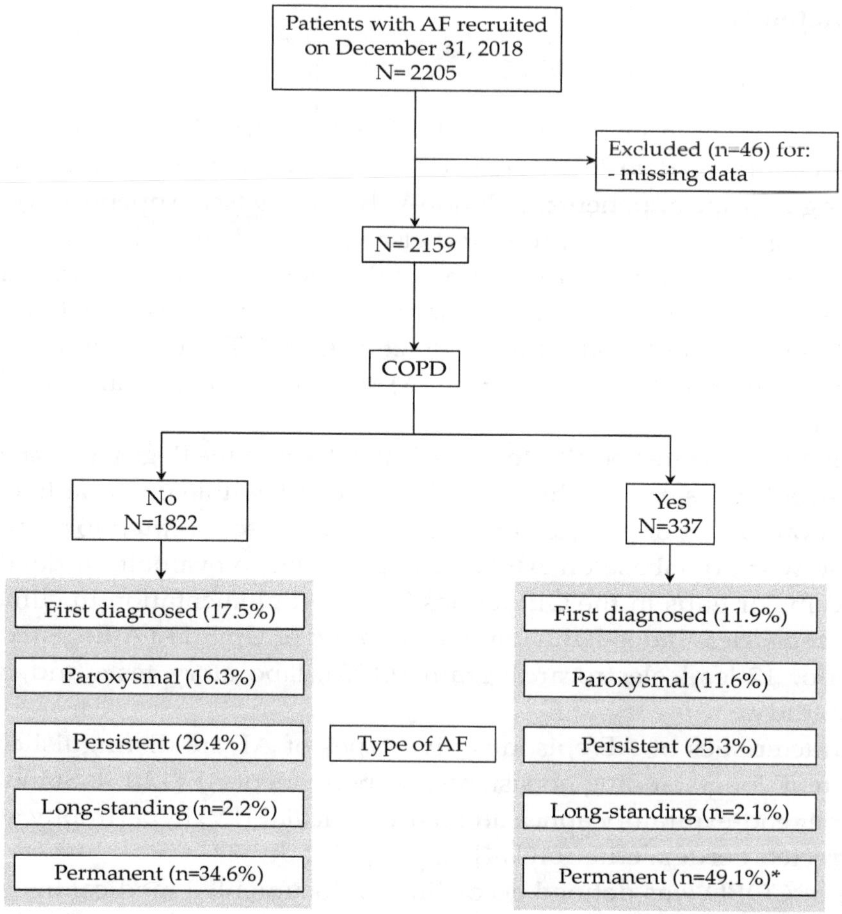

Figure 1. Flow chart of patients through the study. Types of atrial fibrillation are also depicted. * $p < 0.0001$ vs. patients without chronic obstructive pulmonary disease (COPD).

Table 1. Baseline characteristics of patients included in the analysis.

Variable	Overall (n = 2159)	COPD No (1822)	COPD Yes (n = 3 37)	p
Age (years)	75.6 ± 11.2	74.9 ± 11.5	79.2 ± 8.4	<0.0001
Sex (female, %)	44.5	46.3	34.7	0.0001
BMI (Kg/m^2)	26.8 ± 13.7	26.5 ± 11.9	28.5 ± 20.9	0.0153
Systolic BP (mmHg)	130 ± 18	131 ± 18	127 ± 16	0.0016
Diastolic BP (mmHg)	77 ± 11	77 ± 11	75 ± 11	0.0008
Pulse pressure (mmHg)	53 ± 15	53 ± 15	52 ± 15	0.1960
Heart rate (b.p.m.)	78 ± 22	77 ± 21	82 ± 23	0.0037
Risk factors and comorbid conditions				
Current smoker (%)	6.7	5.8	11.6	<0.0001
Hypertension (%)	80.9	81.2	79.8	0.561
Diabetes (%)	19.7	18.4	26.7	<0.0001
Chronic kidney disease (%) *	29.6	28.1	38.0	<0.0001
Peripheral artery disease (%)	6.1	4.7	13.9	<0.0001
Previous vascular events				
Coronary artery disease (%)	17.8	16.6	24.6	<0.0001
Acute coronary syndrome (%)	14.2	13.5	17.8	0.037
Heart failure (%)	21.1	17.4	40.9	<0.0001
Stroke/Transient ischemic attack (%)	18.1	17.3	22.3	0.029
Pulmonary embolism (%)	1.5	1.5	1.2	0.625

Legend: BMI = body mass index; BP = blood pressure; * eGFR < 60 mL/min/1.73m^2.

Similar results were obtained for history of previous vascular events: COPD was significantly associated with a higher prevalence of acute coronary syndrome, stroke/transient ischemic attack, and heart failure (HF, all $p < 0.05$). Of note, COPD patients showed an impressive 2.5-fold increase in the frequency of prior HF requiring hospitalization when compared to AF patients without COPD (40.9% vs. 17.4%, $p < 0.0001$). Such different distributions of HF among the two groups translated in lower BP values measured in COPD patients due to LV systolic dysfunction. Indeed, after exclusion of patients with HF from both groups (COPD and non-COPD), none of blood pressure (BP) components showed statistically significant differences between the groups (all $p \geq 0.05$).

Routine laboratory data are reported in Table 2. As expected, COPD patients had a lower estimated glomerular filtration rate (eGFR, computed using the CKD-EPI formulas [15]) compared to patients without COPD. Distributions of eGFR classes in the two groups are depicted in Figure 2.

Table 2. Laboratory data of patients included in the analysis.

Variable	Overall (n = 2159)	COPD No (1822)	COPD Yes (n = 337)	p
Haemoglobin (g/dL)	13.4 ± 4.3	13.5 ± 4.6	12.9 ± 2.0	0.0179
Total cholesterol (mg/dL)	170 ± 43	172 ± 43	162 ± 42	0.0013
LDL cholesterol (mg/dL)	100 ± 35	101 ± 35	93 ± 33	0.0024
Serum glucose (mg/dL)	109 ± 34	108 ± 32	115 ± 43	0.0023
Creatinine (mg/dL)	1.08 ± 0.61	1.06 ± 0.58	1.20 ± 0.76	0.0003
BUN (mg/dL)	52 ± 27	50 ± 26	60 ± 34	<0.0001
eGFR (mL/min/1.73m^2)	67 ± 22	68 ± 22	62 ± 23	0.0001
Uric acid (mg/dL)	6.7 ± 5.3	6.7 ± 5.7	6.8 ± 2.8	0.7657

Legend: LDL=low density lipoprotein; BUN=blood urea nitrogen; eGFR=glomerular filtration rate estimated by Cockcroft-Gault equation.

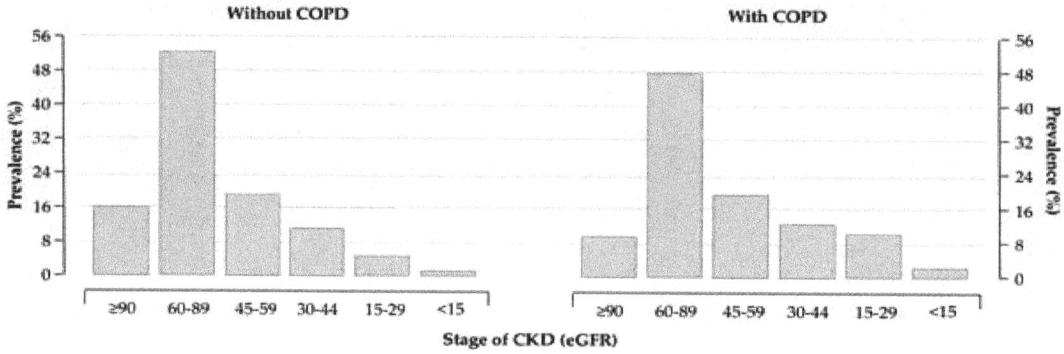

Figure 2. Distribution of chronic kidney disease (CKD) stages in patients without (left panel) and with (right panel) COPD; 28% and 38% of patients without and with COPD had an estimated glomerular filtration rate (eGFR) < 60 mL/min/1.73 m^2, respectively ($p < 0.0001$).

Of note, COPD influenced the history of previous anemia (24% for COPD patients vs. 14% for patients without COPD, $p < 0.0001$) with mean values of hemoglobin of 12.9 g/dL and 13.5 g/dL for patients with and without COPD at the baseline examination (Table 2), respectively.

The thromboembolic and bleeding risk, as reflected by the CHA_2DS_2VASc [16] (4.3 ± 0.09 vs. 3.6 ± 0.04, $p < 0.0001$) and HAS-BLED [17] (1.9 ± 0.06 vs. 1.5 ± 0.02, $p < 0.0001$) scores, were higher in patients with COPD. About 96% of patients with COPD had the recommendation to be treated with oral anticoagulants according to current Guidelines [12,13] (Figure 3).

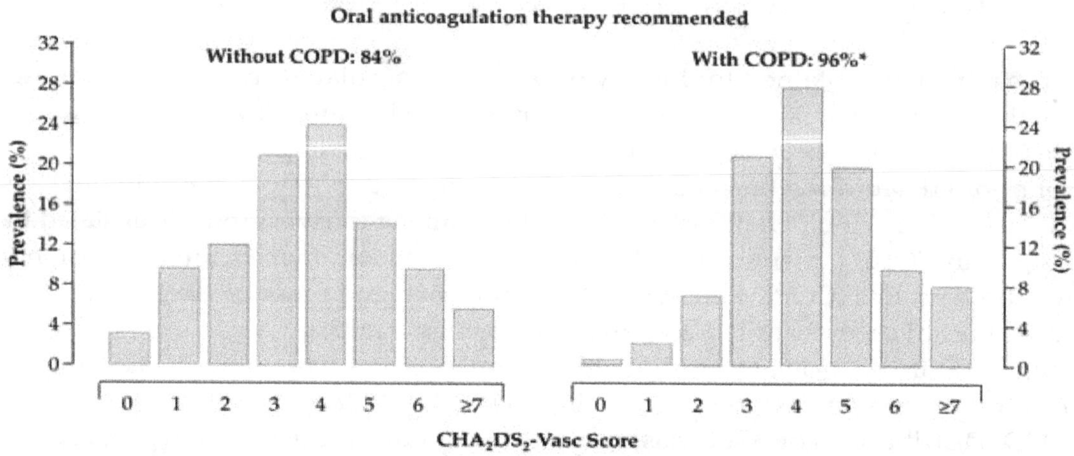

Figure 3. Distribution of CHA_2DS_2VASc score in patients without (left panel) and with (right panel) COPD; 84% and 96% of patients without and with COPD had the recommendation to be treated with oral anticoagulants, respectively; * $p < 0.05$ vs. patients without COPD.

Among ECG characteristics, 71% of patients with COPD had AF at entry-ECG with a mean heart rate equal to 82 ± 23 b.p.m. In the control group of patients without COPD, 57% showed AF at baseline with a mean heart rate of 77 ± 21 b.p.m. ($p = 0.0037$ vs. patients with COPD). Interestingly, patients with COPD were more likely to have LV hypertrophy at standard ECG than individuals forming the cohort without COPD (45% vs. 38%, $p = 0.018$).

4. Discussion

COPD is a major cause of morbidity and mortality and its prevalence is steadily rising resulting in a significant economic and social burden [2]. Although COPD is a predominantly respiratory disease, it has been recently recognized as a systemic disease with significant clinical extra-pulmonary effects and manifestations, leading to a worsening cardiovascular prognosis [7].

A recent study conducted in 7441 patients (mean age 64, 49% women, 92% Caucasian) demonstrated that COPD is an independent predictor of AF onset and progression [3,18]. More specifically, the increased likelihood of AF associated to the presence of COPD remained significant ($p < 0.0001$) after adjusting for several confounders including age, gender, tobacco use, obesity, hypertension, coronary artery disease, HF, diabetes, anemia, cancer, CKD, and rate/rhythm control medications [3].

A wide variety of mechanisms for arrhythmias in COPD seems to exists. In particular, experimental models showed that COPD-related inflammatory responses and hypoxia are implicated in AF development and perpetuation as well [19–21]. Furthermore, the coexistence of AF and COPD is a stronger predictor of vascular events than AF only or COPD only [5,7–10]. Huang et al. reported that the presence of COPD in patients with AF is an independent risk factor for one-year all-cause and cardiovascular mortality [22]; similarly, in the EURObservational Research Programme-Atrial Fibrillation General Registry Pilot Phase (EORP-AF Pilot), COPD was highly prevalent in European AF patients, and was associated with higher rates of cardiovascular death, all-cause death, and the composite outcome of any thromboembolic event/bleeding/cardiovascular death [23]. Furthermore, The Atrial Fibrillation in the Emergency Room (AFTER) Study, derived and validated a complex and a simplified model for the prediction of mortality in the emergency department patients with AF. Of note, both the models that included COPD as a risk variable have been shown to predict mortality after an emergency visit for AF [24].

Nonetheless, the relationships between these two disorders and how they simultaneously act in increasing the risk of vascular events are not completely understood. Taking advantage of the unique features of Umbria-AF registry [11], we tried to elucidate in a large cohort of AF patients the potential mechanisms explaining the increased vascular risk related to COPD. Results of our cross-sectional analysis highlighted the notion that AF patients with COPD have a higher risk of cardio- and cerebro-vascular complications than AF patients without this lung disease. Moreover, our analysis identified potential markers and mediators of high vascular risk that can be easily measured in clinical practice. They include LV hypertrophy, reduced renal function, anemia, and atherosclerosis of large arteries. As summarized below, all these conditions play a central part in the prediction and development of vascular complications (Figure 4).

LV hypertrophy is a powerful and independent predictor of all-cause mortality and major cardiac and cerebrovascular events [25,26]. Experimental evidence is accumulating that several factors. which promote progression of atherosclerosis through plaque growth and destabilization can also induce LV hypertrophy by acting on myocyte and interstitium [25,27]. LV hypertrophy may also be a causative factor for myocardial ischemia and reduced pumping performance and arrhythmias [25,28]. In other words, LV hypertrophy is a marker of cardiovascular risk because it reflects and integrates the long-term level of activity of factors inducing progression of atherosclerosis.

In this context, it is worth mentioning that atherosclerosis of large arteries, as reflected by a wide pulse pressure is significantly related to the risk of major cardiovascular events [29–31] and a progressive stiffening of large elastic arteries have been observed in early stages of renal dysfunction [32]. Various studies showed a strong association between the markers of CKD (typically the reduced eGFR) and cardiovascular morbidity and mortality [33–35]; more specifically, eGFR is indirectly related to the elevated probability of death and cardiovascular disease [33–35]. A recent meta-analysis of clinical studies including 7 million participants reported an increased risk of vascular events and all-cause mortality by 20–30% with a 30% decrease in eGFR [34]. It also suggested that around 20% of vascular events among those over 70 years is attributable to renal dysfunction [34]. Importantly, the complex association of CKD with cardiovascular disease is due to clustering of several cardiovascular risk factors, including "traditional risk factors" (i.e., advanced age, hypertension, diabetes mellitus, and dyslipidemia) and "nontraditional risk factors" that are specific to CKD (i.e., volume overload and anemia). Of note, the presence of anemia may lead to adverse cardiovascular consequences. In the Atherosclerosis Risk in Communities study (ARIC), anemia was associated with cardiovascular outcomes [36], and a significant interaction between anemia and the presence of CKD was documented [37,38]. From a pathophysiological point of view, chronic anemia may increase preload, reduce afterload, and lead to increased cardiac output. In the long term, this may also exacerbate cardiac ischemia as a result of decreased supply or increased demand for oxygen, such as in patients with underlying coronary disease or those with LV hypertrophy, respectively [39].

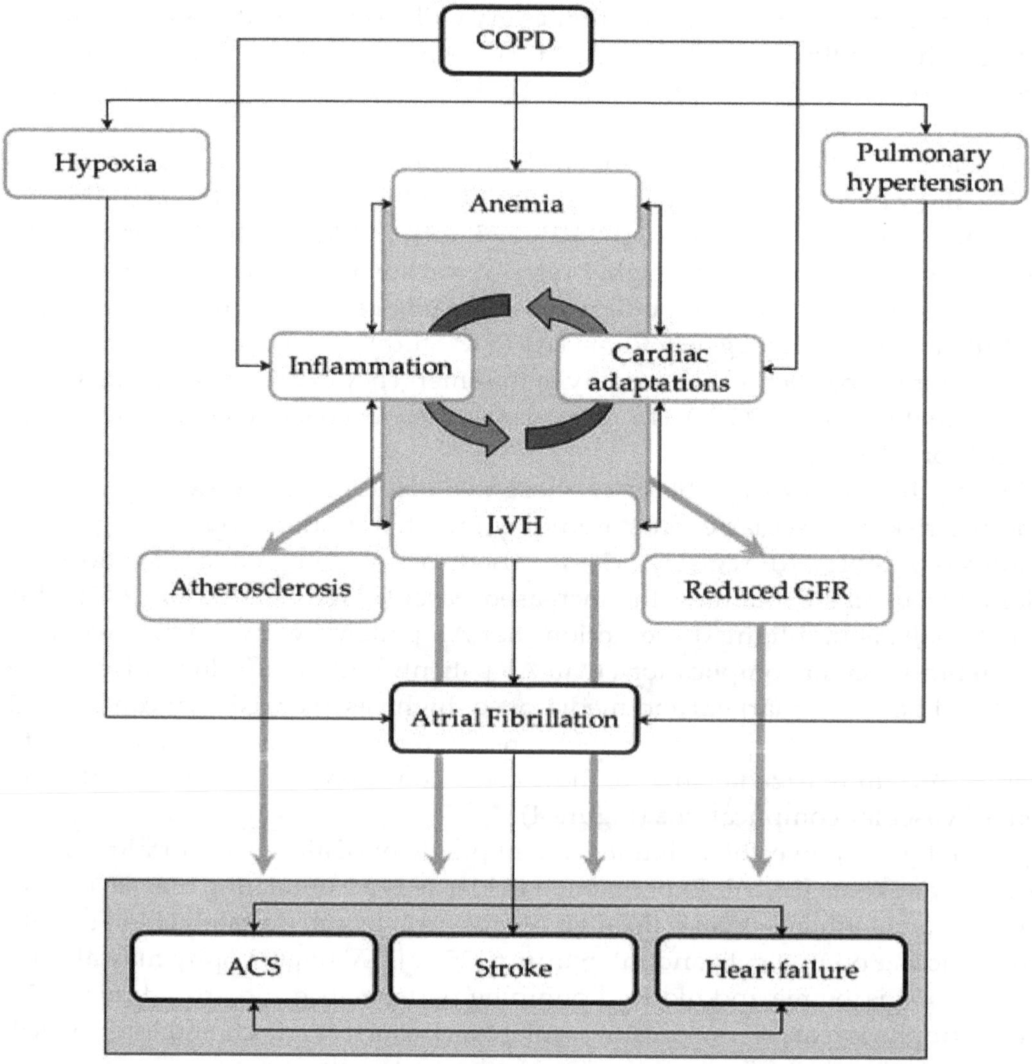

Figure 4. Graphical representation of the potential interplays between atrial fibrillation (AF) and COPD. LVH = left ventricular hypertrophy; ACS = acute coronary syndrome; GFR = glomerular filtration rate.

Taken together, these observations suggest that implications of our results are obvious but clinically relevant at the same time. The elucidation of underlying mechanisms affecting the risk of adverse outcome of AF patients with COPD offers the possibility for better therapeutic options and surveillance strategies. Treatment of AF patients with concomitant COPD should not be the same as those without COPD and physicians need to increase monitoring and early intervention for COPD patients to treat AF.

Our cross-sectional analysis has some limitations. Since white subjects were 99%, caution is needed in extrapolating results to different ethnic groups. Presence or absence of COPD was acknowledged into the electronic case report form reporting the presence/absence of the condition, but with no further details on its severity and lung function testing parameters. The absence of any further details about clinical and severity of COPD is a major limitation. Finally, markers of inflammation are not routinely collected in our Registry. Thus, we are unable to explore the relationships between a pro-inflammatory state and COPD.

5. Conclusions

COPD is one of the leading causes of mortality and morbidity worldwide. COPD is an independent risk factor for AF. The coexistence of COPD and AF significantly affects the risk of mortality and vascular events. Thus, it is important to understand the relationship between these two disorders and appropriately manage both these co-morbidities for improved outcomes.

Our cross-sectional analysis produced several findings. First, we highlighted the point that the estimated risk of cardiovascular complications is markedly higher in AF patients with COPD than in those without COPD. Second, we identified markers and mediators of high vascular risk that can be easily measured in clinical practice. Finally, our analysis suggests that specific surveillance strategies and early intervention for COPD patients with AF should be urgently implemented.

Author Contributions: Conceptualization, F.A., G.R., M.T. and P.V.; Data curation, F.A., G.R., M.T., A.A. and P.V.; Formal analysis, F.A., G.R., M.T. and P.V.; Funding acquisition, P.V.; Investigation, F.A., G.R., M.T., A.A., G.A. and P.V.; Methodology, F.A., G.R., M.T. and P.V.; Project administration, F.A., G.R. and P.V.; Supervision, F.A., G.R. and P.V.; Writing—Original draft, F.A., G.R., M.T. and P.V.; Writing—Review & Editing, F.A., G.R., M.T. and P.V.

Appendix A

Umbria-Atrial fibrillation study group (www.umbriafa.it)

Steering Committee: Giancarlo Agnelli; Giuseppe Ambrosio; Fabio Angeli; Claudio Cavallini; Adriano Murrone; Gianpaolo Reboldi; Paolo Verdecchia (Chairperson); Gianluca Zingarini.

No-profit Sponsor: Fondazione Umbra Cuore e Ipertensione—ONLUS.

Scientific Secretary: Fabio Angeli.

Participating Investigators: Hospital of Ancona and University of Ancona, Department of Cardiology (A. Capucci, F. Guerra, G. Ciliberti); Hospital of Ascoli Piceno, Department of Cardiology (L. Moretti, P. Marchese, F. Gennaro, G. Mazzotta); Hospital of Fabriano, Department of Cardiology (S. Coiro, M. Politano, P. Scipione); Hospital of Amelia, Department of Cardiology (M.L. Suadoni, S. Bergonzini); Hospital of Narni, Department of Medicine (P. Rinaldi); Hospital of Assisi, Department of Medicine (P. Verdecchia, G. Molini, A. Aita); Hospital of Branca, Department of Medicine (S. Radicchia, O. Cazzato); Hospital of Branca, Department of Cardiology (E. Capponi, D. Cosmi, G. Mazzotta); Hospital of Branca, Department of Neurology (D. Giannandrea); Hospital of Città di Castello, Department of Neurology (S. Ricci, M.R. Condurso, L. Greco); Hospital of Città di Castello, Department of Cardiology (A. Murrone, A. Contine, L. Marinacci, K. Mboumi); Hospital of Castiglione del Lago (C. Dembech, N. Sacchi, M. Guerrieri, M. Martinelli); Hospital of Perugia and University of Perugia, Medicina Interna e Vascolare (G. Agnelli, M.G. De Natale, C. Becattini, M.C. Vedovati); Hospital of Perugia and University of Perugia, Cardiologia e Fisiopatologia Cardiovascolare (F. Angeli, F. Scavelli, M. Reccia, G. Giuffrè); Hospital of Perugia and University of Perugia, Medicina Interna (M. Pirro, V. Bianconi, A. Labate); Hospital of Perugia, Struttura Complessa di Cardiologia (C. Cavallini, G.L. Zingarini, F. Notaristefano, C. Riccini); Hospital of Perugia, Struttura Complessa di Pronto Soccorso (P. Groff, V. Mommi); Hospital of Foligno, Struttura Complessa di Cardiologia (G. Bagliani, C. Andreoli, C. Mangialasche); Hospital of Orvieto, Struttura Complessa di Cardiologia (R. Di Cristofaro); USL Umbria 1, Cardiologia Ambulatoriale 1 (M.G. Pinzagli); USL Umbria 2, Cardiologia Ambulatoriale 2 (L. Filippucci, A. Faleburle); USL Umbria 2, Cardiologia Ambulatoriale (S. Repaci), USL Umbria 2, Cardiologia Ambulatoriale (G. Proietti); Hospital Media Valle del Tevere, Struttura Complessa di Medicina (U. Paliani, C. Fuoco, M.G. Conti, A. Cardona, C. Bartolini); Hospital of Terni, Struttura Complessa di Cardiologia (G. Carreras, E. Boschetti, C. Poltronieri, A. Crocetti, G. Tilocca, G. Khoury); Hospital of Terni, Medicina Interna (G. Vaudo, G. Pucci, L. Sanesi, R. Sgariglia, S. Alessio, A. Cerasari, I. Dominioni).

References

1. Vogelmeier, C.F.; Criner, G.J.; Martinez, F.J.; Anzueto, A.; Barnes, P.J.; Bourbeau, J.; Celli, B.R.; Chen, R.; Decramer, M.; Fabbri, L.M.; et al. Global strategy for the diagnosis, management, and prevention of chronic obstructive lung disease 2017 report: GOLD executive summary. *Eur. Respir. J.* **2017**, *49*. [CrossRef]
2. Adeloye, D.; Chua, S.; Lee, C.; Basquill, C.; Papana, A.; Theodoratou, E.; Nair, H.; Gasevic, D.; Sridhar, D.; Campbell, H.; et al. Global health epidemiology reference, global and regional estimates of COPD prevalence: Systematic review and meta-analysis. *J. Glob. Health.* **2015**, *5*, 020415. [CrossRef] [PubMed]
3. Konecny, T.; Park, J.Y.; Somers, K.R.; Konecny, D.; Orban, M.; Soucek, F.; Parker, K.O.; Scanlon, P.D.; Asirvatham, S.J.; Brady, P.A.; et al. Relation of chronic obstructive pulmonary disease to atrial and ventricular arrhythmias. *Am. J. Cardiol.* **2014**, *114*, 272–277. [CrossRef] [PubMed]
4. Li, J.; Agarwal, S.K.; Alonso, A.; Blecker, S.; Chamberlain, A.M.; London, S.J.; Loehr, L.R.; McNeill, A.M.; Poole, C.; Soliman, E.Z.; et al. Airflow obstruction, lung function, and incidence of atrial fibrillation: The atherosclerosis risk in communities (ARIC) study. *Circulation* **2014**, *129*, 971–980. [CrossRef] [PubMed]
5. Chen, X.; Wang, W. The progression in atrial fibrillation patients with COPD: A systematic review and meta-analysis. *Oncotarget* **2017**, *8*. [CrossRef] [PubMed]
6. Chen, C.Y.; Liao, K.M. The impact of atrial fibrillation in patients with COPD during hospitalization. *Int. J. Chron. Obstruct. Pulmon. Dis.* **2018**, *13*, 2105–2112. [CrossRef] [PubMed]
7. Goudis, C.A. Chronic obstructive pulmonary disease and atrial fibrillation: An unknown relationship. *J. Cardiol.* **2017**, *69*, 699–705. [CrossRef]
8. Chen, L.Y.; Sotoodehnia, N.; Buzkova, P.; Lopez, F.L.; Yee, L.M.; Heckbert, S.R.; Prineas, R.; Soliman, E.Z.; Adabag, S.; Konety, S.; et al. Atrial fibrillation and the risk of sudden cardiac death: The atherosclerosis risk in communities study and cardiovascular health study. *JAMA Intern. Med.* **2013**, *173*, 29–35. [CrossRef]
9. Durheim, M.T.; Cyr, D.D.; Lopes, R.D.; Thomas, L.E.; Tsuang, W.M.; Gersh, B.J.; Held, C.; Wallentin, L.; Granger, C.B.; Palmer, S.M.; et al. Chronic obstructive pulmonary disease in patients with atrial fibrillation: Insights from the ARISTOTLE trial. *Int. J. Cardiol.* **2016**, *202*, 589–594. [CrossRef]
10. Pokorney, S.D.; Piccini, J.P.; Stevens, S.R.; Patel, M.R.; Pieper, K.S.; Halperin, J.L.; Breithardt, G.; Singer, D.E.; Hankey, G.J.; Hacke, W.; et al. Committee, investigators, and R.A.S.C. investigators, Cause of death and predictors of all-cause mortality in anticoagulated patients with nonvalvular atrial fibrillation: Data from ROCKET AF. *J. Am. Heart Assoc.* **2016**, *5*, e002197. [CrossRef]
11. Angeli, F.; Verdecchia, P.; Cavallini, C.; Aita, A.; Turturiello, D.; Mazzotta, G.; Trapasso, M.; de Fano, M.; Reboldi, G. Electrocardiography for diagnosis of left ventricular hypertrophy in hypertensive patients with atrial fibrillation. *Int. J. Cardiol. Hypertens.* **2019**. [CrossRef]
12. Steffel, J.; Verhamme, P.; Potpara, T.S.; Albaladejo, P.; Antz, M.; Desteghe, L.; Haeusler, K.G.; Oldgren, J.; Reinecke, H.; Roldan-Schilling, V.; et al. The 2018 European Heart Rhythm Association practical guide on the use of non-vitamin K antagonist oral anticoagulants in patients with atrial fibrillation. *Eur. Heart J.* **2018**, *39*, 1330–1393. [CrossRef] [PubMed]
13. Kirchhof, P.; Benussi, S.; Kotecha, D.; Ahlsson, A.; Atar, D.; Casadei, B.; Castella, M.; Diener, H.C.; Heidbuchel, H.; Hendriks, J.; et al. 2016 ESC Guidelines for the management of atrial fibrillation developed in collaboration with EACTS. *Eur. Heart J.* **2016**, *37*, 2893–2962. [CrossRef] [PubMed]
14. Angeli, F.; Verdecchia, P.; Iacobellis, G.; Reboldi, G. Usefulness of QRS voltage correction by body mass index to improve electrocardiographic detection of left ventricular hypertrophy in patients with systemic hypertension. *Am. J. Cardiol.* **2014**, *114*, 427–432. [CrossRef] [PubMed]
15. Levey, A.S.; Stevens, L.A.; Schmid, C.H.; Zhang, Y.L.; Castro, A.F., 3rd; Feldman, H.I.; Kusek, J.W.; Eggers, P.; van Lente, F.; Greene, T.; et al. A new equation to estimate glomerular filtration rate. *Ann. Intern. Med.* **2009**, *150*, 604–612. [CrossRef] [PubMed]
16. Lip, G.Y.; Nieuwlaat, R.; Pisters, R.; Lane, D.A.; Crijns, H.J. Refining clinical risk stratification for predicting stroke and thromboembolism in atrial fibrillation using a novel risk factor-based approach: the euro heart survey on atrial fibrillation. *Chest* **2010**, *137*, 263–272. [CrossRef]
17. Pisters, R.; Lane, D.A.; Nieuwlaat, R.; de Vos, C.B.; Crijns, H.J.; Lip, G.Y. A novel user-friendly score (HAS-BLED) to assess 1-year risk of major bleeding in patients with atrial fibrillation: The Euro heart survey. *Chest* **2010**, *138*, 1093–1100. [CrossRef] [PubMed]

18. Bhatt, S.P.; Dransfield, M.T. Chronic obstructive pulmonary disease and cardiovascular disease. *Transl. Res.* **2013**, *162*, 237–251. [CrossRef]
19. Harada, M.; van Wagoner, D.R.; Nattel, S. Role of inflammation in atrial fibrillation pathophysiology and management. *Circ. J.* **2015**, *79*, 495–502. [CrossRef]
20. Lammers, W.J.; Kirchhof, C.; Bonke, F.I.; Allessie, M.A. Vulnerability of rabbit atrium to reentry by hypoxia. Role of inhomogeneity in conduction and wavelength. *Am. J. Physiol.* **1992**, *262*, H47–H55. [CrossRef]
21. Angeli, F.; Reboldi, G.; Verdecchia, P. Hypertension, inflammation and atrial fibrillation. *J. Hypertens.* **2014**, *32*, 480–483. [CrossRef] [PubMed]
22. Huang, B.; Yang, Y.; Zhu, J.; Liang, Y.; Zhang, H.; Tian, L.; Shao, X.; Wang, J. Clinical characteristics and prognostic significance of chronic obstructive pulmonary disease in patients with atrial fibrillation: results from a multicenter atrial fibrillation registry study. *J. Am. Med. Dir. Assoc.* **2014**, *15*, 576–581. [CrossRef] [PubMed]
23. Proietti, M.; Laroche, C.; Drozd, M.; Vijgen, J.; Cozma, D.C.; Drozdz, J.; Maggioni, A.P.; Boriani, G.; Lip, G.Y.; EORP-AF Investigators. Impact of chronic obstructive pulmonary disease on prognosis in atrial fibrillation: A report from the EUR observational research programme pilot survey on atrial fibrillation (EORP-AF) general registry. *Am. Heart J.* **2016**, *181*, 83–91. [CrossRef] [PubMed]
24. Atzema, C.L.; Dorian, P.; Fang, J.; Tu, J.V.; Lee, D.S.; Chong, A.S.; Austin, P.C. A Clinical decision instrument for 30-day death after an emergency department visit for atrial fibrillation: The atrial fibrillation in the emergency room (AFTER) study. *Ann. Emerg. Med.* **2015**, *66*, 658–668. [CrossRef] [PubMed]
25. Angeli, F.; Reboldi, G.; Poltronieri, C.; Stefanetti, E.; Bartolini, C.; Verdecchia, P.; Investigators, M. The prognostic legacy of left ventricular hypertrophy: cumulative evidence after the MAVI study. *J. Hypertens.* **2015**, *33*, 2322–2330. [CrossRef] [PubMed]
26. Hijazi, Z.; Verdecchia, P.; Oldgren, J.; Andersson, U.; Reboldi, G.; di Pasquale, G.; Mazzotta, G.; Angeli, F.; Eikelboom, J.W.; Ezekowitz, D.M.; et al. Cardiac biomarkers and Left ventricular hypertrophy in relation to outcomes in patients with atrial fibrillation: experiences from the RE—LY Trial. *J. Am. Heart Assoc.* **2019**, *8*, e010107. [CrossRef]
27. Angeli, F.; Reboldi, G.; Verdecchia, P. Microcirculation and left-ventricular hypertrophy. *J. Hypertens.* **2012**, *30*, 477–481. [CrossRef]
28. Angeli, F.; Verdecchia, P.; Trapasso, M.; Reboldi, G. Left ventricular hypertrophy and coronary artery calcifications: a dangerous duet? *Am. J. Hypertens.* **2018**, *31*, 287–289. [CrossRef]
29. Angeli, F.; Angeli, E.; Ambrosio, G.; Mazzotta, G.; Cavallini, C.; Reboldi, G.; Verdecchia, P. Neutrophil count and ambulatory pulse pressure as predictors of cardiovascular adverse events in postmenopausal women with hypertension. *Am. J. Hypertens.* **2011**, *24*, 591–598. [CrossRef]
30. Angeli, F.; Reboldi, G.; Verdecchia, P. More than a reason to use arterial stiffness as risk marker and therapeutic target in hypertension. *Hypertens. Res.* **2011**, *34*, 445–457. [CrossRef]
31. Angeli, F.; Reboldi, G.; Verdecchia, P. Heart failure, pulse pressure and heart rate: Refining risk stratification. *Int. J. Cardiol.* **2018**, *271*, 206–208. [CrossRef] [PubMed]
32. Olechnowicz-Tietz, S.; Gluba, A.; Paradowska, A.; Banach, M.; Rysz, J. The risk of atherosclerosis in patients with chronic kidney disease. *Int. Urol. Nephrol.* **2013**, *45*, 1605–1612. [CrossRef] [PubMed]
33. Hillege, H.L.; van Gilst, W.H.; van Veldhuisen, D.J.; Navis, G.; Grobbee, D.E.; de Graeff, P.A.; de Zeeuw, D.; Trial, C.R. Accelerated decline and prognostic impact of renal function after myocardial infarction and the benefits of ACE inhibition: the CATS randomized trial. *Eur. Heart J.* **2003**, *24*, 412–420. [CrossRef]
34. Mafham, M.; Emberson, J.; Landray, M.J.; Wen, C.P.; Baigent, C. Estimated glomerular filtration rate and the risk of major vascular events and all-cause mortality: a meta-analysis. *PLoS ONE* **2011**, *6*, e25920. [CrossRef] [PubMed]
35. Van der Velde, M.; Matsushita, K.; Coresh, J.; Astor, B.C.; Woodward, M.; Levey, A.; de Jong, P.; Gansevoort, R.T.; Chronic, C.; van der Velde, M.; et al. Lower estimated glomerular filtration rate and higher albuminuria are associated with all-cause and cardiovascular mortality. A collaborative meta-analysis of high-risk population cohorts. *Kidney Int.* **2011**, *79*, 1341–1352. [CrossRef] [PubMed]
36. Sarnak, M.J.; Tighiouart, H.; Manjunath, G.; MacLeod, B.; Griffith, J.; Salem, D.; Levey, A.S. Anemia as a risk factor for cardiovascular disease in The atherosclerosis risk in communities (ARIC) study. *J. Am. Coll. Cardiol.* **2002**, *40*, 27–33. [CrossRef]

37. Abramson, J.L.; Jurkovitz, C.T.; Vaccarino, V.; Weintraub, W.S.; McClellan, W. Chronic kidney disease, anemia, and incident stroke in a middle-aged, community-based population: the ARIC Study. *Kidney Int.* **2003**, *64*, 610–615. [CrossRef]
38. Jurkovitz, C.T.; Abramson, J.L.; Vaccarino, L.V.; Weintraub, W.S.; McClellan, W.M. Association of high serum creatinine and anemia increases the risk of coronary events: results from the prospective community-based atherosclerosis risk in communities (ARIC) study. *J. Am. Soc. Nephrol.* **2003**, *14*, 2919–2925. [CrossRef]
39. Anand, I.S.; Chandrashekhar, Y.; Ferrari, R.; Poole-Wilson, P.A.; Harris, P.C. Pathogenesis of oedema in chronic severe anaemia: studies of body water and sodium, renal function, haemodynamic variables, and plasma hormones. *Br. Heart J.* **1993**, *70*, 357–362. [CrossRef]

12

Atrial Fibrillation and Stroke: A Review on the Use of Vitamin K Antagonists and Novel Oral Anticoagulants

Alfredo Caturano, Raffaele Galiero and Pia Clara Pafundi *

Department of Advanced Medical and Surgical Sciences, University of Campania "Luigi Vanvitelli", Piazza Luigi Miraglia 2, IT-80138 Naples, Italy; alfredo.caturano@virgilio.it (A.C.); raffaele_ga@outlook.it (R.G.)

* Correspondence: piaclara.pafundi@unicampania.it

Abstract: Atrial fibrillation (AF) is the most common arrhythmia, ranging from 0.1% in patients <55 years to >9% in octogenarian patients. One important issue is represented by the 5-fold increased ischemic stroke risk in AF patients. Hence, the role of anticoagulation is central. Until a few years ago, vitamin K antagonists (VKAs) and low molecular weight heparin represented the only option to prevent thromboembolisms, though with risks. Novel oral anticoagulants (NOACs) have radically changed the management of AF patients, improving both life expectancy and life quality. This review aims to summarize the most recent literature on the use of VKAs and NOACs in AF, in light of the new findings.

Keywords: NOACs; non vitamin K oral anticoagulants; atrial fibrillation; stroke; oral anticoagulation

1. Introduction

Atrial fibrillation (AF) is the most common arrhythmia, ranging from 0.1% in patients aged <55 years to >9% in octogenarian patients. One of the most important issues is represented by the 5-fold increased risk of ischemic stroke in AF patients [1].

Atria are excited in a chaotic, disorganized manner, with a frequency of activation variable from 400 to 650 beats/min. The atrioventricular node (AVN) receives much more impulses from the atrium than it is able to conduct, thus exercising a filter function which transmits a not excessively high number of beats to the ventricles. In fact, numerous impulses penetrate only partially into the AVN and then they are trapped inside.

The patient is often symptomatic at onset. The most common symptom is palpitation, but, in the case of the concomitant presence of an organic heart disease, the loss of effective atrial systole, as well as tachycardia, favor a hemodynamic decompensation. Less frequently, AF runs asymptomatic.

The diagnostic suspicion may already arise at the evaluation of the radial pulse and/or the cardiac auscultation, and then confirmed by an electrocardiogram (ECG) characterized by the absence of regular and morphologically similar atrial activation waves, with a totally irregular interval of the QRS complexes of ventricular activation.

AF treatment has 4 main approaches:

1. Heart rate control with either beta blockers (Bisoprolol, Metoprolol), non-dihydropyridine calcium antagonists (Verapamil, Diltiazem), digoxin (less used due to the possible risk of toxicity, especially in patients with renal insufficiency) or, as a last resort, Amiodarone;
2. Either electrical or pharmacological cardioversion with class antiarrhythmics III (Amiodarone, Ibutilide) or I-C (Flecainide, propafenone, in the absence of cardiac structural damage);

3. AF deletion through catheter ablation, either by acting on its trigger points or by altering the arrhythmogenic substrate. In either case, the risk of relapse still persists, especially during the first 6–12 months after the procedure;
4. The control of thrombo-embolic complications by using anticoagulants (novel oral anticoagulants (NOACs), vitamin K antagonists (VKAs), heparin).

A more in-depth analysis of the latter point, in fact, shows that the reduction of blood flow in the atrial chambers, caused by the reduced ventricular depletion (consequent to the reduction of diastolic time and the loss of atrial contraction, as well as, sometimes, the reduction of myocardial contractility secondary to tachycardia) makes more likely the formation of thrombi in the left atrium (LA), including the left atrial appendage (LAA).

The occurrence of this condition significantly increases when arrhythmia lasts for over 48 h, with an embolic thrombus risk increased even more significantly at the reestablishment of the sinus rhythm. A risk stratification in these patients may be estimated by using the CHA2DS2-VASc score, for which a score is assigned to each risk factor, finally providing a sum which represents the overall risk of stroke per year for the patients (Table 1).

Table 1. Risk stratification of stroke by the CHA2DS2-VASc score [2].

Risk Factors	Score	CHA2DS2-VASc Score	Stroke Risk Per Year
Congestive Heart Failure	1	0	0%
LV Dysfunction	1	1	1.3%
Hypertension	1	2	2.2%
Age ≥ 75 years	2	3	3.2%
Diabetes Mellitus	1	4	4.0%
Stroke/TIA/Thromboembolism	2	5	6.7%
Vascular Disease	1	6	9.8%
Age 65–74	1	7	9.6%
Female	1	8	6.7%
Total	9	9	15.2%

LV: Left Ventricle, TIA: Transient Ischemic Attack.

2. Atrial Fibrillation (FA) Cardioversion and Anticoagulation

Current ESC guidelines for patients with AF, for less than 48 h, with a CHA2DS2-VASc score of either 0 in men or 1 in women, recommend the administration of heparin, a factor Xa inhibitor or a direct thrombin inhibitor, versus no anticoagulant therapy, without the need for post-cardioversion oral anticoagulation. Conversely, an AF for 48 h or more, needs an appropriate anticoagulation for at least 3 weeks or a negative transesophageal echocardiogram (TEE), followed by 4 weeks anticoagulation after cardioversion. In the case of a rescue cardioversion due to hemodynamic instability, anticoagulation should be initiated as soon as possible and continued for at least 4 weeks after cardioversion, unless contraindicated [2].

A recent meta-analysis comparing warfarin and novel oral anticoagulants (NOACs) on 7588 AF patients undergoing electric cardioversion (CV) showed overlapping risks of ischemic stroke, major bleeding, mortality and hemorrhagic stroke [3]. In this subset of patients, several real-world studies have confirmed a favorable clinical outcome [4–8].

Though an appropriate therapy, the risk of systemic embolism in elective cardioversion is still present. In fact, a transesophageal echocardiogram may highlight the presence of a thrombus in LA or LAA in 5% of patients, despite adequate anticoagulation with both vitamin K antagonists (VKAs) or NOACs [9]. Data from real-world studies have highlighted a similar incidence of LA thrombus before performing CV, both among the use of different NOACs and in the case of VKA treatment [10,11]. Additionally, the importance of practicing TEE in patients at high risk of LA/LAA thrombus (e.g., CHA2DS2-VASc score >3) has been pointed out [12].

The average stroke rate <1% makes it reasonable to assume a lower prevalence of thromboembolism during cardioversion or, maybe, that not every stroke is clinically diagnosed. Moreover, it is not surprising that patients with a very high-risk score for thromboembolism could be refractory to standard anticoagulation [12].

The use of NOACs compared to VKAs treatment has shown, both in trials and in real-world settings, a reduction in the timing to CV, with a consequent higher satisfaction of patients and cost savings for clinical facilities [13–15].

In patients in whom sinus rhythm has been restored, the same drugs used for cardioversion may be used to prevent arrhythmia relapses. Among these drugs, amiodarone has been shown to be the most effective antiarrhythmic, though not without long term side effects [16].

3. Oral Anticoagulation with Vitamin K Antagonists

VKAs were the first anticoagulants used in AF patients. Their discovery was completely random and dates back to the 1920s, when in the U.S., sweet clover was used to feed livestock, which was stored in silos. The fermentation of the clover produced bis-hydroxycoumarin. The anticoagulant effect of this by-product determined the consistent death of herds of cattle on farms in Wisconsin, due to hemorrhagic syndromes. The fear that warfarin could be excessively toxic to humans initially led to only being used as rat poison. The drug with the trade name of Coumadin was approved only in 1954, though the skepticism of the medical community remained until 1955, when President Eisenhower, struck by coronary artery disease (CAD), requested to be treated with the most powerful "antithrombotic" drug of the time.

VKAs (warfarin and acenocoumarol) are indirect anticoagulants, which interfere with the hepatic production of dependent vitamin K coagulation factors. The lag time between drug intake and pharmacological action varies between 3 and 7 days, the time required for activated coagulation factors to be deleted and/or exhausted. On the other hand, prothrombin time (PT) can be lengthened in a short time due to the inhibition of short-life coagulation factors, such as factor VII.

The dosage of oral anticoagulants, due to the individual variability of their pharmacokinetics and pharmacodynamics, should be established based on the determination of the International Normalized Ratio (INR), given by the ratio between the PT of each patient and the PT of a healthy subject. In the case of AF, INR must be maintained between 2 and 3 [2].

Vitamin K represents the antidote of dicoumarols in the case of major bleeding, but it can also be found in several vegetables (e.g., tomatoes, spinach, cabbages, turnip greens), as well as in some dairy and animal products. Therefore, a reduction of the intake of these foods is strongly recommended to improve the time in therapeutic range (TTR).

The use of VKAs is limited by the narrow therapeutic interval, which needs frequent monitoring, dose adjustments and attention to drugs interaction (e.g., nonsteroidal anti-inflammatory drugs (NSAIDs) may lead to hemorrhage due to pharmacokinetic interactions and to their antiplatelet effect) [2].

VKAs efficacy and safety have been established over time and all over the world by several studies [17,18], and currently represent the first-choice treatment in AF patients with rheumatic mitral valve disease and/or a mechanical heart valve prosthesis [19]. Conversely, the use of NOACs in AF patients undergoing valves replacement and transcatheter aortic valve replacement (TAVR) is only supported by few and limited data [1,20].

In a meta-analysis, patients under VKAs therapy showed a relative risk reduction of ischemic stroke of 67%, with no significant difference between primary and secondary prevention, and 25% of all-cause mortality rate compared to controls (either aspirin or placebo). Also, the risk of intracranial hemorrhage was mild [21].

The fact that antiplatelet agents may play a preventive role during AF has been investigated by several studies. For example, Lip et al. [22], in a meta-analysis, demonstrated a 22% relative reduction in the risk of thromboembolism in AF with AP monotherapy compared to placebo. In addition, the authors also showed a 36% risk reduction with warfarin compared to aspirin. Several studies have compared warfarin to AP monotherapy and dual AP therapy (aspirin + clopidogrel), with a lower effectiveness of AP therapy and either a similar or increased risk of bleeding [23–25].

Thus, the most recent ESC guidelines have discouraged a routine use of AP monotherapy for stroke prevention in AF patients [26].

The Garfield AF registry shows how the administration of AP monotherapy in newly diagnosed AF has slowed down over the years, though a consistent number of patients are still under treatment (about 20% of the 51,270 patients analyzed are under AP monotherapy with no indication) [27].

Furthermore, AF patients cannot be treated with indirect anticoagulants if they are pregnant or breastfeeding, if they have bleeding diathesis or in the case of invasive surgical procedures. In addition, in fragile and/or cardiac and/or hepatic insufficient patients, closer INR controls are required.

4. Novel Oral Anticoagulants (NOACs): A Future Already Present

Until a few years ago, as shown in the previous sections, anticoagulant therapy with VKAs represented, along with the use of low molecular weight heparin (LMWH), the only therapeutic aid to reduce thromboembolic risk [28].

NOACs selectively inhibit only one factor of the coagulation cascade: thrombin, in the case of dabigatran, or activated factor X (Xa), in the case of rivaroxaban, apixaban and edoxaban.

Their pharmacodynamics are predictable, with little variability even at the individual level and there are no relevant interactions with both food and drugs. The half-life is well defined, but its increase with age and with the reduction of the renal filtrate should always be considered.

Their action is fast and their effect quickly ends after interruption and, in either case, can be predicted based on a few easily calculable variables (mainly the time from the last dose taken, type of molecule, age and the glomerular filtrate).

These characteristics make the monitoring of the coagulative structure superfluous (and confounding). In this way, the induction of the anticoagulant effect is eased without having to resort to the administration of heparin [28,29]. Moreover, both the safety and efficacy of NOACs have been positively tested in a randomized clinical trial [30] and confirmed by several clinical real-world casuistries [1,31–35].

For this reason, in recent years, NOACs have become a valid alternative to VKAs to prevent stroke in AF patients and have emerged as the first choice, especially in patients who are new to anticoagulants.

It is of fundamental importance to remember how some specific subpopulations of AF patients cannot be treated with NOACs. Among these are the wearers of cardiac mechanical prostheses, patients with severe mitral stenosis on a rheumatic basis and patients with aneurysms [22]. However, subjects with biological valve prostheses, subjected to mitral valvuloplasty three months after implantation, and those with hypertrophic cardiomyopathy have been granted by the 2018 EHRA PRACTICAL GUIDE update and 2016 ESC guidelines, the possibility of using NOACs [22,36].

Four large phase III trials assessed the non-inferiority of NOACs compared to VKAs. The overall assessment of the findings from the four trials allowed for establishing how NOACs are able to, with respect to conventional VKAs therapy, further reduce the combined risk of stroke and embolic events by 19% and the risk of all-cause mortality.

The prescription of the most appropriate NOAC must be based on the knowledge of the clinical characteristics of each patient and of the pharmacological characteristics of the different NOACs.

The recommended dosages for the treatment of AF patients are listed in Figure 1. To understand the profile of each NOAC, it is necessary to know the findings from the most important clinical trials which led to their registration.

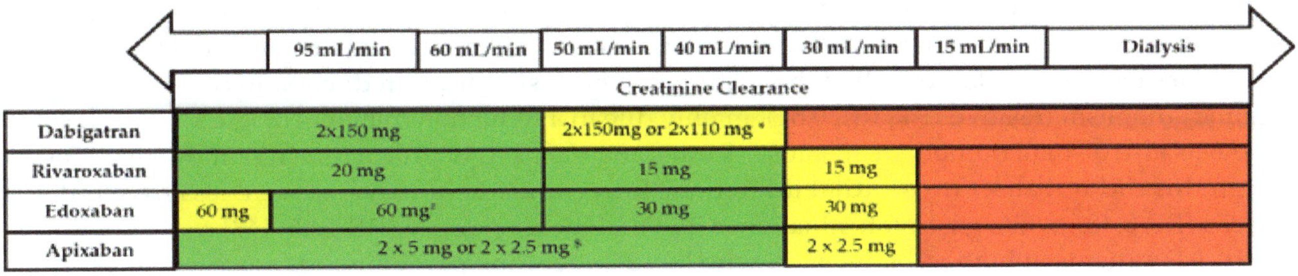

Figure 1. Use of non-vitamin K antagonists (VKAs) according to renal function. * 2 × 110 mg in patients at high risk of bleeding (per SmPc). # Other dose reduction criteria may apply (weight ≤60 kg, concomitant potent P-Gp inhibitor therapy). $ 2 × 2.5 mg only if at least two out of three fulfilled: age ≥80 years, body weight ≤60 kg, creatinine ≥1.5 mg/dL (133 mmol/L). Orange arrows indicate cautionary use (dabigatran in moderate renal insufficiency, FXa inhibitors in severe renal insufficiency, edoxaban in 'supranormal' renal function). [36].

The randomized open-label RE-LY clinical trial assessed the non-inferiority of dabigatran 150 mg bid (reduced to a 110 mg bid in elderly patients and in those with reduced renal function) compared to warfarin (INR 2 to 3) in AF patients. The study showed a statistically significant reduction in systemic stroke/embolism, hemorrhagic stroke and vascular mortality. The major bleeding rates were, instead, comparable. In addition, a significant reduction in the total number of bleedings, life-threatening bleeding for the patient and intracranial bleeding, as well as a statistically significant increase in gastrointestinal major bleeding with dabigatran 150 mg were observed [37].

In the ROCKET-AF double-blind randomized clinical trial, rivaroxaban was shown to be not inferior to Warfarin in the prevention of either stroke or systemic embolism, without significant difference between the two groups for overall mortality or differences between two drugs in the risk of major bleeding or major bleeding plus the clinically relevant ones. Even in the ROCKET-AF, however, a statistically significant increase in gastrointestinal major bleeding was observed [38].

Two trials, ARISTOTLE and AVERROES, instead assessed the efficacy and safety of apixaban 5 mg bid (reduced to 2.5 mg bid in elderly patients and in those with reduced renal function). Apixaban emerged statistically superior to Warfarin in the prevention of stroke and systemic embolisms, major bleeding, including intracranial ones, and no major clinically relevant ones, as well as in reducing all-cause mortality. Comparable outcomes emerged for major gastrointestinal bleeding [39,40].

Finally, edoxaban. The ENGAGE AF-TIMI 48 trial demonstrated the non-inferiority of edoxaban 60 mg vs. warfarin in preventing stroke or systemic embolic events, with a statistically significant reduction in hemorrhagic stroke, vascular mortality, major bleeding and the number of intracranial bleedings and a statistically significant increase in major gastrointestinal bleedings [41].

The meta-analysis of Dentali et al. states that all NOACs directly act on the final phase of the coagulation cascade, and therefore, differ from the VKAs mechanism of action [42].

In the prevention of stroke during AF, NOACs overall, compared to VKAs, significantly reduce (1) stroke and systemic embolism, (2) major bleeding, (3) intracranial bleeding, (4) cardiovascular and (5) global mortality.

Despite the several advantages of NOACs with respect to VKAs therapy, a careful decision-making process is required in each case to ensure the safety of the choice of one option over another.

As more findings emerge from clinical studies and real-world evidence, the use of NOACs is becoming increasingly varied, replacing VKAs therapy in many contexts as a safe, reliable and effective therapeutic approach [9,12,16–18,21,43]. However, VKAs still play an important role in countless contexts, including situations where NOACs are contraindicated [36].

At present, the difference between each NOAC depends on the preferences of the physician (evaluating the risk profile of each patient compared to that present in the groups treated in each study), the pros and cons of each molecule, and the costs. An indirect comparison between the four drugs can lead to the suggestion of which one would be preferred for each individual patient. A recent meta-analysis, including all of the four major clinical trials, showed that NOACs reduce ischemic events compared to warfarin in patients with AF, but at the cost of increased gastrointestinal bleeding [44]. The comprehensive results from all of these studies show a significant reduction in cases of stroke and systemic embolism (relative risk, RR, 0.81), mainly due to a reduction in hemorrhagic strokes (RR 0.49). There was also a small number of all-cause deaths, compared to warfarin, during follow-up (RR 0.90), though this did not affect myocardial infarction. Intracranial hemorrhages were less frequent with NOACs (RR 0.48), while gastrointestinal ones had a higher incidence (RR 1.25) [43].

In AF patients at high ischemic risk, who have undergone percutaneous coronary intervention (PCI) with stenting for acute coronary syndrome (ACS), dabigatran etexilate 110 mg twice daily versus VKAs, in association with DAPT (aspirin plus clopidogrel) showed a safer profile and a lower cumulative incidence of major bleeding, as well as a lower hospitalization rate for cardiovascular events in real-world settings [45,46].

5. Bridging Therapy

Perioperative management of AF patients receiving NOACs is an extremely sensitive issue. The strategy not to initiate the so-called "bridge therapy" is comparable to "bridge therapy" in terms of prevention of thromboembolic events, though it translates into a greater reduction in the risk of major bleeding. This requires a more in-depth consideration of the advantages of both pharmacokinetic and pharmacodynamic aspects of the different anticoagulation regimens in each individual patient [36].

Therefore, the management of patients who need to interrupt oral anticoagulant therapy (OAT) to undergo either surgery or invasive procedures is particularly complex and requires collaboration among the different medical figures. The American College of Cardiology Anticoagulation Work Group, in order to assess the current clinical practice, devised a specific survey. Several professionals, including cardiologists (in different sub-specialties), internists, gastroenterologists and orthopedists, were asked how to manage patients taking oral anticoagulant therapy (OAT), candidates for invasive procedures and surgical procedures [47].

With the advent of NOACs in most recent years, the decision-making process has become even more complicated, since guidelines on this issue only provide general recommendations. The BRIDGE study, published in the New England Journal of Medicine, attempted to address this issue. The study found that the no bridging strategy was inferior to the low molecular weight heparin bridging therapy for the prevention of thromboembolic events, while at the same time, it determined a reduction in the risk of major bleedings [48].

In particular, the BRIDGE study assessed how the different professional figures managed, in the common clinical practice, patients taking OAT as candidates for invasive procedures. From the findings of the study, the most frequently involved professional class was that of cardiologists. The study also showed that among the most commonly used parameters to identify patients with an increased risk of thromboembolic events during OAT interruption is the presence of a mechanical heart valve, a history of previous stroke or transient ischemic attack (TIA) and an elevated CHA2DS2-VASc score. With regard to this latter finding, it was emphasized that, frequently, this score is used in clinical practice to refer patients to the use of bridge therapy, though this approach has never been validated in this field. Despite many patients at low risk of thromboembolic events, that are referred to invasive procedures, being considered as low risk for bleeding without OAT interruption, the study showed that several doctors still prefer bridge therapy, exposing patients to a high risk of bleeding. Moreover, the variability in the choice of both dose and duration of parenteral anticoagulant therapy was also confirmed.

The study also underlined the problem of the management of patients on anticoagulant therapy with NOACs. A similar use of bridging therapy was observed for patients who were candidates for either surgical interventions or invasive procedures, treated with VKAs and with NOACs despite the extremely different pharmacokinetic characteristics of the drugs. In patients taking NOACs, however, in the case of an intermediate risk of thromboembolic events and in procedures with a low risk of bleeding, bridging therapy was used infrequently. Conversely, the use of parenteral anticoagulant therapy in high-risk patients treated with NOACs subjected to procedures with a higher risk of bleeding, requiring the interruption of anticoagulant therapy for a long period, has remained uncertain [49].

One of the drugs usable in the case of urgent procedures in subjects treated with dabigatran, who either had severe bleeding or required an urgent procedure, is the idarucizumab monoclonal antibody, studied in a trial of 503 patients, in the RE-VERSE AD study. Idarucizumab has received full FDA approval [50]. In addition, Andexanet alfa, a genetically modified and recombinant protein designed to serve as an antidote against direct factor Xa inhibitors, has also been reported to reverse the effects of rivaroxaban and apixaban and was approved according to the FDA's accelerated approval process, based on the effects in healthy volunteers [51].

Furthermore, in a special subpopulation of patients undergoing coronary angiography with or without PCI, a meta-analysis by Kowalewski et al. showed a comparable safety of uninterrupted (UAC) and interrupted OAT (IAC). This safety also appeared higher in the case of IAC with bridging [52].

6. Anticoagulant Therapy: An Upcoming Challenge

AF is commonly diagnosed in the setting of active malignancy [53]. Cancer is associated with the hypercoagulable state, with an increased risk of thromboembolism, regardless of the CHA2DS2-VASc score [54]. Moreover, these patients, in particular the ones affected by either primary or metastatic intracranial tumors or hematological malignancies, also present an increased risk of bleeding. Other important issues should also be taken into account, such as drug–drug interaction with cancer treatment, changes in renal and hepatic function, dietary and nutritional status, chemotherapeutic toxicity and disease state. All these conditions may determine a fluctuation of INR values.

Up until now, VKAs have represented the gold standard in long term treatment. However, this class of drugs is burdened by the need to maintain the INR at target. In the last few years, with the advent of NOACs, several studies have assessed the safety and efficacy in this specific population [32,55–58]. Nevertheless, the limited sample size and the wide spectrum of malignancies render it necessary to conduct further in-depth studies.

Thus, anticoagulation with both NOACs and VKAs for AF related thromboembolism in patients affected by malignancies is challenging.

7. Conclusions

In conclusion, given the extreme complexity of this scenario, which involves multiple professional figures, it would be worthwhile establishing standardized protocols and research models oriented towards the development of clinical pathways. In this way we could improve the management of patients under OAT, candidates for interventions surgical and invasive procedures, especially in light of the new commercial oral anticoagulants.

Author Contributions: Conception and design: A.C.; Analysis and interpretation of the data: A.C., R.G., P.C.P.; Drafting of the article: A.C., R.G., P.C.P.; Critical revision for important intellectual content: A.C., R.G., P.C.P.; Provision of study materials or patients: A.C., R.G., P.C.P.; Statistical expertise: P.C.P.; Collection and assembly of data: A.C., R.G., P.C.P.; Final approval of the article: A.C., R.G., P.C.P.

References

1. Russo, V.; Attena, E.; Mazzone, C.; Melillo, E.; Rago, A.; Galasso, G.; Riegler, L.; Parisi, V.; Rotunno, R.; Nigro, G.; et al. Real-life Performance of Edoxaban in Elderly Patients with Atrial Fibrillation: A Multicenter Propensity Score-Matched Cohort Study. *Clin. Ther.* **2019**, *41*, 1598–1604. [CrossRef] [PubMed]

2. January, C.T.; Wann, L.S.; Calkins, H.; Field, M.E.; Chen, L.Y.; Furie, K.L.; Cigarroa, J.E.; Heidenreich, P.A.; Cleveland, J.C., Jr.; Murray, K.T.; et al. 2019 AHA/ACC/HRS Focused Update of the 2014 AHA/ACC/HRS Guideline for the Management of Patients with Atrial Fibrillation: A Report of the American College of Cardiology/American Heart Association Task Force on Clinical Practice Guidelines and the Heart Rhythm Society. *Heart Rhythm* **2019**, *140*, 125–151.
3. Telles-Garcia, N.; Dahal, K.; Kocherla, C.; Lip, G.Y.H.; Reddy, P.; Dominic, P. Non-vitamin K antagonists oral anticoagulants are as safe and effective as warfarin for cardioversion of atrial fibrillation: A systematic review and meta-analysis. *Int. J. Cardiol.* **2018**, *268*, 143–148. [CrossRef] [PubMed]
4. Gibson, C.M.; Basto, A.N.; Howard, M.L. Direct Oral Anticoagulants in Cardioversion: A Review of Current Evidence. *Ann. Pharm.* **2018**, *52*, 277–284. [CrossRef] [PubMed]
5. Russo, V.; Rago, A.; Proietti, R.; Di Meo, F.; Antonio Papa, A.; Calabrò, P.; D'onofrio, A.; Nigro, G.; AlTurki, A. Efficacy and safety of the target-specific oral anticoagulants for stroke prevention in atrial fibrillation: The real-life evidence. *Ther. Adv. Drug Saf.* **2017**, *8*, 67–75. [CrossRef] [PubMed]
6. Rago, A.; Papa, A.A.; Cassese, A.; Arena, G.; Magliocca, M.C.G.; D'onofrio, A.; Golino, P.; Nigro, G.; Russo, V. Clinical Performance of Apixaban vs. Vitamin K Antagonists in Patients with Atrial Fibrillation Undergoing Direct Electrical Current Cardioversion: A Prospective Propensity Score-Matched Cohort Study. *Am. J. Cardiovasc. Drugs* **2019**, *19*, 421–427. [CrossRef]
7. Russo, V.; Rago, A.; Papa, A.A.; D'onofrio, A.; Golino, P.; Nigro, G. Efficacy and safety of dabigatran in patients with atrial fibrillation scheduled for transoesophageal echocardiogram-guided direct electrical current cardioversion: A prospective propensity score-matched cohort study. *J. Thromb. Thrombolysis* **2018**, *45*, 206–212. [CrossRef]
8. Russo, V.; Di Napoli, L.; Bianchi, V.; Tavoletta, V.; De Vivo, S.; Cavallaro, C.; Vecchione, F.; Rago, A.; Sarubbi, B.; Calabrò, P.; et al. A new integrated strategy for direct current cardioversion in non-valvular atrial fibrillation patients using short-term rivaroxaban administration: The MonaldiVert real life experience. *Int. J. Cardiol* **2016**, *224*, 454–455. [CrossRef]
9. Reers, S.; Karanatsios, G.; Borowski, M.; Kellner, M.; Reppel, M.; Waltenberger, J. Frequency of atrial thrombus formation in patients with atrial fibrillation under treatment with non-vitamin K oral anticoagulants in comparison to vitamin K antagonists: A systematic review and meta-analysis. *Eur. J. Med. Res.* **2018**, *23*, 49. [CrossRef]
10. Klein, A.L.; Murray, R.D.; Grimm, R.A. Role of transesophageal echocardiography-guided cardioversion of patients with atrial fibrillation. *J. Am. Coll. Cardiol.* **2001**, *37*, 691–704. [CrossRef]
11. Stabile, G.; Russo, V.; Rapacciuolo, A.; De Divitiis, M.; De Simone, A.; Solimene, F.; D'onofrio, A.; Iuliano, A.; Maresca, G.; Esposito, F.; et al. Transesophageal echocardiograpy in patients with persistent atrial fibrillation undergoing electrical cardioversion on new oral anticoagulants: A multi center registry. *Int. J. Cardiol.* **2015**, *184*, 283–284. [CrossRef] [PubMed]
12. Bertaglia, E.; Anselmino, M.; Zorzi, A.; Russo, V.; Toso, E.; Peruzza, F.; Rapacciuolo, A.; Migliore, F.; Gaita, F.; Cucchini, U.; et al. NOACs and atrial fibrillation: Incidence and predictors of left atrial thrombus in the real world. *Int. J. Cardiol.* **2017**, *249*, 179–183. [CrossRef] [PubMed]
13. Frederiksen, A.S.; Albertsen, A.E.; Christesen, A.M.S.; Vinter, N.; Frost, L.; Møller, D.S. Cardioversion of atrial fibrillation in a real-world setting: Non-vitamin K antagonist oral anticoagulants ensure a fast and safe strategy compared to warfarin. *Europace* **2018**, *20*, 1078–1085. [CrossRef] [PubMed]
14. Hohnloser, S.H.; Cappato, R.; Ezekowitz, M.D.; Evers, T.; Sahin, K.; Kirchhof, P.; Meng, I.L.; van Eickels, M.; Camm, A.J. X-VeRT Steering Committee and Investigators. Patient-reported treatment satisfaction and budget impact with rivaroxaban vs. standard therapy in elective cardioversion of atrial fibrillation: A post hoc analysis of the X-VeRT trial. *Europace* **2016**, *18*, 184–190. [CrossRef] [PubMed]
15. Russo, V.; Rago, A.; Papa, A.A.; Bianchi, V.; Tavoletta, V.; DE Vivo, S.; Cavallaro, C.; Nigro, G.; D'onofrio, A. Budget impact analysis of rivaroxaban vs. warfarin anticoagulation strategy for direct current cardioversion in non-valvular atrial fibrillation patients: The MonaldiVert Economic Study. *Minerva Cardioangiol.* **2018**, *66*, 1–5. [PubMed]
16. Grosu, A.I.; Radulescu, D.; Grosu, L.C.; Pop, D. Remodelling in atrial fibrillation: The impact of amiodarone. *Cardiovasc. J. Afr.* **2019**, *30*, 1–7. [CrossRef] [PubMed]

17. Raunso, J.; Selmer, C.; Olesen, J.B.; Charlot, M.G.; Olsen, A.M.; Bretler, D.M.; Nielsen, J.D.; Dominguez, H.; Gadsbøll, N.; Køber, L.; et al. Increased short-term risk of thrombo-embolism or death after interruption of warfarin treatment in patients with atrial fibrillation. *Eur. Heart J.* **2012**, *33*, 1886–1892. [CrossRef] [PubMed]
18. Sjogren, V.; Grzymala-Lubanski, B.; Renlund, H.; Friberg, L.; Lip, G.Y.; Svensson, P.J.; Själander, A. Safety and efficacy of well managed warfarin. A report from the Swedish quality register Auricula. *Thromb. Haemost.* **2015**, *113*, 1370–1377. [CrossRef] [PubMed]
19. Eikelboom, J.W.; Connolly, S.J.; Brueckmann, M.; Granger, C.B.; Kappetein, A.P.; Mack, M.J.; Blatchford, J.; Devenny, K.; Friedman, J.; Guiver, K.; et al. Dabigatran versus warfarin in patients with mechanical heart valves. *N. Engl. J. Med.* **2013**, *369*, 1206–1214. [CrossRef]
20. Carnicelli, A.P.; De Caterina, R.; Halperin, J.L.; Renda, G.; Ruff, C.T.; Trevisan, M.; Nordio, F.; Mercuri, M.F.; Antman, E.; Giugliano, R.P.; et al. Edoxaban for the prevention of thromboembolism in patients with atrial fibrillation and bioprosthetic valves. *Circulation* **2017**, *135*, 1273–1275. [CrossRef]
21. Hart, R.G.; Pearce, L.A.; Aguilar, M.I. Meta-analysis: Antithrombotic therapy to prevent stroke in patients who have nonvalvular atrial fibrillation. *Ann. Intern. Med.* **2007**, *146*, 857–867. [CrossRef] [PubMed]
22. Lip, G.Y.; Hart, R.G.; Conway, D.S. Antithrombotic therapy for atrial fibrillation. *BMJ.* **2002**, *325*, 1022–1025. [CrossRef] [PubMed]
23. ACTIVE Writing Group of the ACTIVE Investigators; Connolly, S.; Pogue, J.; Hart, R.; Pfeffer, M.; Hohnloser, S.; Chrolavicius, S.; Pfeffer, M.; Hohnloser, S.; Yusuf, S. Clopidogrel plus aspirin versus oral anticoagulation for atrial fibrillation in the Atrial fibrillation Clopidogrel Trial with Irbesartan for prevention of Vascular Events (ACTIVE W): A randomised controlled trial. *Lancet* **2006**, *367*, 1903–1912. [PubMed]
24. Mant, J.; Hobbs, F.D.; Fletcher, K.; Roalfe, A.; Fitzmaurice, D.; Lip, G.Y.; Murray, E. BAFTA investigators; Midland Research Practices Network (MidReC). Warfarin versus aspirin for stroke prevention in an elderly community population with atrial fibrillation (the Birmingham Atrial Fibrillation Treatment of the Aged Study, BAFTA): A randomised controlled trial. *Lancet* **2007**, *370*, 493–503.
25. ACTIVE Investigators; Connolly, S.J.; Pogue, J.; Hart, R.G.; Hohnloser, S.H.; Pfeffer, M.; Chrolavicius, S.; Yusuf, S. Effect of clopidogrel added to aspirin in patients with atrial fibrillation. *N. Engl. J. Med.* **2009**, *360*, 2066–2078. [PubMed]
26. Kirchhof, P.; Benussi, S.; Kotecha, D.; Ahlsson, A.; Atar, D.; Casadei, B.; Castellá, M.; Diener, H.C.; Heidbuchel, H.; Hendriks, J.; et al. 2016 ESC Guidelines for the management of atrial fibrillation developed in collaboration with EACTS. *Europace* **2016**, *18*, 1609–1678. [CrossRef] [PubMed]
27. Verheugt, F.W.A.; Gao, H.; Al Mahmeed, W.; Ambrosio, G.; Angchaisuksiri, P.; Atar, D.; Bassand, J.P.; Camm, A.J.; Cools, F.; Eikelboom, J.; et al. Characteristics of patients with atrial fibrillation prescribed antiplatelet monotherapy compared with those on anticoagulants: Insights from the GARFIELD-AF registry. *Eur. Heart J.* **2018**, *39*, 464–473. [CrossRef]
28. Pignatelli, P.; Pastori, P.; Violi, F. Antithrombotic therapy in atrial fibrillation: Tailoring the choice. *Giornale Italiano Dell'Arteriosclerosi* **2017**, *8*, 52–64.
29. Lip, G.Y.; Banerjee, A.; Boriani, G.; Chiang, C.E.; Fargo, R.; Freedman, B.; Lane, D.A.; Ruff, C.T.; Turakhia, M.; Werring, D.; et al. Antithrombotic Therapy for Atrial Fibrillation: CHEST Guideline and Expert Panel Report. *Chest* **2018**, *154*, 1121–1201. [CrossRef]
30. Ruff, C.T.; Giugliano, R.P.; Braunwald, E.; Hoffman, E.B.; Deenadayalu, N.; Ezekowitz, M.D.; Camm, A.J.; Weitz, J.I.; Lewis, B.S.; Parkhomenko, A.; et al. Comparison of the efficacy and safety of new oral anticoagulants with warfarin in patients with atrial fibrillation: A meta-analysis of randomised trials. *Lancet* **2014**, *383*, 955–962. [CrossRef]
31. Russo, V.; Bianchi, V.; Cavallaro, C.; Vecchione, F.; De Vivo, S.; Santangelo, L.; Sarubbi, B.; Calabrò, P.; Nigro, G.; D'onofrio, A. Efficacy and safety of dabigatran in a "real-life" population at high thromboembolic and hemorrhagic risk: Data from MonaldiCare registry. *Eur. Rev. Med. Pharmacol. Sci.* **2015**, *19*, 3961–3967.
32. Russo, V.; Rago, A.; Papa, A.A.; Meo, F.D.; Attena, E.; Golino, P.; D'onofrio, A.; Nigro, G. Use of Non-Vitamin K Antagonist Oral Anticoagulants in Atrial Fibrillation Patients with Malignancy: Clinical Practice Experience in a Single Institution and Literature Review. *Semin. Thromb. Hemost.* **2018**, *44*, 370–376.
33. Verdecchia, P.; D'onofrio, A.; Russo, V.; Fedele, F.; Adamo, F.; Benedetti, G.; Ferrante, F.; Lodigiani, C.; Paciullo, F.; Aita, A.; et al. Persistence on apixaban in atrial fibrillation patients: A retrospective multicentre study. *J. Cardiovasc. Med.* **2019**, *20*, 66–73. [CrossRef] [PubMed]

34. Russo, V.; Bottino, R.; Rago, A.; Micco, P.D.; D'onofrio, A.; Liccardo, B.; Golino, P.; Nigro, G. Atrial Fibrillation and Malignancy: The Clinical Performance of Non-Vitamin K Oral Anticoagulants-A Systematic Review. *Semin. Thromb. Hemost.* **2019**, *45*, 205–214. [PubMed]
35. Russo, V.; Carbone, A.; Rago, A.; Golino, P.; Nigro, G. Direct Oral Anticoagulants in octogenarians with atrial fibrillation: It's never too late. *J. Cardiovasc. Pharmacol.* **2019**, *73*, 207–214. [CrossRef] [PubMed]
36. Steffel, J.; Verhamme, P.; Potpara, T.S.; Albaladejo, P.; Antz, M.; Desteghe, L.; Haeusler, K.G.; Oldgren, J.; Reinecke, H.; Roldan-Schilling, V.; et al. The 2018 European Heart Rhythm Association Practical Guide on the use of non-vitamin K antagonist oral anticoagulants in patients with atrial fibrillation. *Eur. Heart J.* **2018**, *39*, 1330–1393. [CrossRef]
37. Connolly, S.J.; Ezekowitz, M.D.; Yusuf, S.; Eikelboom, J.; Oldgren, J.; Parekh, A.; Pogue, J.; Reilly, P.A.; Themeles, E.; Varrone, J.; et al. Dabigatran versus warfarin in patients with atrial fibrillation. *N. Engl. J. Med.* **2009**, *361*, 1139–1151. [CrossRef]
38. Patel, M.R.; Mahaffey, K.W.; Garg, J.; Pan, G.; Singer, D.E.; Hacke, W.; Breithardt, G.; Halperin, J.L.; Hankey, G.J.; Piccini, J.P.; et al. Rivaroxaban versus warfarin in nonvalvular atrial fibrillation. *N. Engl. J. Med.* **2011**, *365*, 883–891. [CrossRef]
39. Granger, C.B.; Alexander, J.H.; McMurray, J.J.; Lopes, R.D.; Hylek, E.M.; Hanna, M.; Al-Khalidi, H.R.; Ansell, J.; Atar, D.; Avezum, A.; et al. Apixaban versus warfarin in patients with atrial fibrillation. *N. Engl. J. Med.* **2011**, *365*, 981–992. [CrossRef]
40. Connolly, S.J.; Eikelboom, J.; Joyner, C.; Diener, H.C.; Hart, R.; Golitsyn, S.; Flaker, G.; Avezum, A.; Hohnloser, S.H.; Diaz, R.; et al. Apixaban in patients with atrial fibrillation. *N. Engl. J. Med.* **2011**, *364*, 806–817. [CrossRef]
41. Giugliano, R.P.; Ruff, C.T.; Braunwald, E.; Murphy, S.A.; Wiviott, S.D.; Halperin, J.L.; Waldo, A.L.; Ezekowitz, M.D.; Weitz, J.I.; Špinar, J.; et al. Edoxaban versus warfarin in patients with atrial fibrillation. *N. Engl. J. Med.* **2013**, *369*, 2093–2104. [CrossRef]
42. Dentali, F.; Riva, N.; Crowther, M.; Turpie, A.G.; Lip, G.Y.; Ageno, W. Efficacy and safety of the novel oral anticoagulants in atrial fibrillation: A systematic review and meta-analysis of the literature. *Circulation* **2012**, *126*, 2381–2391. [CrossRef]
43. Kimachi, M.; Furukawa, T.A.; Kimachi, K.; Goto, Y.; Fukuma, S.; Fukuhara, S. Direct oral anticoagulants versus warfarin for preventing stroke and systemic embolic events among atrial fibrillation patients with chronic kidney disease. *Cochrane Database Syst. Rev.* **2017**, *11*, CD011373. [CrossRef]
44. Loo, S.Y.; Dell'Aniello, S.; Huiart, L.; Renoux, C. Trends in the prescription of novel oral anticoagulants in UK primary care: Novel oral anticoagulant prescription trends. *Br. J. Clin. Pharmacol.* **2017**, *83*, 2096–2106. [CrossRef]
45. Russo, V.; Rago, A.; D'onofrio, A.; Nigro, G. The clinical performance of dabigatran in the Italian real-life experience. *J. Cardiovasc. Med. (Hagerstown)* **2017**, *18*, 922–923. [CrossRef]
46. Russo, V.; Rago, A.; Proietti, R.; Attena, E.; Rainone, C.; Crisci, M.; Papa, A.A.; Calabrò, P.; D'onofrio, A.; Golino, P.; et al. Safety and Efficacy of Triple Antithrombotic Therapy with Dabigatran versus Vitamin KAntagonist in Atrial Fibrillation Patients: A Pilot Study. *Biomed. Res. Int.* **2019**, *13*, 5473240.
47. Flaker, G.C.; Theriot, P.; Binder, L.G.; Dobesh, P.P.; Cuker, A.; Doherty, J.U. Management of Periprocedural Anticoagulation: A Survey of Contemporary Practice. *J. Am. Coll. Cardiol.* **2016**, *68*, 217–226. [CrossRef]
48. Douketis, J.D.; Spyropoulos, A.C.; Kaatz, S.; Becker, R.C.; Caprini, J.A.; Dunn, A.S.; Garcia, D.A.; Jacobson, A.; Jaffer, A.K.; Kong, D.F.; et al. Perioperative bridging anticoagulation in patients with atrial fibrillation. *N. Engl. J. Med.* **2015**, *373*, 823–833. [CrossRef]
49. Beyer-Westendorf, J.; Gelbricht, V.; Forster, K.; Ebertz, F.; Köhler, C.; Werth, S.; Kuhlisch, E.; Stange, T.; Thieme, C.; Daschkow, K.; et al. Peri-interventional management of novel oral anticoagulants in daily care: Results from the prospective Dresden NOAC registry. *Eur. Heart J.* **2014**, *35*, 1888–1896. [CrossRef]
50. Pollack, C.V., Jr.; Reilly, P.A.; van Ryn, J.; Eikelboom, J.W.; Glund, S.; Bernstein, R.A.; Dubiel, R.; Huisman, M.V.; Hylek, E.M.; Kam, C.W.; et al. Idarucizumab for dabigatran reversal—Full cohort analysis. *N. Engl. J. Med.* **2017**, *377*, 431–441. [CrossRef]
51. Siegal, D.M.; Curnutte, J.T.; Connolly, S.J.; Lu, G.; Conley, P.B.; Wiens, B.L.; Mathur, V.S.; Castillo, J.; Bronson, M.D.; Leeds, J.M.; et al. Andexanet alfa for the reversal of factor Xa inhibitor activity. *N. Engl. J. Med.* **2015**, *373*, 2413–2424. [CrossRef]

52. Kowalewski, M.; Suwalski, P.; Raffa, G.M.; Słomka, A.; Kowalkowska, M.E.; Szwed, K.; Borkowska, A.; Kowalewski, J.; Malvindi, P.G.; Undas, A.; et al. Meta-analysis of uninterrupted as compared to interrupted oral anticoagulation with or without bridging in patients undergoing coronary angiography with or without percutaneous coronary intervention. *Int. J. Cardiol.* **2016**, *223*, 186–194. [CrossRef]
53. Mann, D.L.; Krone, R.J. Cardiac disease in cancer patients: An overview. *Prog. Cardiovasc. Dis.* **2010**, *53*, 80–87. [CrossRef]
54. Falanga, A.; Marchetti, M.; Russo, L. The mechanisms of cancer-associated thrombosis. *Thromb. Res.* **2015**, *135* (Suppl. 1), S8–S11. [CrossRef]
55. Laube, E.S.; Yu, A.; Gupta, D.; Miao, Y.; Samedy, P.; Wills, J.; Harnicar, S.; Soff, G.A.; Mantha, S. Rivaroxaban for Stroke Prevention in Patients with Nonvalvular Atrial Fibrillation and Active Cancer. *Am. J. Cardiol.* **2017**, *120*, 213–217. [CrossRef]
56. Melloni, C.; Dunning, A.; Granger, C.B.; Thomas, L.; Khouri, M.G.; Garcia, D.A.; Hylek, E.M.; Hanna, M.; Wallentin, L.; Gersh, B.J.; et al. Efficacy and Safety of Apixaban Versus Warfarin in Patients with Atrial Fibrillation and a History of Cancer: Insights from the ARISTOTLE Trial. *Am. J. Med.* **2017**, *130*, 1440–1448. [CrossRef]
57. Fanola, C.L.; Ruff, C.T.; Murphy, S.A.; Jin, J.; Duggal, A.; Babilonia, N.A.; Sritara, P.; Mercuri, M.F.; Kamphuisen, P.W.; Antman, E.M.; et al. Efficacy and Safety of Edoxaban in Patients with Active Malignancy and Atrial Fibrillation: Analysis of the ENGAGE AF—TIMI 48 Trial. *J. Am. Heart Assoc.* **2018**, *7*, e008987. [CrossRef]
58. Melloni, C.; Shrader, P.; Carver, J.; Piccini, J.P.; Thomas, L.; Fonarow, G.C.; Ansell, J.; Gersh, B.; Go, A.S.; Hylek, E.; et al. Management and outcomes of patients with atrial fibrillation and a history of cancer: The ORBIT-AF registry. *Eur. Heart J. Qual. Care Clin. Outcomes* **2017**, *3*, 192–197. [CrossRef]

13

Role of Biological Markers for Cerebral Bleeding Risk STRATification in Patients with Atrial Fibrillation on Oral Anticoagulants for Primary or Secondary Prevention of Ischemic Stroke (Strat-AF Study)

Anna Poggesi [1,2,3,*], Carmen Barbato [2], Francesco Galmozzi [2], Eleonora Camilleri [4], Francesca Cesari [5], Stefano Chiti [6], Stefano Diciotti [7], Silvia Galora [4], Betti Giusti [4], Anna Maria Gori [4], Chiara Marzi [7], Anna Melone [2], Damiano Mistri [2], Francesca Pescini [1], Giovanni Pracucci [2], Valentina Rinnoci [1,2,3], Cristina Sarti [1,2], Enrico Fainardi [8], Rossella Marcucci [4] and Emilia Salvadori [1,2,3]

1 Stroke Unit, Careggi University Hospital, 50134 Florence, Italy; francesca.pescini@unifi.it (F.P.); valentina.rinnoci@unifi.it (V.R.); cristina.sarti@unifi.it (C.S.); emilia.salvadori@unifi.it (E.S.)

2 NEUROFARBA Department, Neuroscience Section, University of Florence, 50134 Florence, Italy; carmenbarbato88@gmail.com (C.B.); galmo89@icloud.com (F.G.); melone.anna@hotmail.it (A.M.); damiano.mistri@gmail.com (D.M.); giovanni.pracucci@unifi.it (G.P.)

3 IRCCS Don Carlo Gnocchi, 50143 Florence, Italy

4 Department of Experimental and Clinical Medicine, University of Florence, 50134 Florence, Italy; camillerieleonora@gmail.com (E.C.); silviagalora@gmail.com (S.G.); betti.giusti@unifi.it (B.G.); annamaria.gori@unifi.it (A.M.G.); rossella.marcucci@unifi.it (R.M.)

5 Central Laboratory, Careggi University Hospital, 50134 Florence, Italy; francesca.cesari@gmail.com

6 Department Health Professions, U.O.c Research and Development, 50134 Careggi University Hospital, 50134 Florence, Italy; stefano.chiti@gmail.com

7 Department of Electrical, Electronic, and Information Engineering "Guglielmo Marconi", University of Bologna, 40136 Bologna, Italy; stefano.diciotti@unibo.it (S.D.); chiara.marzi3@unibo.it (C.M.)

8 Neuroradiology Unit, Department of Experimental and Clinical Biomedical Sciences, University of Florence, Careggi University Hospital, 50134 Florence, Italy; henryfai@tin.it

* Correspondence: anna.poggesi@unifi.it

Abstract: *Background and Objectives:* In anticoagulated atrial fibrillation (AF) patients, the validity of models recommended for the stratification of the risk ratio between benefits and hemorrhage risk is limited. Cerebral small vessel disease (SVD) represents the pathologic substrate for primary intracerebral hemorrhage and ischemic stroke. We hypothesize that biological markers—both circulating and imaging-based—and their possible interaction, might improve the prediction of bleeding risk in AF patients under treatment with any type of oral anticoagulant. *Materials and Methods*: The Strat-AF study is an observational, prospective, single-center hospital-based study enrolling patients with AF, aged 65 years or older, and with no contraindications to magnetic resonance imaging (MRI), referring to Center of Thrombosis outpatient clinic of our University Hospital for the management of oral anticoagulation therapy. Recruited patients are evaluated by means of a comprehensive protocol, with clinical, cerebral MRI, and circulating biomarkers assessment at baseline and after 18 months. The main outcome is SVD progression—particularly microbleeds—as a selective surrogate marker of hemorrhagic complication. Stroke occurrence (ischemic or hemorrhagic) and the progression of functional, cognitive, and motor status will be evaluated as secondary outcomes. Circulating biomarkers may further improve predictive potentials. *Results*: Starting from September 2017, 194 patients (mean age 78.1 ± 6.7, range 65–97; 61% males) were enrolled. The type of AF was paroxysmal in 93 patients (48%), and persistent or permanent in the remaining patients. Concerning the type of oral anticoagulant, 57 patients (29%) were on vitamin K antagonists, and 137 (71%) were on direct oral anticoagulants. Follow-up clinical evaluation and brain MRI are ongoing. *Conclusions*: The Strat-AF study may be an essential step towards the exploration of the role of a combined clinical biomarker or multiple biomarker models in predicting stroke risk in AF, and might sustain the incorporation of such new markers in the existing stroke prediction schemes by the demonstration of a greater incremental value in predicting stroke risk and improvement in clinical outcomes in a cost-effective fashion.

Keywords: atrial fibrillation; anticoagulation; stroke; intracerebral hemorrhage; cerebral small vessel disease; brain MRI; circulating biomarkers

1. Introduction

Thromboprophylaxis with oral anticoagulation effectively reduces stroke risk in patients with atrial fibrillation (AF). Benefits must be balanced against the risk of bleeding, with intracranial hemorrhage being the most feared. Stroke and bleeding risk stratification schemes are aimed at identifying patients who may benefit most from different types of oral anticoagulation (vitamin K antagonists vs. direct oral anticoagulants). Currently, such schemes (e.g., CHADS2VASC2 and HASBLED scores) rely only on clinical information, the validity of which remains controversial and needs to be improved. In AF patients, advanced imaging technology such as magnetic resonance imaging (MRI), has led to the increased detection of asymptomatic brain changes, mainly those related to small vessel disease (SVD), which is the pathologic substrate for primary intracerebral hemorrhage (ICH) [1–6]. These changes have also been proven to strongly predict stroke risk [2,5]. Such imaging findings, obtained both at baseline and in terms of lesion progression over time, could be used as additional markers for risk stratification [3,7]. Furthermore, markers of coagulation activation, including prothrombin fragment 1+2, thrombin–antithrombin complex, D-dimer, time in therapeutic range for warfarin, and drug dosage for new anticoagulants, may be also studied as cofactors. Preliminary data suggest that circulating biomarkers of endothelial dysfunction, hypercoagulable state, and inflammation may further enhance risk prediction [4].

The validity of the currently recommended models for the stratification of risk ratio between benefits and hemorrhagic risk in anticoagulated AF patients is limited. These models do not specifically take intracranial hemorrhage into account, which is indeed the most severe hemorrhagic complication [8]. Our hypothesis is that biological markers—both circulating and imaging-based, and their possible interaction—might improve the prediction of bleeding risk in AF patients treated with any type of oral anticoagulant. Neuroimaging biomarkers of SVD—particularly microbleeds—may serve as a selective surrogate marker of hemorrhagic complications. Circulating biomarkers assessed together with imaging may further improve predictive potentials.

In this scenario, we set up the prospective observational Strat-AF study, primarily aimed at investigating circulating biomarkers and MRI markers (baseline and progression) of SVD as surrogate markers for the prediction of cerebral bleeding in a cohort of patients with AF on oral anticoagulants. Secondary outcomes included stroke occurrence (either ischemic or hemorrhagic) and the progression of functional, cognitive, and motor status.

2. Materials and Methods

Stratification of Cerebral Bleeding Risk in AF, Strat-AF, Strat-AF is an observational, prospective, single-center hospital-based study enrolling patients with AF, referring to the Center of Thrombosis outpatient clinic of our University Hospital for the management of oral anticoagulation therapy.

2.1. Inclusion Criteria

- Diagnosis of AF and ongoing oral anticoagulation therapy;
- Aged ≥ 65 years;
- No contraindications to MRI.

2.2. Exclusion Criteria

- Inability or refusal to undergo cerebral MRI;
- Inability to give an informed consent.

All subjects gave their informed consent for inclusion before they participated in the study. The study was conducted in accordance with the Declaration of Helsinki, and the protocol was approved by the Ethics Committee of the Careggi University Hospital (Project identification code 16RFAP, approved on March 2017).

Sample size was estimated based on a feasibility criterion (i.e., the real flow of patients to the Thrombosis outpatient clinic of Careggi Hospital). Yearly, approximately 600 patients with AF on oral anticoagulation refer to the outpatient clinic. Considering a foreseeable rate of ineligible patients and refusals, we originally estimated to contact approximately 300 patients in one year fulfilling the inclusion criteria. Starting from September 2017, consecutive eligible patients were invited to participate in the study. The initial foreseen period for enrollment was 12 months, but in order to augment the number of included patients, we extended the enrollment period to 18 months.

2.3. Clinical Assessment

All enrolled patients were assessed at baseline by means of a standard clinical/functional protocol collecting information on vascular risk factors (particularly hypertension and diabetes), dietary habits, previous cerebrovascular events, general neurological and functional status, cognitive performances, mood and gait disorders, and general neurological examination.

In detail, clinical data were collected about social and medical history; a standard cardiovascular and neurological examination, including office blood pressure measurement, were performed. Functional status was assessed using the Activities of Daily Living scale and the Instrumental Activities of Daily Living scale [9,10]; mood assessment using the Geriatric Depression Scale [11]; motor performance using the Short Physical Performance Battery [12]; daytime sleepiness using the Epworth Sleepiness Scale [13]; and quality of life using the EuroQol Visual Analog Scale [14]. Dietary habits were assessed by means of the questionnaire on the adherence to the Mediterranean diet [15].

A comprehensive multi-domain cognitive assessment, including global functioning, orientation, memory, attention, executive functions, language, speed, and motor control was administered to each included patient.

The cognitive domains assessed by means of the extensive battery of tests were as follows:

- <u>Global cognitive efficiency,</u> by means of the Montreal Cognitive Assessment (MoCA): it is a 10-minute cognitive screening tool created to detect mild cognitive impairment (MCI), suggested from the harmonization standards of the National Institute of Neurological Disorders and Stroke—Canadian Stroke Network (NINDS-CSN) and thought to be specifically sensitive to frontal, attention, and executive deficits [16–18]. It covers eight cognitive domains: short-term and delayed verbal memory; visuospatial abilities; executive functions; attention; concentration; working memory; language; and orientation (score range 0–30)
- <u>Verbal memory,</u> by means of the Rey Auditory-Verbal Learning Test (RAVLT) and the Short Story Recall Test [19,20]. The RAVLT and Short Story Recall Test measure several components of verbal memory, such as immediate free recall, verbal learning, and retention of information after a certain period of time. Two scores are obtained from the RAVLT: immediate free recall (range 0–75) and delayed free recall (range 0–15). The Short Story Recall Test has a total score obtained by the

mean number of elements correctly remembered on the immediate and delayed recalls (score range 0–28).

- Attention, by means of the Visual Search test [21]. This is a number cancellation task that requires visual selectivity at fast speed, and assesses the capacity for sustained attention and accuracy of visual scanning (score range 0–60). The Colour Word Stroop test was also used [22]. It is a measure of concentration effectiveness and deals with response inhibition and selective attention. The activity required by this test is a selective processing of only one visual feature while continuously blocking out the processing of others. The execution time and the errors committed are recorded.
- Language, by means of:

  i. Semantic verbal fluency test: a test allowing the semantic evaluation of lexical access [23]. Three categories were tested: car brands, fruits, and animals. The total score was given by the sum of the number of words produced for each category in one minute.
  ii. Sentence construction test: a test used to evaluate the verbal ability to construct a meaningful sentence starting from a set of two or three words (score range 0–25) [19].

All raw test scores were demographically corrected according to Italian population normative data, and adjusted scores were then recoded as normal, borderline, or abnormal according to equivalent scores (ES) methodology [24]. ES methodology is a non-parametric norming method based on percentiles and is independent from the distribution form. ES is an ordinal 5-point scale (ranging from 0 to 4), and the main point of ES methodology is to fix the outer tolerance limit of the left queue of the adjusted scores so that it is possible to assess, with a known risk of error (<5%), the cut-off splitting the bottom 5% of the population and representing pathological performance (ES = 0). At the other end of the scale, ES = 4 indicates an optimal performance (equal to or better than the median). ES = 1 indicates a borderline performance (an adjusted score between the outer and inner confidence limits for the fifth centile of the normal population), while the remaining ES scores of 2 and 3 represent normal performances.

The diagnosis of MCI requires at least one altered score (ES = 0) plus one borderline score (ES = 1) in any cognitive test included in the neuropsychological battery.

2.4. Cerebral Magnetic Resonance Imaging Assessment

Cerebral MRI scans were performed at baseline, and again 18 months after enrollment. The brain imaging protocol was planned and set up by imaging personnel with different expertise and skills, as suggested by current guidelines [25].

Baseline and follow-up MRI examinations are performed on an Ingenia 1.5-Tesla MRI unit (Philips Healthcare, Eindhoven, The Netherlands). Our standardized MRI protocol consisted of the following sequences: sagittal T1-weighted spin-echo (repetition time (TR) = 547 ms; echo time (TE) = 12 ms; slice thickness = 5 mm; interslice spacing = 0.5 mm; matrix size = 320 × 250; field of view (FOV) = 23 cm × 23 cm; number of signals averaged (NSA) = 1), coronal T2-weighted fast spin-echo (TR = 3347 ms; TE = 110 ms; slice thickness = 5 mm; interslice spacing = 0.5 mm; matrix size = 512 × 322; FOV = 22 cm × 22 cm; NSA = 2); axial fluid-attenuated inversion recovery (FLAIR) (TR = 11,000 ms; TE = 125 ms; inversion time (TI) = 2800 ms; slice thickness = 5 mm; interslice spacing = 0.5 mm; matrix size = 384 × 204; FOV = 23 cm × 23 cm; NSA = 2); axial gradient-echo T2* (GRE) (TR = 534 ms; TE = 23 ms; flip angle (FA) = 18; slice thickness = 5 mm; interslice spacing = 0.5 mm; matrix size = 256 × 185; FOV = 23 cm × 23 cm; NSA = 1); axial diffusion-weighted imaging (DWI) (TR = 3891 ms; TE = 75 ms; slice thickness = 5 mm; interslice spacing = 0.5 mm; matrix size = 164 × 162; FOV = 23 cm × 23 cm; NSA = 2); gradient-echo 3D T1-weighted (TR = 7.5 ms; TE = 3.4 ms; TI = 950, slice thickness = 1 mm; matrix size = 256 × 241; FOV = 25.6 cm × 25.6 cm; NSA = 1) followed by multiplanar reconstruction (MPR) in axial, coronal, and sagittal planes. DWI images were obtained by single-shot echo-planar spin-echo sequences according to the Stejskal–Tanner method. The diffusion gradients were applied in three orthogonal directions (x, y, z) with two b-values (0 and 1000 s/mm^2) to form the isotropic DWI images at b 1000 s/mm^2. Apparent diffusion coefficient (ADC) maps were generated automatically by the software provided by the manufacturer from isotropic DWI images and concurrent images with a b value of 0 s/mm^2 by using the following equation: ADC = -ln [S(b)/S(0)]/b, where b indicates the b value and S(b) and S(0) are the signal intensities of images with b values equal to 1000 and 0, respectively.

Each MRI scan was evaluated by an expert neuroradiologist, and a written medical report was provided to patients. Neurologists involved in the project revised the report before returning it to patients, so that any incidental findings could be handled according to individual needs.

Qualitative and quantitative analyses of SVD-related features on MRI are under way.

The following features related to SVD will be assessed: i) lacunar infarcts, either silent or not; ii). white matter hyperintensities; iii) microbleeds; iv) dilated perivascular spaces; v) cortical and subcortical atrophy; vi) superficial siderosis [5].

Non-lacunar infarcts will be visually assessed in terms of number and location of lesions.

2.5. Circulating Biomarker Assessment

Venous blood samples were collected after enrollment and placed at -80 °C for long-term storage.

Besides routine parameters (complete blood count (CBC), prothrombin time (PT), activated partial thromboplastin time (APTT), D-dimer, fibrinogen, low-density lipoprotein (LDL), high-density lipoprotein (HDL), triglycerides, glucose, creatinine, glomerular filtration rate (GFR), alanine aminotransferase, C-reactive protein (CRP), N Terminal pro B-type natriuretic peptide, Lp(a), troponin), several circulating biomarkers will be evaluated:

- Endothelial function biomarkers;
- Pro- and anti-inflammatory molecules;
- Metalloproteinases and their inhibitors;
- Markers of renal function;
- Markers of blood clotting activation and of fibrinolytic system of coagulation activation, including prothrombin fragment 1+2, thrombin–antithrombin complex, D-dimer, and endogenous thrombin potentials;
- Genetic polymorphisms that may influence the effect of anticoagulants and plasmatic microRNA profile.

The list of biomarkers under investigation is detailed in Table 1. The biological material (serum, plasma, DNA) is properly conserved to allow the evaluation of further biomarkers by specific or global assessment strategies (e.g., metabolomics profiling, targeted or whole-exome sequencing).

Proteomic and genetic biomarkers will be evaluated with high-multiplex immunoassays or high-throughput technologies such as Bio-Plex Multiplex Immunoassay System (BioRad), Proximity Extension Assay (Olink) technology, H-nuclear magnetic resonance spectroscopy (Bruker BioSpin), real-time PCR (Life Technologies), droplet digital PCR (BioRad), and high-throughput sequencing (Illumina).

Biosamples were processed using standard and harmonized operating procedures.

Clinical data are registered electronically in the web-based registry (http://www.strat-af.it/). Quality controls are done on a weekly basis. Imaging data are instantly checked for protocol conformity.

The same clinical/functional assessment and brain MRI will be repeated 18 months after enrollment. An interim telephone follow-up interview will be scheduled approximately three months before the final clinical assessment.

Table 1. Circulating biomarkers under investigation in the Strat-AF study.

Category	Biomarkers Name
Markers of endothelial function	- von Willebrand Factor (vWF) - Tissue Factor Pathway Inhibitor (TFPI)
Pro- and anti-inflammatory molecules	- Chemokine (C-C motif) ligand 3 (CCL3) - Interleukin (IL)-1β (IL-1β), - IL-1 Receptor antagonist (IL-1RA) - IL-2 - IL-6 - IL-8 - IL-10 - IL-12 P40 - Tumor Necrosis Factor Alpha (TNF-Alfa) - Intercellular Adhesion Molecule-1 (ICAM-1) - Vascular cell adhesion molecule-1 (VCAM-1) - Vascular Endothelial Factor (VEGF)
Metalloproteinases	- Matrix metalloproteinase (MMP)-2, MMP-8, MMP-9, MMP-12 - Tissue Inhibitor of Metalloproteinases (TIMP)-1, TIMP-2, TIMP-3, TIMP-4
Markers of coagulation activation	- Endogenous thrombin potential (ETP) - Plasminogen activator inhibitor-1 (PAI-1) antigen - Prothrombin fragment 1+2 (F1+2) - Thrombin antithrombin complexes (TAT) - Tissue factor - Plasminogen Activator Inhibitor-1 (PAI-1) antigen - Clot lysis time (CLT)
Genetic polymorphisms and plasmatic miRNA	- CES1 rs2244613 - CES1 rs8192935 - ABCB1 rs148738 - VKORC1 G3673A or −1639G>A rs9923231 - CYP2C9*2 rs1799853 - CYP2C9*3 rs1057910 - CYP2C9*5 rs28371686 - CYP2C9*6 rs9332131 - CYP4F2 V433M rs2108622 C>T - GGCX rs11676382 - Plasmatic miRNA profiling by real-time PCR

2.6. *Primary Endpoint*

The primary study endpoint will be SVD progression, evaluated by means of the control MRI performed 18 months after enrollment. The progression of lacunar infarcts and microbleeds will be evaluated as the appearance of at least one new lesion, respectively. White matter hyperintensities progression will be rated by means of the visual Rotterdam Progression Scale (score range from 0 to 9) [26]. Absence or presence of progression (0 or 1, respectively) will be rated in three periventricular regions (frontal caps, occipital caps, bands), four subcortical white matter regions (frontal, parietal, occipital, temporal), basal ganglia, and the infratentorial region. Post-processing and ratings will be centralized and performed by expert and reliable observers, blinded to clinical data.

2.7. *Secondary Endpoints*

Secondary endpoints will be:

1. Stroke occurrence (ischemic or hemorrhagic).
2. Considering data from medical history and available laboratory and imaging exams, new major cerebrovascular events will be recorded as ischemic or hemorrhagic strokes. Ischemic strokes will

be further categorized in subtypes according to the TOAST classification system [27]. Hemorrhagic strokes will be classified according to lesion type and location.

3. Progression of global functioning, cognitive, and motor performances.
4. Progression in cognitive status will be determined by the occurrence of a diagnosis of MCI or dementia, and defined according to performances on the comprehensive neuropsychological test battery (evaluated as normal or abnormal by means of national normative data), and functional status.
5. The change in global functional status will be based on the Activities of Daily Living and Instrumental Activities of Daily Living scales, and the worsened condition will be defined as the loss of at least one item (i.e., the patient became dependent for an item function that was preserved at baseline evaluation).
6. Motor status will be evaluated by means of the Short Physical Performance Battery. Based on the total score (range 0–12), at each visit individuals will be categorized as having normal (SPPB $\geq$ 11) or impaired mobility (SPPB $\leq$ 10), and variations in performance categories over time (baseline vs. 18 months) will be evaluated for each patient.

2.8. Statistical Analyses

Multivariate regression analyses will be performed in order to identify independent predictors of SVD and its progression. Among the variables of interest, apart from the clinical ones and those assessed by means of conventional MRI, special attention will be paid to the relationship with advanced neuroimaging features and circulating biological markers.

Cerebral SVD and its progression—particularly microbleeds, which are considered the main expression of a bleeding-prone state—will be studied as outcome variables in multivariate regression models, considering the independent effect of all relevant markers, including major vascular risk factors and anticoagulant treatment with different types of anticoagulants (vitamin K antagonists vs. direct thrombin antagonists or factor Xa antagonists), and circulating biomarkers.

Interactions of circulating biomarkers with imaging markers, and types of oral anticoagulants will also be analyzed. Bonferroni correction will be applied in multivariate models to counteract the problem of multiple comparisons.

The multivariable prediction of the risk of SVD progression in this cohort of AF patients on oral anticoagulants will be studied as the methodological background for clinical research in the setting of stroke prevention in patients with AF (i.e., for designing and sample sizing studies potentially adopting the above indicated biomarkers as surrogate markers of the clinical outcomes).

3. Results

Starting from September 2017 until March 2019, 617 patients referring to the outpatient clinic of the Center of Thrombosis for oral anticoagulants therapy control were screened for inclusion in the study. As shown in Figure 1, 423 patients (68%) were excluded because of MRI contraindications (n = 227) or refusal (n = 196). The remaining 194 patients were enrolled. Demographic and clinical characteristics of the baseline sample are shown in Table 2: mean age was 78.1 ± 6.7 (range 65–97) years, 118 (61%) were males, and mean education was 9.1 ± 4.3 (range 2–19) years. The type of AF was paroxysmal in 93 patients (48%), and persistent or permanent in the remaining patients. Concerning the type of oral anticoagulant, 57 patients (29%) were on vitamin K antagonists, and 137 (71%) were on direct oral anticoagulants. Follow-up clinical evaluation and brain MR are ongoing.

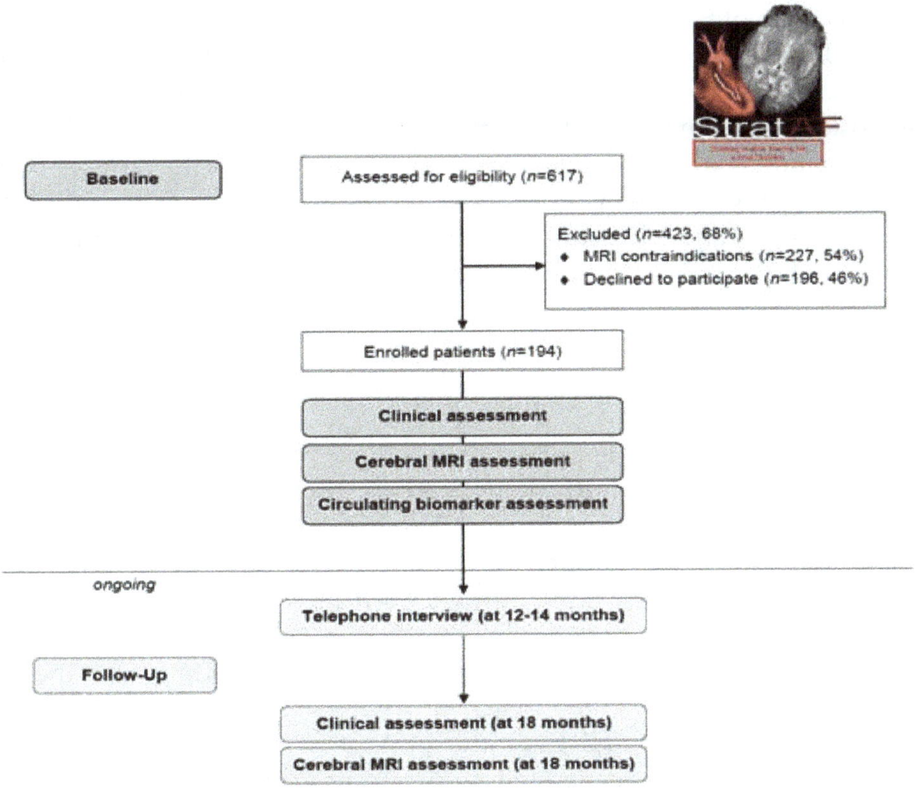

Figure 1. Strat-AF flow diagram.

Table 2. Baseline sample demographic and clinical characteristics.

	Min–Max	Baseline Sample $n = 194$
Age, years (mean ± SD)	65–97	78.1 ± 6.7
Years of education	2–19	9.1 ± 4.3
Sex (% males)	-	61% ($n = 118$)
Hypertension	-	82% ($n = 159$)
Hypercholesterolemia	-	48% ($n = 94$)
Diabetes	-	13% ($n = 25$)
Smoking habits	-	61% ($n = 119$)
History of stroke	-	22% ($n = 42$)
Alcohol consumption	-	51% ($n = 100$)
Paroxysmal AF	-	48% ($n = 93$)
Type of oral anticoagulant		
Vitamin K antagonists	-	29% ($n = 57$)
Direct oral anticoagulants	-	71% ($n = 137$)

4. Discussion

The Strat-AF study is an ongoing, single-center, longitudinal observation study evaluating elderly patients with AF on oral anticoagulation for primary or secondary prevention of stroke. The project foresees, in consecutive elderly patients with AF attending the Center for Thrombosis outpatient clinic of Careggi University Hospital for management of oral anticoagulation therapy, the implementation of a comprehensive neurological, neuropsychological, and functional evaluation together with blood sample collection for the determination of circulating biological markers (in relation to the hemorrhagic risk profile) and brain MRI for the determination of brain parenchyma lesions as surrogate markers of a bleeding-prone state. The Strat-AF cohort will allow the evaluation of the possible role of biological markers, including clinical, circulating, and neuroimaging-based, and their interaction, on the prediction of bleeding risk in AF patients under treatment with any type of oral anticoagulant.

Neuroimaging biomarkers of SVD, particularly microbleeds, will be tested as a selective surrogate marker of such complication. Circulating biomarkers assessed together with imaging might further improve the predictive potentials. Active enrollment started from September 2017 and ended in March 2019. The baseline study cohort included 194 elderly patients. Follow-up assessments are now ongoing.

One first major comment arises from the fact that in order to reach the number of enrolled patients, more than 600 patients had to be screened. Of these, more than half were excluded. Main reasons for exclusion were refusal (46%) and MRI contraindications (54%). Thus, the method under evaluation (i.e., brain MRI) will not be feasible for all AF patients, but just for those without contraindication. According to our experience, about one-quarter of patients would not be included in such a new stratification risk schema.

Overall, the study protocol seems feasible, and nearly all included patients completed the evaluation.

Our results will provide a unique opportunity to achieve preliminary data about SVD progression as a surrogate marker of the effect of antithrombotic treatments used for stroke prevention in patients with AF. The longitudinal design of the study may also provide clues about the possible association of SVD and its progression with clinical endpoints. Thrombo-embolic and bleeding risk will be assessed using the clinical risk scores CHADS2VASC2 and HAS-BLED respectively. Such predictive models will be completed studying the effect of neuroimaging features, particularly those related to SVD, and circulating biological markers, in order to provide preliminary knowledge about the incremental value of such markers.

Conclusive evidence about the predictive value of these markers in single patients can only come from adequately powered large prospective follow-up studies, and few efforts are already under way. Prospective multicenter studies such as the CROMIS 2 (clinical relevance of microbleeds in stroke; ClinicalTrials.gov Identifier NCT02513316), ICH because of oral anticoagulants: prediction of the risk by MRI (HERO, Hirulog Early Reperfusion/Occlusion Trial; ClinicalTrials.gov Identifier NCT02238470), and CMB-NOW (CMBs during NOACs or warfarin therapy in non-valvular AF patients with acute ischemic stroke; ClinicalTrials.gov Identifier NCT02356432) are ongoing. Main results from CROMIS-2 have been recently published: among the 1490 patients with AF enrolled after their ischemic stroke, the presence of CMBs significantly increased the risk of symptomatic ICH (adjusted hazard ratio 3.67, 95% CI 1.27–10.60), confirming that CMBs are independently associated with symptomatic ICH risk, and could be used to inform anti-coagulation decisions. In this study, after 24 months of follow-up, 14 patients had an intracerebral hemorrhage. The very low number of events did not allow the establishment of whether a CMBs threshold exists. Moreover, the study does not foresee a control MRI, so no information is available concerning the possible role of CMBs progression. A recent meta-analysis assessed the association between CMBs and future ICH risk in ischemic stroke patients with AF taking oral anticoagulants. The authors concluded that the presence of CMBs on MRI and the dichotomized cutoff of ≥5 CMBs might identify subgroups of patients with high ICH risk [28], but these data need to be confirmed before they can be used in clinical practice.

5. Conclusions

Long-term oral anticoagulation is the mainstay therapy for ischemic stroke prevention in patients with AF. Available stroke and bleeding risk stratification schemes are aimed at identifying patients who may benefit most from oral anticoagulation [29]. Such schemes (e.g., CHADS2VASC2, HAS-BLED scores) currently rely only on clinical information, the validity of which remains controversial and needs to be improved. Attempts have been made to refine the risk stratification scores by the addition of various biomarkers (blood, urine, cardiac, and cerebral imaging), but data are still inconclusive as to whether the costs are justified [30].

The Strat-AF study may be an essential step towards the exploration of the role of a combined clinical biomarker or multiple biomarker models in predicting stroke risk in AF, and might sustain the incorporation of such new markers in the existing stroke prediction schemes by the demonstration of a greater incremental value in predicting stroke risk and improvement in clinical outcomes in a cost-effective fashion.

Author Contributions: Conceptualization, A.P., F.C., S.D., B.G., A.M.G., R.M., E.S.; methodology, A.P., F.C., S.C., S.D., B.G., A.M.G., G.P., E.F., R.M., E.S.; formal analysis, A.P., G.P., E.S.; investigation, A.P., C.B., F.G., E.C., S.G., C.M., A.M., D.M., V.R., E.F., R.M., E.S.; data curation, A.P., G.P., E.S.; writing—original draft preparation, A.P., C.B., F.G., E.S.; writing—review and editing, A.P., C.B., F.G., E.C., F.C., S.C., S.D., S.G., B.G., A.M.G., A.M., D.M., F.P., G.P., V.R., C.S., E.F., R.M., E.S.; supervision, A.P.; project administration, A.P., F.C., S.D., F.P, R.M., E.S.; funding acquisition, A.P., F.C., S.D., F.P, E.S.

Acknowledgments: The authors would like to thank Graziella Terranova and the staff of Careggi office for the administrative support.

References

1. Haeusler, K.G.; Wilson, D.; Fiebach, J.B.; Kirchhof, P.; Werring, D.J. Brain MRI to personalise atrial fibrillation therapy: Current evidence and perspectives. *Heart* **2014**, *100*, 1408–1413. [CrossRef]
2. Inzitari, D. Leukoaraiosis: An independent risk factor for stroke? *Stroke* **2003**, *34*, 2067–2071. [CrossRef] [PubMed]
3. Kirchhof, P.; Breithardt, G.; Aliot, E.; Al Khatib, S.; Apostolakis, S.; Auricchio, A.; Bailleul, C.; Bax, J.; Benninger, G.; Blomstrom-Lundqvist, C.; et al. Personalized management of atrial fibrillation: Proceedings from the fourth Atrial Fibrillation competence NETwork/European Heart Rhythm Association consensus conference. *Europace* **2013**, *15*, 1540–1556. [CrossRef] [PubMed]
4. Vílchez, J.A.; Roldán, V.; Hernández-Romero, D.; Valdés, M.; Lip, G.Y.; Marín, F. Biomarkers in atrial fibrillation: An overview. *Int. J. Clin. Pract.* **2014**, *68*, 434–443. [CrossRef] [PubMed]
5. Wardlaw, J.M.; Smith, E.E.; Biessels, G.J.; Cordonnier, C.; Fazekas, F.; Frayne, R.; Lindley, R.I.; O'Brien, J.T.; Barkhof, F.; Benavente, O.R.; et al. Neuroimaging standards for research into small vessel disease and its contribution to ageing and neurodegeneration. *Lancet Neurol.* **2013**, *12*, 822–838. [CrossRef]
6. Wilson, D.; Charidimou, A.; Werring, D.J. Use of MRI for risk stratification in anticoagulation decision making in atrial fibrillation: promising, but more data are needed for a robust algorithm. *Front. Neurol.* **2014**, *5*, 3. [CrossRef] [PubMed]
7. Charidimou, A.; Shakeshaft, C.; Werring, D.J. Cerebral microbleeds on magnetic resonance imaging and anticoagulant-associated intracerebral hemorrhage risk. *Front. Neurol.* **2012**, *3*, 133. [CrossRef] [PubMed]
8. Fisher, M. MRI screening for chronic anticoagulation in atrial fibrillation. *Front. Neurol.* **2013**, *4*, 137. [CrossRef]
9. Katz, S.; Ford, A.B.; Moskowitz, R.W.; Jackson, B.A.; Jaffe, M.W. Studies of illness in the aged. The index of ADL: A standardized measure of biological and psychosocial function. *JAMA* **1963**, *185*, 914–919. [CrossRef]
10. Lawton, M.P.; Brody, E.M. Assessment of older people: Self-maintaining and instrumental activities of daily living. *Gerontologist* **1969**, *9*, 179–186. [CrossRef]
11. Yesavage, J.A. Geriatric depression scale. *Psychopharmacol. Bull.* **1988**, *24*, 709–711. [PubMed]
12. Guralnik, J.M.; Simonsick, E.M.; Ferrucci, L.; Glynn, R.J.; Berkman, L.F.; Blazer, D.G.; Scherr, P.A.; Wallace, R.B. A short physical performance battery assessing lower extremity function: Association with self-reported disability and prediction of mortality and nursing home admission. *J. Gerontol.* **1994**, *49*, 85–94. [CrossRef] [PubMed]
13. Johns, M.W. A new method for measuring daytime sleepiness: The Epworth sleepiness scale. *Sleep* **1991**, *14*, 540–545. [CrossRef] [PubMed]
14. Rabin, R.; de Charro, F. EQ-5D: A measure of health status from the EuroQol Group. *Ann. Med.* **2001**, *33*, 337–343. [CrossRef] [PubMed]
15. Sofi, F.; Dinu, M.; Pagliai, G.; Marcucci, R.; Casini, A. Validation of a literature-based adherence score to Mediterranean diet: The MEDI-LITE score. *Int. J. Food Sci. Nutr.* **2017**, *68*, 757–762. [CrossRef] [PubMed]
16. Nasreddine, Z.S.; Phillips, N.A.; Bédirian, V.; Charbonneau, S.; Whitehead, V.; Collin, I.; Cummings, J.L.; Chertkow, H. The Montreal Cognitive Assessment, MoCA: A brief screening tool for mild cognitive impairment. *J. Am. Geriatr. Soc.* **2005**, *53*, 695–699. [CrossRef] [PubMed]

17. Hachinski, V.; Iadecola, C.; Petersen, R.C.; Breteler, M.M.; Nyenhuis, D.L.; Black, S.E.; Powers, W.J.; DeCarli, C.; Merino, J.G.; Kalaria, R.N.; et al. National institute of neurological disorders and stroke-Canadian stroke network vascular cognitive impairment harmonization standards. *Stroke* **2006**, *37*, 2220–2241. [CrossRef]
18. Conti, S.; Bonazzi, S.; Laiacona, M.; Masina, M.; Coralli, M.V. Montreal cognitive assessment (MoCA)-Italian version: Regression based norms and equivalent scores. *Neurol. Sci.* **2015**, *36*, 209–214. [CrossRef]
19. Carlesimo, G.A.; Caltagirone, C.; Gainotti, G. The mental deterioration battery: Normative data, diagnostic reliability and qualitative analyses of cognitive impairment. The group for the standardization of the mental deterioration battery. *Eur. Neurol.* **1996**, *36*, 378–384. [CrossRef]
20. Novelli, G.; Papagno, C.; Capitani, E.; Laiacona, M.; Cappa, S.F.; Vallar, G. Tre test clinici di memoria a lungo termine. *Arch. Psicol. Neurol. Psichiatr.* **1986**, *47*, 278–296.
21. Della Sala, S.; Laiacona, M.; Spinnler, H.; Ubezio, C. A cancellation test: Its reliability in assessing attentional deficit in Alzheimer's disease. *Psychol. Med.* **1992**, *22*, 885–901. [CrossRef]
22. Caffarra, P.; Vezzadini, G.; Dieci, F.; Zonato, F.; Venneri, A. Una versione abbreviata del test di Stroop. Dati normativi nella popolazione italiana. *Nuova Riv. Neurol.* **2002**, *12*, 111–115.
23. Novelli, G.; Papagno, C.; Capitani, E.; Laiacona, M. Tre test clinici di ricerca e produzione lessicale. Taratura su soggetti normali. *Arch. Psicol. Neurol. Psichiatr.* **1986**, *47*, 477–506.
24. Capitani, E.; Laiacona, M. Composite neuropsychological batteries and demographic correction: Standardization based on equivalent scores, with a review of published data. The Italian Group for the Neuropsychological Study of Ageing. *J. Clin. Exp. Neuropsychol.* **1997**, *19*, 795–809. [CrossRef]
25. Wiseman, S.J.; Meijboom, R.; Valdés Hernández, M.D.C.; Pernet, C.; Sakka, E.; Job, D.; Waldman, A.D.; Wardlaw, J.M. Longitudinal multi-centre brain imaging studies: Guidelines and practical tips for accurate and reproducible imaging endpoints and data sharing. *Trials* **2019**, *20*, 21. [CrossRef]
26. Schmidt, R.; Berghold, A.; Jokinen, H.; Gouw, A.A.; van der Flier, W.M.; Barkhof, F.; Scheltens, P.; Petrovic, K.; Madureira, S.; Verdelho, A.; et al. White matter lesion progression in LADIS: Frequency, clinical effects, and sample size calculations. *Stroke* **2012**, *43*, 2643–2647. [CrossRef]
27. Adams, H.P., Jr.; Bendixen, B.H.; Kappelle, L.J.; Biller, J.; Love, B.B.; Gordon, D.L.; Marsh, E.E. Classification of subtype of acute ischemic stroke. Definitions for use in a multicenter clinical trial. TOAST. Trial of Org 10172 in Acute Stroke Treatment. *Stroke* **1993**, *24*, 35–41. [CrossRef]
28. Charidimou, A.; Karayiannis, C.; Song, T.J.; Orken, D.N.; Thijs, V.; Lemmens, R.; Kim, J.; Goh, S.M.; Phan, T.G.; Soufan, C.; et al. Brain microbleeds, anticoagulation, and hemorrhage risk: Meta-analysis in stroke patients with AF. *Neurology* **2017**, *89*, 2317–2326. [CrossRef]
29. Lip, G.Y.; Lane, D.A. Stroke prevention in atrial fibrillation: A systematic review. *JAMA* **2015**, *313*, 1950–1962. [CrossRef]
30. Lip, G.Y. Stroke and bleeding risk assessment in atrial fibrillation: When, how, and why? *Eur. Heart J.* **2013**, *34*, 1041–1049. [CrossRef]

14

Left Atrial Function after Atrial Fibrillation Cryoablation Concomitant to Minimally Invasive Mitral Valve Repair

Matteo Anselmino [1,*], Chiara Rovera [2], Giovanni Marchetto [3], Davide Castagno [1], Mara Morello [1], Simone Frea [1], Fiorenzo Gaita [4], Mauro Rinaldi [3] and Gaetano Maria De Ferrari [1]

1. Division of Cardiology, "Città della Salute e della Scienza di Torino" Hospital, Department of Medical Sciences, University of Turin, 10124 Torino, Italy; davide.castagno@unito.it (D.C.); mara.morello@unito.it (M.M.); frea.simone@gmail.com (S.F.); gaetanomaria.deferrari@unito.it (G.M.D.F.)
2. Cardiology Unit, "Ospedale Civico", Chivasso, 10034 Torino, Italy; roverachiara@gmail.com
3. Division of Cardiac Surgery, "Città della Salute e della Scienza di Torino" Hospital, University of Turin, 10124 Torino, Italy; giovanni.marchetto@libero.it (G.M.); mauro.rinaldi@unito.it (M.R.)
4. Cardiology Department, Clinica Pinna Pintor, 10129 Torino, Italy; fiorenzo.gaita@unito.it

* Correspondence: matteo.anselmino@unito.it

Abstract: *Background and Objectives:* Surgical atrial fibrillation (AF) ablation concomitant to minimally invasive mitral valve repair has been proven to offer improved short- and long-term sinus rhythm (SR) maintenance compared to mitral valve surgery only. The objective of the present study was to explore, by thorough echocardiographic assessment, long-term morphological and functional left atrial (LA) outcomes after this combined surgical procedure. *Materials and Methods*: From October 2006 to November 2015, 48 patients underwent minimally invasive mitral valve repair and concomitant surgical AF cryoablation. *Results:* After 3.8 ± 2.2 years, 30 (71.4%) of those completing the follow-up (n = 42, 87.5%) presented SR. During follow-up, four (9.5%) patients suffered from cerebrovascular accidents and two of these subjects had a long-standing persistent AF relapse and were in AF at the time of the event, while the other two were in SR. An echocardiographic study focused on LA characteristics was performed in 29 patients (69.0%). Atrial morphology and function (e.g., maximal LA volume indexed to body surface area and total LA emptying fraction derived from volumes) in patients with stable SR (60.6 ± 13.1 mL/mq and 25.1 ± 7.3%) were significantly better than in those with AF relapses (76.8 ± 16.2 mL/mq and 17.5 ± 7.4%; respectively, p = 0.008 and p = 0.015). At follow-up, patients who suffered from ischemic cerebral events had maximal LA volume indexed to body surface area 61 ± 17.8 mL/mq, with total LA emptying fraction derived from volumes 23.6 ± 13.7%; patients with strokes in SR showed very enlarged LA volume (>70 mL/mq). *Conclusions*: AF cryoablation concomitant with minimally invasive mitral valve repair provides a high rate of SR maintenance and this relates to improved long-term morphological and functional LA outcomes. Further prospective studies are needed to define the cut-off values determining an increase in the risk for thromboembolic complications in patients with restored stable SR.

Keywords: atrial fibrillation; surgical cryoablation; left atrial function; minimally invasive mitral valve repair; echocardiography; ischemic cerebral events

1. Introduction

Atrial fibrillation (AF) prevalence in patients with indication for mitral valve surgery is about 30–54% [1], it has a strong impact on hemodynamics [2], and it has been demonstrated to significantly affect the mortality rate [3,4].

Concomitant surgical AF ablation to video-assisted minimally invasive mitral valve surgery (MIMVS) [5–7] has been proven to offer improved short- and long-term sinus rhythm (SR) maintenance compared to patients undergoing mitral valve surgery only (73% versus 43% of SR maintenance at 12 months' follow-up) [8] without increasing complications [9,10].

Therefore, SR maintenance seems achievable, but does this reflect in an improved atrial function? It has been demonstrated that SR maintenance is related to reduced left atrial volumes [11], but little is known about left atrial (LA) functional properties in this clinical setting. In fact, an organized atrial activity is not always accompanied by an effective mechanical atrial contraction [12].

In patients with underlying mitral valve diseases, atrial remodeling is remarkable: longstanding volume overload to the LA results in chronic stretching and atrophy of atrial myocytes, interstitial fibrosis, overall thinning, and dilatation of the LA wall, which may relate to functional alterations despite the underling electrical activity.

To date, however, it remains unknown to which degree "the residual atrial function" after a successful AF ablation predicts clinical outcome. For example, which level of contractility is required to avoid the increased thromboembolic risk of a "static" LA, despite SR?

The aim of the present study was therefore to describe, by a thorough echocardiographic assessment, long term LA morphology and function in patients submitted to surgical ablation of persistent/long-term persistent AF concomitant to MIMVS.

2. Materials and Methods

2.1. Surgical Procedure

According to current guidelines, patients referred to our Cardiac Surgery Division for mitral valve disease and AF resistant to antiarrhythmic therapy, when technically feasible, were proposed video-assisted MIMVS via right mini-thoracotomy through the fourth intercostal space and concomitant left sided AF cryoablation. All enrolled patients were retrospectively identified, starting since October 2006. Patients that had already performed a cardiac surgical procedure or a previous transcatheter AF ablation were not included in this series. Each patient in our study signed a written informed consent for inclusion. The study was conducted in accordance with the Declaration of Helsinki, was observational and retrospective, did not add treatment or modify conventional surgical procedure for the specific clinical indication and was approved by the local Institutional Review Board (Project Identification "CryoMIMS—Concomitant Cryoablation to Video-assisted Minimally INvasive Mitral Valve Surgery", code 9718; date of approval 1 February 2016).

Surgical technique has already been described [13].

Concomitant left sided AF cryoablation (Argon based Cryomaze, Cryoflex Medtronic, Minneapolis, MN, USA) consisted of isolation of the pulmonary veins (PVs) and of the posterior LA wall between the veins by a "U" encircling cryolesion connected to the surgical paraseptal LA incision performed for mitral exposure, eventually creating the so-called "box lesion". In addition, a linear cryolesion was performed from the previously created box lesion to the mitral valve annulus to block conduction across the left atrial isthmus ("mitral line") [6,14]. The surgical procedure performed was the same in every patient included in the study.

2.2. Echocardiographic Analysis

Complete echocardiographic assessment was performed in patients undergoing mitral valve repair by the MIMVS approach and concomitant left sided AF cryoablation. The echocardiographic assessment was performed at 4.0 ± 2.1 years after the surgical procedure. Subjects who underwent mitral valve replacement with biological or mechanical prosthesis were excluded due to distortions related to the presence of the prosthetic scaffold.

Echocardiographic scans were performed by a Philips ultrasound system (iE33 xMATRIX, Andover, MA, USA) with S5-1 sector array probe and X3-1 3D probe. All the examinations were carried out by the same operator. Standard measurements were computed based on the American Society of Echocardiography guidelines. Maximum left atrial diameter (LAD max), minimum (LAD min) and at the beginning of atrial contraction (LAD pre-A) antero-posterior diameters were measured in the parasternal long axis view by either B-mode or M-mode technique (Figure 1A).

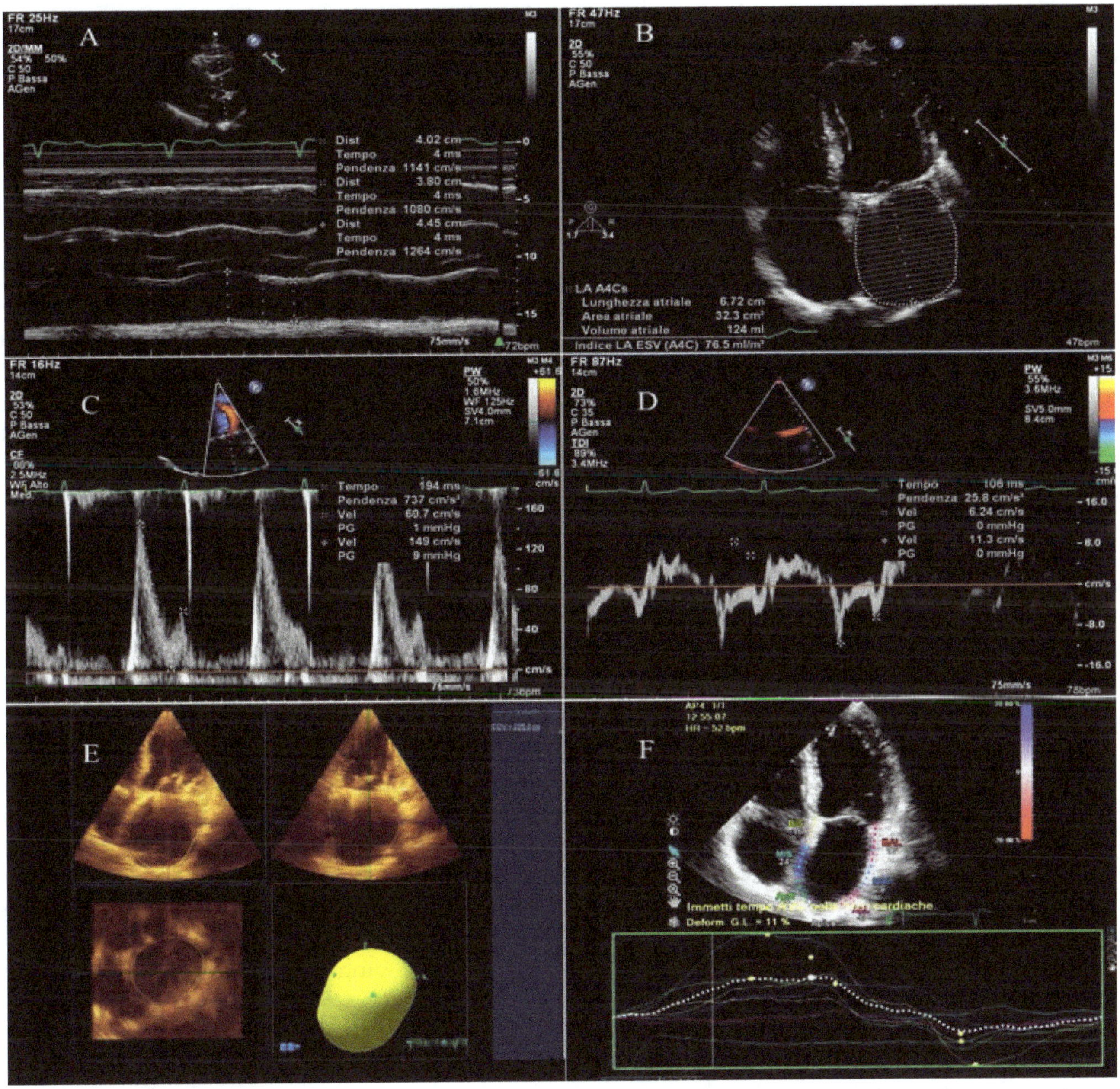

Figure 1. Echocardiographic evaluation of left atrial function: (**A**) measurement of antero-posterior diameters; (**B**) evaluations of areas and volumes and measurement of maximum supero-inferior diameter; (**C**) measurement of transmitral peak velocity of the late filling wave (A wave); (**D**) measurement of lateral mitral annulus peak velocity related to atrial contraction (a' wave) and evaluation of atrial conduction delay; (**E**) calculation of maximum 3D volume; (**F**) evaluation of global longitudinal atrial strain.

The apical four chamber view was used to measure maximum left atrial supero-inferior diameter (Figure 1B).

The left atrial volumes were evaluated by modified Simpson's method using the apical four chamber view at the tele-systolic frame preceding the mitral valve opening (maximum volume, LAV max), at the tele-diastolic frame preceding mitral valve closure (minimum volume, LAV min), and at the beginning of the P wave for the subjects not in AF at the moment of the exam (pre A volume, LAV pre-A) (Figure 1B).

Volumes were subsequently indexed on the body surface area.

From the above-mentioned linear measurements and volumes, the following parameters defining different components of LA function were calculated:

- Left atrial active emptying fraction, related to the LA booster pump function;
- Left atrial passive emptying fraction, describing the LA conduit function;
- Left atrial total emptying fraction, defining the LA reservoir function.

Similarly, the LA areas (maximal, minimal, and at the beginning of the P wave) were measured (Figure 1B). The LA ejection fraction was calculated from maximal and minimal areas, being reduced if ≤45% [15].

Left atrial 3D maximum volume was calculated using the QLAB-3D Quantification (3DQ) Advanced application (Figure 1E).

The transmitral flow velocity was measured by pulsed Doppler echocardiography. Peak velocity of the early filling wave (E wave) and of the late filling wave (A wave) were determined (Figure 1C), considering a peak A wave velocity ≥10 cm/s an indicator of the presence of some atrial contraction [16].

The lateral and septal mitral annulus peak velocities related to early relaxation (e' wave) and to atrial contraction (a' wave) were evaluated by tissue Doppler imaging (TDI, Figure 1D). A TDI a' ≤7 cm/s was considered an index of anomalous LA active contractile function [17].

Furthermore, atrial conduction time was measured: the PA-TDI interval was calculated, defined as the time interval between the beginning of the P wave and the TDI a' wave (Figure 1D). The standard deviation of PA-TDI measurements performed on all segments was also calculated for every single patient.

Eventually, LA global longitudinal strain by two-dimensional speckle tracking was calculated for every patient by QLAB CMQ Cardiac Motion Quantification (Figure 1F).

2.3. *Clinical Follow-Up and Event Definition*

After discharge patients were followed by outpatient visits, including clinical examinations and ECG at 3, 6, and 12 months and then yearly. At least once a year, 24 h ECG Holter monitoring was performed. In case of symptoms recurrence between follow-up visits, patients were reassessed by clinical examination, ECG, and Holter monitoring. Electrophysiological study and transcatheter AF ablation were performed when indicated. All patients in the study were followed for at least six months.

A blanking period of three months was considered; following this interval any AF episode, persistent or paroxysmal, was accounted as an event.

2.4. *Statistical Analysis*

Categorical variables are reported as counts and percentages, while continuous variables as means and standard deviations (SDs). Correlations between parameters and study groups were tested in cross tabulation tables by means of the Pearson Chi-Square or Fisher's exact test and by one-way ANOVA, respectively, for categorical and continuous variables. McNemar's test was used on paired categorical variables. Kaplan Meier curves were computed to describe AF free survival over time. A two-sided p-value < 0.05 was considered statistically significant; all analyses were performed on SPSS 20.0 (IBM Corp., Armonk, NY, USA).

3. Results

From October 2006 to November 2015, 48 patients were submitted to minimally invasive mitral valve repair and concomitant AF cryoablation. The baseline characteristics of the study population are listed in Table 1.

Table 1. Preoperative characteristics of the study population stratified by AF relapses at follow-up. (AF, atrial fibrillation; AP, antero-posterior; BMI, body mass index; BSA, body surface area; COPD, chronic obstructive pulmonary disease; LS, long-standing; MV, mitral valve; NYHA, New York Heart Association functional class; PAPs, systolic pulmonary artery pressure; SI, supero-inferior; SR, sinus rhythm; TV, tricuspid valve).

	N = 48	AF Relapse (N = 12/42 28.6%)	SR Maintenance (N = 30/42 71.4%)	*p*-Value
Age (years)	67.7 ± 9.8	69.0 ± 6.9	66.7 ± 11.3	0.516
Male gender (N,%)	31 (64.6%)	5 (41.7%)	20 (66.7%)	0.127
NYHA class ≥III (N,%)	31 (64.6%)	10 (83.3%)	17 (56.7%)	0.054
BSA (mq)	1.8 ± 0.19	1.78 ± 0.21	1.82 ± 0.19	0.502
Obesity (BMI > 30) (N,%)	14 (29.2%)	4 (33.3%)	9 (30.0%)	0.619
COPD (N,%)	8 (16.7%)	2 (16.7%)	5 (16.7%)	0.615
Hypertension (N,%)	32 (66.7%)	9 (75.0%)	21 (70.0%)	0.496
Diabetes (N,%)	5 (10.4%)	1 (8.3%)	4 (13.3%)	0.488
Dysthyroidism (N,%)	11 (22.9%)	2 (16.7%)	9 (30.0%)	0.231
Previous cerebrovascular accidents (N,%)	5 (10.4%)	1 (8.3%)	4 (13.3%)	0.488
CHADS2 score	2.29 ± 1.17	2.12 ± 0.93	2.33 ± 1.27	0.542
CHA2DS2VASc score	3.41 ± 1.52	3.47 ± 1.28	3.37 ± 1.63	0.825
Antiarrhythmic therapy at the time of surgery (N,%)	17 (35.4%)	5 (41.7%)	12 (40.0%)	0.473
Type of AF				
Paroxysmal (N,%)	7 (14.6%)	0 (0.0%)	7 (23.3%)	0.001
Persitent/LS persistent (N%)	40 (83.3%)	12 (100%)	22 (73.3%)	
AF duration (days)	1077.6 ± 2052.4	1317.9 ± 2406.3	550.4 ± 849.9	0.127
Left ventricular ejection fraction (%)	57.1 ± 10.5	57.5 ± 10.1	57.6 ± 11.0	0.984
Etiology of MV disease				
Degenerative	32 (66.7%)	7 (58.3%)	22 (73.3%)	0.289
Rheumatic	1 (2.1%)	1 (8.3%)	0 (0.0%)	
Functional	13 (27.1%)	4 (33.3%)	6 (20.0%)	
Left atrial AP diameter (mm)	50.9 ± 10.0	51.1 ± 7.0	51.8 ± 12.1	0.899
Left atrial SI diameter (mm)	65.5 ± 9.1	68.3 ± 10.4	66.6 ± 8.1	0.754
PAPs (mmHg)	43.2 ± 14.1	42.9 ± 12.0	44.1 ± 15.8	0.822

Twenty (41.7%) patients underwent simple valve repair while 28 (58.3%) were submitted to complex valve repair. Seven subjects (14.6%) received concomitant tricuspid valve surgery. Only one procedure was electively converted to full sternotomy (2.1%) due to unexpected severe pleural adhesions. Total clamp time was 99.5 ± 25.6 min. There was no reopening for any cause.

About one third of the study population (18, 37.5%) suffered AF relapses during hospitalization, while 39 (81.3%) patients were discharged in SR. One patient (2.1%) required PM implantation in the subacute phase. Early mortality was 2.1% (one patient died due to respiratory complications following cardiac arrest resuscitated in the ward).

By April 2016, 42 (87.5%) patients completed the follow-up after a mean of 3.8 ± 2.2 years from the procedure. The study flow chart is depicted in Figure 2.

Except the patient who died few days after surgery, the remaining four deaths were not due to cardiovascular causes.

In this time frame no patient required redo surgery.

NYHA functional class showed a significant improvement (NYHA ≥ 3 patients decreased from 64.6% pre-surgery to 4.8% at follow-up, $p < 0.001$). Three (7.1%) patients required PM implantation during follow-up.

Thirty patients (71.4%) maintained SR throughout the follow-up. Out of the 12 (28.6%) patients suffering AF relapses, three (25%) had paroxysmal episodes, while nine (75%) developed persistent AF (Figure 2). Five (41.7%) patients relapsed with an atypical atrial flutter, while the remaining seven (58.3%) as AF. Out of all patients, one patient (8.3%) suffered symptomatic recurrences and was referred for electrophysiological study and transcatheter redo ablation. Following transcatheter ablation he relapsed with an asymptomatic focal atrial tachycardia. A total of 16 (38%) patients were on antiarrhythmic therapy at follow-up; this percentage did not significantly vary between patients maintaining SR (10, 33%) or suffering AF relapses (6, 50%; $p = 0.315$). Oral anticoagulation was discontinued, instead, in 16 patients (53%) maintaining stable SR at the follow-up end, whereas it was continued in all the patients with documentation of AF relapses.

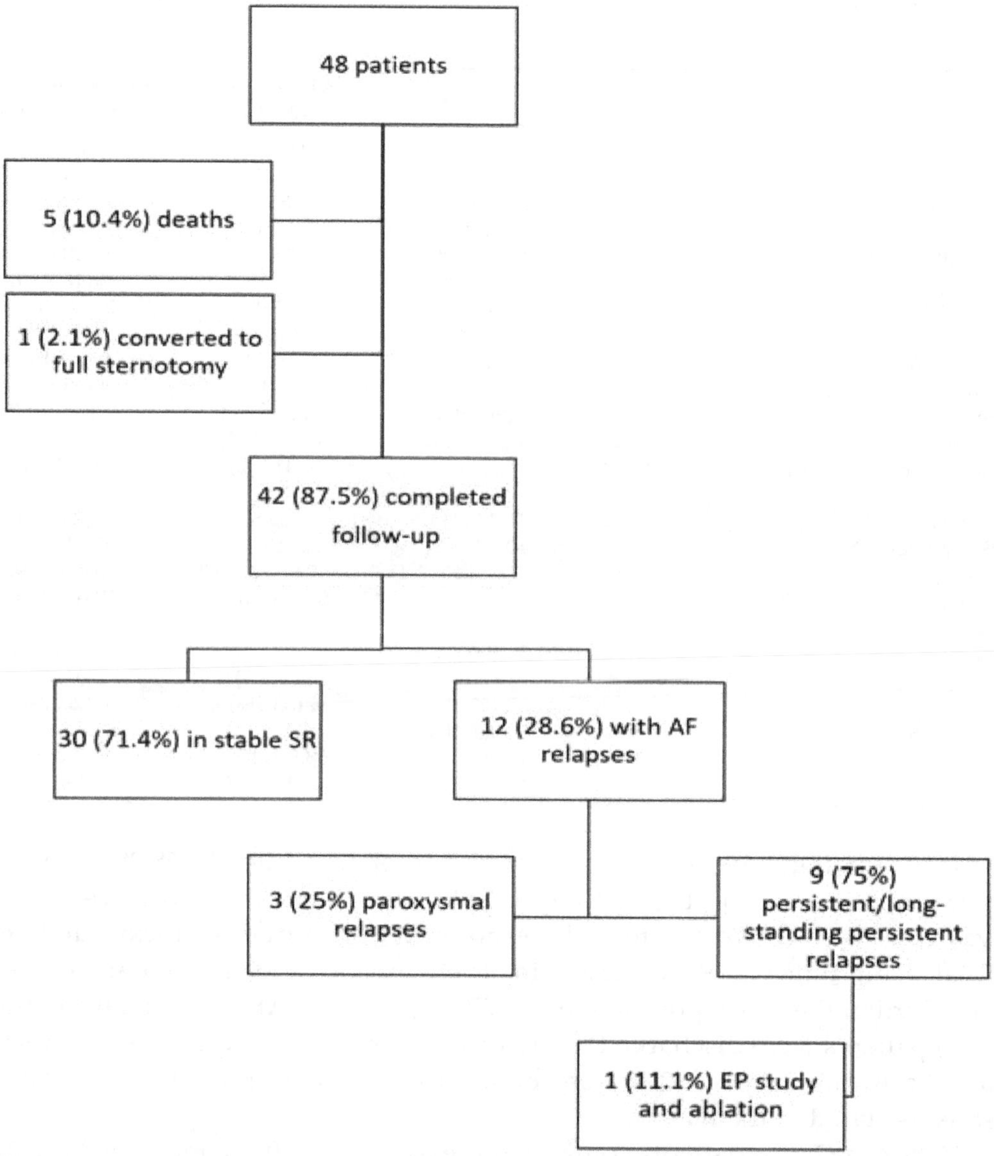

Figure 2. Study flow chart. AF: atrial fibrillation; EP: electrophysiological; SR: sinus rhythm.

Freedom from arrhythmias is reported in Figure 3, showing a 91.7% one-year freedom from AF relapses.

During follow-up, four (9.5%) patients suffered from cerebrovascular accidents; two of these subjects had a long-standing persistent AF relapse and were in AF at the time of the event, while the other two were in SR.

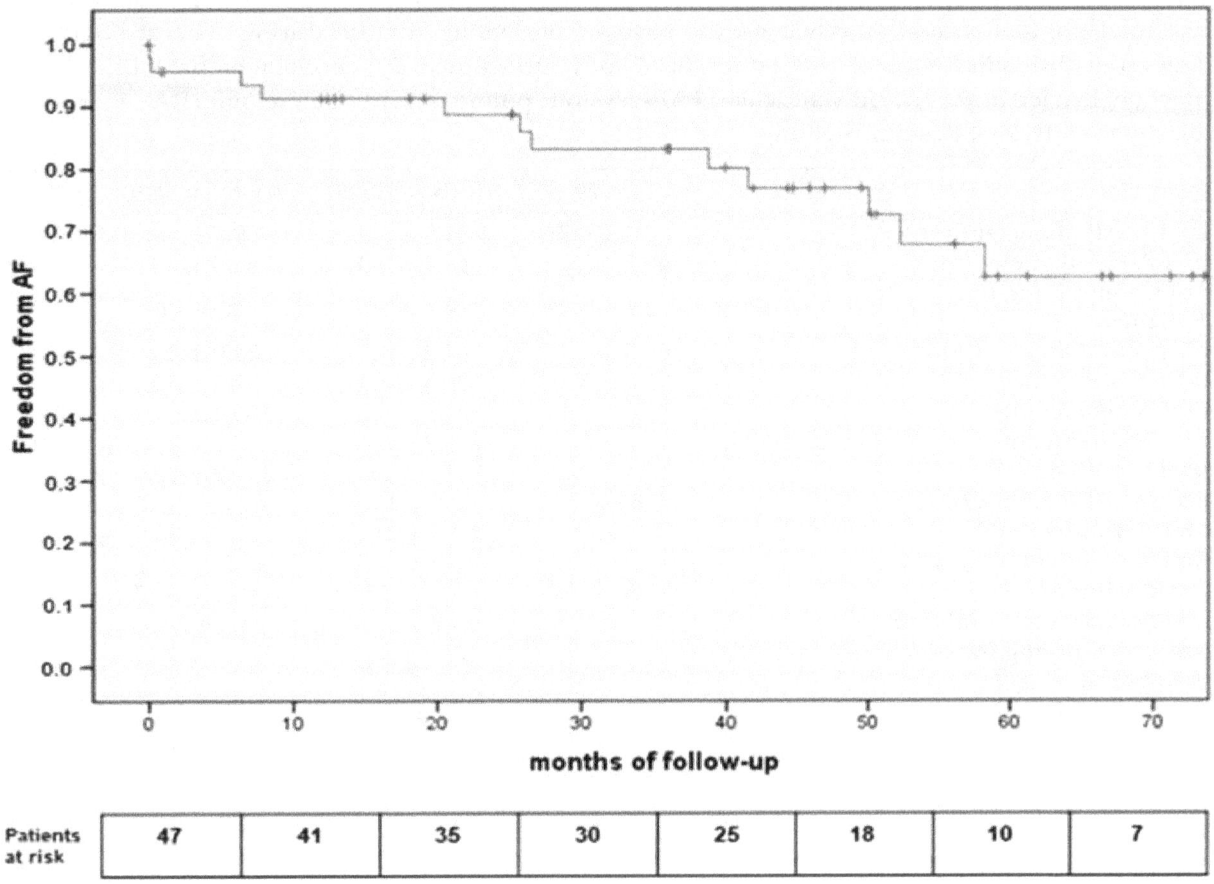

Figure 3. Kaplan Meier curves for freedom from AF relapses.

Thorough LA morphology and function was assessed at follow-up within 29 patients (69.0%) treated by mitral repair; out of the other 19 patients submitted to mitral valve repair who did not undergo the LA focused echocardiographic evaluation, one (2.1%) was converted to full sternotomy, five (10.4%) died (two of cancer, two of other non-cardiac causes, and only one due to respiratory complications following cardiac arrest), and the remaining 13 patients (27.1%) were contacted only by telephone or fax, owing to problems of access due to long distances between the medical center and the patients' residences, being our hospital a reference center for surgery.

Among the 29 patients, four (13.8%) had paroxysmal AF, whereas 25 (86.2%) had persistent/long-standing persistent AF at baseline.

In this subset, 22 patients (75.9%) presented a good outcome of mitral repair with a residual mitral regurgitation absent or trivial in 15 subjects (68.2%) and mild in seven (31.8%).

At the moment of the echocardiographic scan, 22 subjects (75.9%) were in SR, while six (20.7%) were in atrial fibrillation/atypical atrial flutter, and one (3.4%) presented an atrial paced rhythm. At univariate analysis the residual mitral regurgitation did not relate to AF relapses ($p = 0.103$).

Table 2 shows details concerning all measurements and functional parameters stratified by heart rhythm at the time of the echo scan. Patients suffering relapses reported more enlarged left atria and more significantly impaired LA function.

Similar trends emerged, as shown in Table 3, if measurements and functional parameters were stratified by heart rhythm during follow-up: 20 (69.0%) SR and nine (31.0%) AF recurrences.

Table 2. Echocardiographic parameters and atrial functional evaluations, expressed as mean of the total population and stratified on the basis of presenting rhythm during echocardiography. (AF, atrial fibrillation; AP, antero-posterior; BSA, body surface area; DT, deceleration time; EF, ejection fraction; LA, left atrial; LV, left ventricular; PAPs, systolic pulmonary arterial pressure; RA, right atrial; SI, supero-inferior; SR, sinus rhythm).

	N = 29	SR (N = 22/29)	AF (N = 6/29)	*p*-Value
Max LA AP diameter (mm)	53.4 ± 6.7	51.5 ± 5.9	59.8 ± 6.0	0.018
Min LA AP diameter (mm)	46.7 ± 7.2	44.4 ± 6.0	55.0 ± 5.1	0.002
Total LA emptying fraction derived from AP diameters (%)	12.7 ± 4.4	14.1 ± 4.1	8.0 ± 1.6	0.006
Max LA SI diameter (mm)	68.3 ± 5.4	67.2 ± 4.6	74.0 ± 3.7	0.003
Max LA area (cmq)	31.8 ± 5.2	30.4 ± 4.3	37.3 ± 5.5	0.010
Min LA area (cmq)	27.0 ± 5.1	25.3 ± 3.8	33.4 ± 4.8	0.001
LA ejection fraction derived from areas (%)	15.5 ± 5.4	16.7 ± 5.3	10.5 ± 2.8	0.028
Max LA volume (mL)	120.4 ± 32.6	111.5 ± 25.9	152.8 ± 39.0	0.016
Max LA volume/BSA (mL/mq)	65.6 ± 15.8	60.9 ± 12.5	80.7 ± 18.2	0.010
Min LA volume (mL)	93.5 ± 28.7	84.4 ± 21.1	127.7 ± 30.9	0.002
Min LA volume/BSA (mL/mq)	60.0 ± 14.5	46.2 ± 11.2	67.5 ± 14.4	0.002
3D LA volume (mL)	111.6 ± 38.2	100.2 ± 25.5	158.1 ± 51.7	0.005
3D LA volume/BSA (mL/mq)	61.1 ± 18.9	54.9 ± 12.4	84.0 ± 24.9	0.003
Total LA emptying fraction derived from volumes (%)	22.7 ± 8.0	24.4 ± 7.9	16.0 ± 5.7	0.061
Global longitudinal LA strain (%)	8.5 ± 3.8	9.7 ± 3.6	5.2 ± 1.7	0.013
E wave (cm/s)	137.2 ± 23.7	136.4 ± 25.8	143.5 ± 14.4	0.552
A wave (cm/s)	56.2 ± 19.8	57.1 ± 19.8		0.286
Inferior septal a′ wave (cm/s)	5.8 ± 2.0	5.9 ± 2.0		0.508
Lateral a′ wave (cm/s)	4.5 ± 1.6	4.6 ± 1.6		0.356
Averaged a′ wave (cm/s)	5.2 ± 1.5	5.2 ± 1.5		0.352
P-lateral a′ wave interval (ms)	110.6 ± 31.9	110.3 ± 32.7		0.866
LV EF (%)	57.3 ± 8.0	57.9 ± 6.8	53.8 ± 11.7	0.352
PAPs (mmHg)	37.7 ± 9.4	37.0 ± 9.6	38.2 ± 9.4	0.479

Table 3 points out the markedly enlarged dimensions of the LA, compared to healthy subjects [18], also in patients who maintained SR during the follow-up: the maximum anteroposterior diameter was 51.4 ± 6.2 mm (versus normal values of <41 mm); the maximum indexed volume 60.6 ± 13.1 mL/mq (versus normal values of 22 ± 6 mL/mq); the minimum indexed volume 45.4 ± 10.9 mL/mq (versus normal values of 11 ± 4 mL/mq); the preA indexed volume 51.3 ± 11.6 mL/mq (versus normal values of 15 ± 5 mL/mq); the maximum indexed 3D volume 56.2 ± 13.2 mL/mq (versus normal values of 15–41 mL/mq). However, these same parameter results significantly increased in patients suffering AF relapses at follow-up.

Similarly, SR patients showed a reduction in atrial function when compared to normal values of healthy controls (transmitral A wave velocity 54.7 ± 20.0 cm/s versus 80 ± 20 cm/s [19]; TDI lateral a′ wave 4.6 ± 1.7 cm/s, septal a′ wave 6.0 ± 2.0 cm/s, averaged a′ wave 5.3 ± 1.5 cm/s versus values >7.3 cm/s [17]; LA ejection fraction by areas 17.2 ± 5.0% versus 45% [15]; total emptying fraction by volumes 25.1 ± 7.3% versus normal values ranging from 45% to 65 ± 9% [18,20,21]; active and passive emptying fractions by volumes 11.4 ± 5.4% and 15.5 ± 6.3% versus 46.6 ± 11.7% and 44.3 ± 12.1% [22], respectively; global strain 9.8 ± 3.8% versus 22.9 ± 11.7% [23]). All these parameters, however, were less severely depressed compared to patients with arrhythmia relapses.

At follow-up, patients who suffered from ischemic cerebral events had maximal LA volume/BSA 61 ± 17.8 mL/mq, minimum LA volume/BSA 45.4 ± 5.2 mL/mq, total LA emptying fraction derived from volumes 23.6 ± 13.7%, lateral a′ wave 4.3 ± 0.2 cm/s, and SD of PA-TDI measurements 0.45 ± 0.08. The two patients with strokes in SR showed, instead, extremely enlarged LA volume (>70 mL/mq). One patient suffering a cerebrovascular event despite SR had discontinued oral anticoagulation therapy. The other three patients were on anticoagulation therapy at the time of stroke.

Table 3. Echocardiographic parameters and atrial functional evaluations, stratified according to SR maintenance and type of AF recurrence during follow-up. (AF, atrial fibrillation; AP, antero-posterior; BSA, body surface area; DT, deceleration time; EF, ejection fraction; LA, left atrial; LS, long-standing; LV, left ventricular; PAPs, systolic pulmonary arterial pressure; RA, right atrial; SD, standard deviation; SI, supero-inferior; SR, sinus rhythm).

	Stable SR (N = 20/29)	AF Relapse (N = 9/29)	Paroxysmal AF Relapse (N = 3/29)	Persistent/LS Persistent AF Relapse (N = 6/29)	*p*-Value
Max LA AP diameter (mm)	51.4 ± 6.2	57.8 ± 5.9	53.7 ± 3.2	59.8 ± 6.0	0.019
Min LA AP diameter (mm)	44.3 ± 6.3	52.2 ± 6.0	46.7 ± 3.2	55.0 ± 5.1	0.002
P wave LA AP diameter (mm)	47.5 ± 6.1		49.7 ± 4.2		0.565
Active LA emptying fraction derived from AP diameters (%)	7.0 ± 3.2		5.9 ± 3.0		0.601
Passive LA emptying fraction derived from AP diameters (%)	7.7 ± 3.4		7.5 ± 2.3		0.945
Total LA emptying fraction derived from AP diameters (%)	14.1 ± 4.2	9.7 ± 3.0	13.1 ± 1.9	8.0 ± 1.6	0.006
Max LA SI diameter (mm)	67.0 ± 4.9	71.4 ± 5.2	66.3 ± 4.0	74.0 ± 3.7	0.009
Max LA area (cmq)	30.1 ± 4.3	35.6 ± 5.3	32.2 ± 3.1	37.3 ± 5.5	0.007
Min LA area (cmq)	24.9 ± 3.8	31.4 ± 4.9	27.5 ± 2.2	33.4 ± 4.8	<0.001
P wave LA area (cmq)	27.0 ± 4.0		28.9 ± 2.2		0.430
LA ejection fraction derived from areas (%)	17.2 ± 5.0	11.8 ± 4.6	14.3 ± 7.2	10.5 ± 2.8	0.022
Max LA volume (mL)	109.9 ± 26.4	143.8 ± 34.4	125.7 ± 13.6	152.8 ± 39.0	0.012
Max LA volume/BSA (mL/mq)	60.6 ± 13.1	76.8 ± 16.2	69.0 ± 9.1	80.7 ± 18.2	0.016
Min LA volume (mL)	82.4 ± 21.0	118.2 ± 28.7	99.3 ± 10.2	127.7 ± 30.9	0.001
Min LA volume/BSA (mL/mq)	45.4 ± 10.9	63.3 ± 14.2	55.0 ± 11.6	67.5 ± 14.4	0.002
P wave LA volume (mL)	92.9 ± 22.7		104.3 ± 8.1		0.402
P wave LA volume/BSA (mL/mq)	51.3 ± 11.6		57.6 ± 10.4		0.380
3D LA volume (mL)	101.6 ± 26.6	134.0 ± 51.6	93.9 ± 11.2	158.1 ± 51.7	0.005
3D LA volume/BSA (mL/mq)	56.2 ± 13.2	71.9 ± 25.6	51.7 ± 8.4	84.0 ± 24.9	0.005
Active LA emptying fraction derived from volumes (%)	11.4 ± 5.4		4.9 ± 3.0		0.057
Passive LA emptying fraction derived from volumes (%)	15.5 ± 6.3		16.5 ± 9.0		0.809
Total LA emptying fraction derived from volumes (%)	25.1 ± 7.3	17.5 ± 7.4	20.4 ± 10.9	16.0 ± 5.7	0.039
Global longitudinal LA strain (%)	9.8 ± 3.8	5.8 ± 1.9	7.0 ± 2.0	5.2 ± 1.7	0.021
E wave (cm/s)	131.4 ± 24.2	150.0 ± 17.6	163.0 ± 18.2	143.5 ± 14.4	0.070
A wave (cm/s)	54.7 ± 20.0		66.1 ± 19.5		0.364
Inferior septal a′ wave (cm/s)	6.0 ± 2.0		4.9 ± 2.2		0.409
Lateral a′ wave (cm/s)	4.6 ± 1.7		3.6 ± 0.8		0.306
Averaged a′ wave (cm/s)	5.3 ± 1.5		4.3 ± 1.5		0.274
P-lateral a′ wave interval (ms)	110.8 ± 28.9		109.0 ± 57.3		0.930
SD P-a′ wave intervals	0.56 ± 0.31		0.63 ± 0.47		0.736
LV EF (%)	58.0 ± 7.2	55.8 ± 9.8	59.7 ± 3.5	53.8 ± 11.7	0.484
PAPs (mmHg)	36.2 ± 9.3	40.7 ± 9.5	45.7 ± 9.0	38.2 ± 9.4	0.284

4. Discussion

It is reasonable to infer that a lack of recovery of an efficient mechanical atrial activity, even potentially in the presence of SR, facilitates intra-atrial thrombus formation and subsequent systemic thromboembolic phenomena.

Previous studies on surgical AF ablation concomitant to valve surgery reported a highly variable incidence, from 21% to 87%, of both SR restoration and atrial contraction recovery [24,25].

Following the classic LA Maze ablation, it has already been proven that, despite successful SR restoration, there is a progressive loss of LA function, especially within patients affected by rheumatic mitral disease [26].

Following the latest less extensive LA ablation protocols, sparing large areas of the LA, instead, data are controversial. On one side, Loardi et al. analyzed 122 patients: based on transmitral peak A velocity as an atrial contraction index, they proved that 76% of the subjects presented SR and a normal atrial function at three months, and this percentage even increased to 98% after two years [27]. Similarly, Reyes et al. [28], out of 33 patients, highlighted the presence of a transmitral flow in 70% of SR patients at six months follow-up. Analogous results were reported by Manasse et al. [29].

On the other side, in patients with stable SR at six months follow-up, Johansson et al. [30] demonstrated a significant reduction in transmitral A wave velocity in 15 subjects submitted to combined surgery procedure as compared with 14 subjects submitted to mitral valve surgery alone. Boyd et al. suggested that the ablation procedure might have been responsible for the atrial dysfunction observed [31]. In addition, Schiros et al., comparing 35 degenerative mitral regurgitation patients undergoing combined surgery to 51 normal controls by means of cardiac magnetic resonance imaging, asserted that LA volumes and function do not return to normal values at one year distance (in particular, total atrial emptying fraction derived from volumes resulted in 45% pre-operative and 42% at one year post-surgery, versus 54% in controls) [32] supporting the relevant role of the underlying intrinsic disease of the atrial myocardium. Similar results were also reported by Kim et al. [33] within 12 patients: at one month follow-up the LA emptying fraction at computed tomography was 16.8 ± 6.3% (significantly lower than in controls, 47.9 ± 11.2%, $p < 0.001$) despite SR, and atrial contractile function did not improve over the following six months.

Lastly, Compier et al. placed emphasis on the fact that, notwithstanding the limited lesion set during concomitant cardiac surgery, LA compliance, transport function and contraction, decreased after ablation, were not restored in approximately half of the patients with post-procedural SR [34].

The present study highlights the markedly enlarged dimensions and reduced LA function also in patients who maintained SR during the entire follow-up period, compared to data reported in the literature for healthy subjects (see Results section). However, these parameters are more severely depressed, compared to healthy subjects, when patients suffer arrhythmia relapses (Table 3). These results support that concomitant AF cryoablation, by SR maintenance, guarantees an advantage, even if in the setting of deteriorated LAs, in terms of reverse remodeling.

Similar results were found in the HESTER (Has Electrical Sinus Translated into Effective Remodelling?) study [35]: in this experience, adjunct surgical maze was associated with the recovery of LA function but with a mean active LA ejection fraction (ALAEF) lower in maze patients than in control subjects. Providing evidence that function is restored after adjunct maze, potential clinical benefits in reducing thromboembolic and heart failure risk will arise. Determining whether patients can safely stop taking anticoagulants after SR is restored by a maze procedure requires, instead, longer term follow-up and stroke surveillance, beyond those of the HESTER study. In any case, the varying rates of LA functional recovery after maze strongly suggest that, at least, it would be judicious to measure LA function before considering anticoagulation withdrawal.

As stated in a previous study of our group [12] we suggest that, at least within patients with severely enlarged left atrium, previous cardiac surgery and catheter or surgical AF ablation, especially if repeated, the assessment of atrial contractility by transthoracic echocardiography should be performed before discontinuing oral anticoagulants (OAC), also in patients who maintain SR, despite confirmation by serial ECG or Holter monitorings. In our opinion, SR and LA contractility recovery represent two sides of the same coin, and both should be weighted carefully with the objective of selecting patients who could benefit from OAC continuation/discontinuation following an AF ablation.

There is a real need for improvement in patient stratification and personalization of care after AF ablation. Our understanding of which patients should continue anticoagulants for stroke prevention needs to be further refined to reduce the number of patients receiving anticoagulation after a successful AF ablation, and consequently lower the number of hemorrhagic complications, while endorsing the continuation of OAC in patients with a higher risk profile, and prevent thromboembolic events. In this context, we believe echocardiographic assessment of the restoration of an efficient LA contractility should be included among decisional criteria.

Further prospective studies are needed to define the LA dimensions and function cut-off values determining an increase in the risk for thromboembolic complications in patients with restored stable SR. Moreover, quantitative assessment of LA function may have clinical utility in guiding early surgical intervention and concomitant ablation in patients with mitral regurgitation and AF [36,37].

Study Limitations

This report is an observational and retrospective study. The limited sample size may have influenced the statistical power of the analysis. A comparison with baseline echocardiographic data is not completely feasible because a detailed echocardiography focused on LA morphology and function was not routinely performed before surgery. In addition, echocardiographic follow-up data were not available for the entire cohort of patients. Despite this limitation, we believe our data are representative and of interest. In fact, despite patients lost to follow-up, echocardiographic parameters concerning atrial function in patients followed and with stable SR, after the combined surgical procedure, proved statistically better than in subjects with AF relapse. Being aware that arrhythmia monitoring based on serial 24 h ECG Holter tracings or, even better, implantable recorders would be more accurate, in a mostly persistent AF setting, consideration of any AF relapse, also those present only once during the follow up, should limit event underestimation.

The present study is a starting point; in any case, we are convinced that the concept introduced by the present manuscript may have wider developments in clinical practice.

5. Conclusions

Surgical AF cryoablation concomitant to minimally invasive mitral valve repair was determined to be highly effective in maintaining SR and reducing AF burden at long-term follow-up.

The present study highlights the markedly enlarged dimensions of the LA also in patients who maintained SR during the entire follow-up period.

However, at the echocardiographic evaluation, data concerning atrial function in patients with stable SR after the combined surgical procedure are significantly better than in subjects with AF relapse at follow-up. This finding supports the implementation of AF cryoablation concomitant to MIMVS.

Author Contributions: Conceptualization, M.A. and G.M.; methodology, M.A.; software, M.A. and D.C.; validation, M.M., F.G., and M.R.; formal analysis, C.R.; investigation, C.R.; resources, G.M., M.M. and S.F.; data curation, C.R.; writing—original draft preparation, C.R.; writing—review and editing, M.A., G.M. and C.R.; visualization, S.F.; supervision, F.G., M.R. and G.M.D.F.; project administration, M.A., D.C.

References

1. Chua, Y.L.; Schaff, H.V.; Orszulak, T.A.; Morris, J.J. Outcome of mitral valve repair in patients with preoperative atrial fibrillation. Should the maze procedure be combined with mitral valvuloplasty? *J. Thorac. Cardiovasc. Surg.* **1994**, *107*, 408–415.

2. Scarsoglio, S.; Saglietto, A.; Gaita, F.; Ridolfi, L.; Anselmino, M. Computational fluid dynamics modelling of left valvular heart diseases during atrial fibrillation. *PeerJ* **2016**, *4*, e2240. [CrossRef] [PubMed]
3. Gaita, F.; Ebrille, E.; Scaglione, M.; Caponi, D.; Garberoglio, L.; Vivalda, L.; Barbone, A.; Gallotti, R. Very long-term results of surgical and transcatheter ablation of long-standing persistent atrial fibrillation. *Ann. Thorac. Surg.* **2013**, *96*, 1273–1278. [CrossRef] [PubMed]
4. Ngaage, D.L.; Schaff, H.V.; Mullany, C.J.; Barnes, S.; Dearani, J.A.; Daly, R.C.; Orszulak, T.A.; Sundt, T.M., III. Influence of preoperative atrial fibrillation on late results of mitral repair: Is concomitant ablation justified? *Ann. Thorac. Surg.* **2007**, *84*, 434–442; discussion 442–443. [CrossRef] [PubMed]
5. Chitwood, W.R., Jr.; Wixon, C.L.; Elbeery, J.R.; Moran, J.F.; Chapman, W.H.; Lust, R.M. Video-assisted minimally invasive mitral valve surgery. *J. Thorac. Cardiovasc. Surg.* **1997**, *114*, 773–780; discussion 780–782. [CrossRef]
6. Marchetto, G.; Anselmino, M.; Rovera, C.; Mancuso, S.; Ricci, D.; Antolini, M.; Morello, M.; Gaita, F.; Rinaldi, M. Results of cryoablation for atrial fibrillation concomitant with video-assisted minimally invasive mitral valve surgery. *Semin. Thorac. Cardiovasc. Surg.* **2016**, *28*, 271–280. [CrossRef]
7. Schaff, H.V. Surgical ablation of atrial fibrillation—When, why, and how? *N. Engl. J. Med.* **2015**, *372*, 1465–1467. [CrossRef]
8. Blomström-Lundqvist, C.; Johansson, B.; Berglin, E.; Nilsson, L.; Jensen, S.M.; Thelin, S.; Holmgren, A.; Edvardsson, N.; Källner, G.; Blomström, P. A randomized doubleblind study of epicardial left atrial cryoablation for permanent atrial fibrillation in patients undergoing mitral valve surgery: The SWEDish Multicentre Atrial Fibrillation study (SWEDMAF). *Eur. Heart J.* **2007**, *28*, 2902–2908. [CrossRef]
9. Phan, K.; Xie, A.; Tian, D.H.; Shaikhrezai, K.; Yan, T.D. Systematic review and meta-analysis of surgical ablation for atrial fibrillation during mitral valve surgery. *Ann. Cardiothorac. Surg.* **2014**, *3*, 3–14.
10. Stulak, J.M.; Schaff, H.V. The cardiac surgeon as electrophysiologist. *J. Thorac. Cardiovasc. Surg.* **2016**, *151*, 298–299. [CrossRef]
11. Jeevanantham, V.; Ntim, W.; Navaneethan, S.D.; Shah, S.; Johnson, A.C.; Hall, B.; Shah, A.; Hundley, W.G.; Daubert, J.P.; Fitzgerald, D. Meta-analysis of the effect of radiofrequency catheter ablation on left atrial size, volumes and function in patients with atrial fibrillation. *Am. J. Cardiol.* **2010**, *105*, 1317–1326. [CrossRef] [PubMed]
12. Anselmino, M.; Rovera, C.; Marchetto, G.; Ferraris, F.; Castagno, D.; Gaita, F. Anticoagulant cessation following atrial fibrillation ablation: Limits of the ECG-guided approach. *Expert Rev. Cardiovasc. Ther.* **2017**, *15*, 473–479. [CrossRef] [PubMed]
13. Barbero, C.; Marchetto, G.; Ricci, D.; El Qarra, S.; Attisani, M.; Filippini, C.; Boffini, M.; Rinaldi, M. Right minithoracotomy for mitral valve surgery: Impact of tailored strategies on early outcome. *Ann. Thorac. Surg.* **2016**, *102*, 1989–1994. [CrossRef] [PubMed]
14. Ad, N.; Holmes, S.D.; Lamont, D.; Shuman, D.J. Left-sided surgical ablation for patients with atrial fibrillation who are undergoing concomitant cardiac surgical procedures. *Ann. Thorac. Surg.* **2017**, *103*, 58–65. [CrossRef]
15. Gutman, J.; Wang, Y.S.; Wahr, D.; Schiller, N.B. Normal left atrial function determined by 2-dimensional echocardiography. *Am. J. Cardiol.* **1983**, *51*, 336–340. [CrossRef]
16. Manning, W.J.; Leeman, D.E.; Gotch, P.J.; Come, P.C. Pulsed Doppler evaluation of atrial mechanical function after electrical cardioversion of atrial fibrillation. *J. Am. Coll. Cardiol.* **1989**, *13*, 617–623. [CrossRef]
17. Wang, M.; Yip, G.W.; Wang, A.Y.; Zhang, Y.; Ho, P.Y.; Tse, M.K.; Lam, P.K.; Sanderson, J.E. Peak early diastolic mitral annulus velocity by tissue Doppler imaging adds independent and incremental prognostic value. *J. Am. Coll. Cardiol.* **2003**, *41*, 820–826. [CrossRef]
18. Lupu, S.; Mitre, A.; Dobreanu, D. Left atrium function assessment by echocardiography—physiological and clinical implications. *Med. Ultrason.* **2014**, *16*, 152–159. [CrossRef]
19. Vasan, R.S.; Larson, M.G.; Levy, D.; Galderisi, M.; Wolf, P.A.; Benjamin, E.J. Doppler transmitral flow indexes and risk of atrial fibrillation (the Framingham Heart Study). *Am. J. Cardiol.* **2003**, *91*, 1079–1083. [CrossRef]
20. Le Bihan, D.C.; Della Togna, D.J.; Barretto, R.B.; Assef, J.E.; Machado, L.R.; Ramos, A.I.; Abdulmassih Neto, C.; Moisés, V.A.; Sousa, A.G.; Campos, O. Early improvement in left atrial remodeling and function after mitral valve repair or replacement in organic symptomatic mitral regurgitation assessed by three-dimensional echocardiography. *Echocardiography* **2015**, *32*, 1122–1130. [CrossRef]
21. Ring, L.; Rana, B.S.; Wells, F.C.; Kydd, A.C.; Dutka, D.P. Atrial function as a guide to timing of intervention in mitral valve prolapse with mitral regurgitation. *JACC Cardiovasc. Imaging* **2014**, *7*, 225–232. [CrossRef] [PubMed]

22. Leischik, R.; Littwitz, H.; Dworrak, B.; Garg, P.; Zhu, M.; Sahn, D.J.; Horlitz, M. Echocardiographic evaluation of left atrial mechanics: Function, history, novel techniques, advantages, and pitfalls. *Biomed. Res. Int.* **2015**, *2015*, 765921. [CrossRef] [PubMed]
23. Hammerstingl, C.; Schwekendiek, M.; Momcilovic, D.; Schueler, R.; Sinning, J.M.; Schrickel, J.W.; Mittmann-Braun, E.; Nickenig, G.; Lickfett, L. Left atrial deformation imaging with ultrasound based two-dimensional speckle-tracking predicts the rate of recurrence of paroxysmal and persistent atrial fibrillation after successful ablation procedures. *J. Cardiovasc. Electrophysiol.* **2012**, *23*, 247–255. [CrossRef] [PubMed]
24. Feinberg, M.S.; Waggoner, A.D.; Kater, K.M.; Cox, J.L.; Lindsay, B.D.; Perez, J.E. Restoration of atrial function after the maze procedure for patients with atrial fibrillation: Assessment by Doppler echocardiography. *Circulation* **1994**, *90*, II285–II292.
25. Yuda, S.; Nakatani, S.; Isobe, F.; Kosakai, Y.; Miyatake, K. Comparative efficacy of the maze procedure for restoration of atrial contraction in patients with and without giant left atrium associated with mitral valve disease. *J. Am. Coll. Cardiol.* **1998**, *31*, 1097–1102. [CrossRef]
26. Kim, H.W.; Moon, M.H.; Jo, K.H.; Song, H.; Lee, J.W. Left atrial and left ventricular diastolic function after the maze procedure for atrial fibrillation in mitral valve disease: Degenerative versus rheumatic. *Indian J. Surg.* **2015**, *77*, 7–15. [CrossRef]
27. Loardi, C.; Alamanni, F.; Galli, C.; Naliato, M.; Veglia, F.; Zanobini, M.; Pepi, M. Surgical treatment of concomitant atrial fibrillation: Focus onto atrial contractility. *Biomed. Res. Int.* **2015**, *2015*, 274817. [CrossRef]
28. Reyes, G.; Benedicto, A.; Bustamante, J.; Sarraj, A.; Nuche, J.M.; Alvarez, P.; Duarte, J. Restoration of atrial contractility after surgical cryoablation: Clinical, electrical and mechanical results. *Interact. Cardiovasc. Thorac. Surg.* **2009**, *9*, 609–612. [CrossRef]
29. Manasse, E.; Gaita, F.; Ghiselli, S.; Barbone, A.; Garberoglio, L.; Citterio, E.; Ornaghi, D.; Gallotti, R. Cryoablation of the left posterior atrial wall: 95 patients and 3 years of mean follow-up. *Eur. J. Cardiothorac. Surg.* **2003**, *24*, 731–740. [CrossRef]
30. Johansson, B.; Bech-Hanssen, O.; Berglin, E.; Blomström, P.; Holmgren, A.; Jensen, S.M.; Källner, G.; Nilsson, L.; Thelin, S.; Karlsson, T.; et al. Atrial function after left atrial epicardial cryoablation for atrial fibrillation in patients undergoing mitral valve surgery. *J. Interv. Card. Electrophysiol.* **2012**, *33*, 85–91. [CrossRef]
31. Boyd, A.C.; Schiller, N.B.; Ross, D.L.; Thomas, L. Differential recovery of regional atrial contraction after restoration of sinus rhythm after intraoperative linear radiofrequency ablation for atrial fibrillation. *Am. J. Cardiol.* **2009**, *103*, 528–534. [CrossRef] [PubMed]
32. Schiros, C.G.; Ahmed, M.I.; McGiffin, D.C.; Zhang, X.; Lloyd, S.C.; Aban, I.; Denney, T.S., Jr.; Dell'Italia, L.J.; Gupta, H. Mitral annular kinetics, left atrial, and left ventricular diastolic function post mitral valve repair in degenerative mitral regurgitation. *Front. Cardiovasc. Med.* **2015**, *2*, 31. [CrossRef] [PubMed]
33. Kim, J.B.; Yang, D.H.; Kang, J.W.; Jung, S.H.; Choo, S.J.; Chung, C.H.; Song, J.K.; Lee, J.W. Left atrial function following surgical ablation of atrial fibrillation: Prospective evaluation using dual-source cardiac computed tomography. *Yonsei Med. J.* **2015**, *56*, 608–616. [CrossRef] [PubMed]
34. Compier, M.G.; Tops, L.F.; Braun, J.; Zeppenfeld, K.; Klautz, R.J.; Schalij, M.J.; Trines, S.A. Limited left atrial surgical ablation effectively treats atrial fibrillation but decreases left atrial function. *Europace* **2017**, *19*, 560–567. [CrossRef]
35. Abu-Omar, Y.; Thorpe, B.S.; Freeman, C.; Mills, C.; Stoneman, V.E.A.; Gopalan, D.; Rana, B.; Spyt, T.J.; Sharples, L.D.; Nashef, S.A.M. Recovery of left atrial contractile function after maze surgery in persistent longstanding atrial fibrillation. *JACC* **2017**, *70*, 2309–2311. [CrossRef]
36. Ring, L.; Abu-Omar, Y.; Kaye, N.; Rana, B.S.; Watson, W.; Dutka, D.P.; Vassiliou, V.S. Left atrial function is associated with earlier need for cardiac surgery in moderate to severe mitral regurgitation: Usefulness in targeting for early surgery. *J. Am. Soc. Echocardiogr.* **2018**, *31*, 983–991. [CrossRef]
37. Anselmino, M.; Gaita, F.; Saglietto, A. Effectiveness of catheter ablation of atrial fibrillation: Are we at the dawn of a new era? *J. Thorac. Dis.* **2017**, *9*, 3630–3634. [CrossRef]

15

Association of Antihyperglycemic Therapy with Risk of Atrial Fibrillation and Stroke in Diabetic Patients

Cristina-Mihaela Lăcătușu [1,2,*], Elena-Daniela Grigorescu [1,*], Cristian Stătescu [3,4], Radu Andy Sascău [3,4], Alina Onofriescu [1,2] and Bogdan-Mircea Mihai [1,2]

1 Diabetes, Nutrition and Metabolic Diseases, "Grigore T. Popa" University of Medicine and Pharmacy, 700115 Iași, Romania
2 "Sf. Spiridon" Emergency Hospital, 700111 Iași, Romania
3 Internal Medicine, "Grigore T. Popa" University of Medicine and Pharmacy, 700115 Iași, Romania
4 "George I.M. Georgescu" Cardiovascular Diseases Institute, Cardiology Department, 700503 Iași, Romania
* Correspondence: cristina.lacatusu@umfiasi.ro (C.-M.L.); elena-daniela-gh-grigorescu@umfiasi.ro (E.-D.G.)

Abstract: Type 2 diabetes mellitus (DM) is associated with an increased risk of cardiovascular disease (CVD). Atrial fibrillation (AF) and stroke are both forms of CVD that have major consequences in terms of disabilities and death among patients with diabetes; however, they are less present in the preoccupations of scientific researchers as a primary endpoint of clinical trials. Several publications have found DM to be associated with a higher risk for both AF and stroke; some of the main drugs used for glycemic control have been found to carry either increased, or decreased risks for AF or for stroke in DM patients. Given the risk for thromboembolic cerebrovascular events seen in AF patients, the question arises as to whether stroke and AF occurring with modified incidences in diabetic individuals under therapy with various classes of antihyperglycemic medications are interrelated and should be considered as a whole. At present, the medical literature lacks studies specifically designed to investigate a cause–effect relationship between the incidences of AF and stroke driven by different antidiabetic agents. In default of such proof, we reviewed the existing evidence correlating the major classes of glucose-controlling drugs with their associated risks for AF and stroke; however, supplementary proof is needed to explore a hypothetically causal relationship between these two, both of which display peculiar features in the setting of specific drug therapies for glycemic control.

Keywords: diabetes mellitus; atrial fibrillation; stroke; metformin; thiazolidinediones; GLP-1 receptor agonists; SGLT-2 inhibitors

---

1. Introduction

Cardiovascular disease (CVD) is the main cause of morbidity and mortality in type 2 diabetes patients. The increased cardiovascular risk seen in diabetic patients cannot be mitigated with a monofactorial intervention of plasma glucose control, requiring a multi-factorial control of all cardiovascular risk factors [1,2]. Some of the newer classes of antihyperglycemic drugs have the potential to improve other risk factors beyond glycemic levels, and to protect against major cardiovascular events. Hence, the presence of CVD has become one of the key decision factors in the international guidelines counseling the choice of second-line antidiabetic medication after metformin [3].

Among all potential clinical forms of diabetes-associated obstructive artery disease, cerebrovascular disease is a serious condition, inducing major disabilities and a shortened life span. In a large meta-analysis of 102 prospective studies, diabetes mellitus was associated with a 2.27-fold increase in the risk for ischemic stroke when compared with a non-diabetic status [4].

Accumulating clinical evidence also seems to connect diabetes mellitus with an increased risk for atrial fibrillation (AF) [5]. Diabetes mellitus may induce structural and electrical alterations of the left atrium (deposition of advanced end-glycation products and connexin-mediated fibrosis), and stimulate the production of pro-coagulant factors (von Willibrand factor, soluble P-selectin, and other molecules exerting pro-inflammatory and pro-oxidative actions or favoring platelet activation and aggregation) [6]. All these changes promote clotting in the left atrial appendage and subsequent thromboembolism [6].

In a turning point in diabetes-related clinical research, several older or newer drugs used to control glycemic values in diabetic patients were recently shown—mostly in observational studies, post-hoc analyses of the major trials, or various meta-analyses—to display different levels of risk for either AF or stroke [7,8]. Such evidence exists for all classes of antidiabetic drugs included in the major international guidelines [3,7,8]. These drugs are summarized in Table 1. The body of evidence accumulating for each of these two new facets of antidiabetic medications is continuously increasing, and may represent far more than a random coincidence, even though no studies have been drafted to investigate a specific cause-effect relationship between the AF and stroke risks associated with use of various antihyperglycemic agents. Therefore, the aim of the present review is to gather, for the first time in the literature, the current knowledge on the risks of each of the antihyperglycemic drugs advised by current guidelines for both AF and stroke, raising the question as to whether they are causally interconnected.

Table 1. Classes of antihyperglycemic drugs included in current guidelines [3].

Drug	Mechanism of Action
Insulin	Activation of insulin receptor; various effects on multiple metabolic pathways
Metformin	Reduced insulin resistance, mostly by decreasing gluconeogenesis
Sulfonylureas (SU)	Insulin secretagogues by activation of SUR (SU receptor) unit of ATP-sensitive potassium channels
Thiazolidinediones (TZD)	Insulin sensitizers by the activation of peroxisome proliferator-activated receptor (PPAR)-γ
Dipeptidyl peptidase-4 (DPP-4) inhibitors	Inhibition of DPP-4 and subsequent conservation of native human GLP-1 in its active form
Glucagon-like peptide-1 (GLP-1) receptor agonists	Activation of GLP-1 receptor at high pharmacological concentrations
Sodium-glucose cotransporter-2 (SGLT-2) inhibitors	Inhibition of active reabsorption of glucose and sodium performed by SGLT-2 in the proximal convoluted tubule

2. Antihyperglycemic Drugs, Atrial Fibrillation and Stroke

Recently published research has frequently depicted various classes of antihyperglycemic agents as being associated with modified levels of risk for either AF or stroke. Stroke episodes in AF patients frequently have a thromboembolic nature; hence, the question arises as to whether a specific risk for AF in one or the other of the antidiabetic drugs would reflect an accordingly modified risk for cerebral thromboembolism, and thus stroke. Unfortunately, the major clinical trials have not yet distinguished between the ischemic or hemorrhagic nature of stroke episodes, and least of all, between the atherothrombotic or thromboembolic etiology of ischemic strokes [9,10]. In the absence of dedicated studies using electrocardiogram (ECG) technologies to monitor the heart rhythm, a high number of asymptomatic AF and/or paroxysmal, recurrent episodes of AF may go unrecognized; this may underlie the inconstant associations between diabetes and incidences of AF or stroke seen in clinical studies, especially those not reporting AF as a specific outcome [11]. We searched Medline and Scopus databases using the logical string "atrial fibrillation" OR "stroke" AND "antihyperglycemic"

AND "diabetes" to identify these key terms in the title or abstract of English-written articles published before June 2019. Clinical studies or trials, meta-analyses, and systematic reviews focusing on human subjects were selected. After eliminating duplicates, this initial search returned 14 results. We screened all titles and abstracts to select papers that could be considered relevant to the aim of our review. This operation led to a further reduction to only 11 titles. A second search using the same algorithm and replacing the key term of "antihyperglycemic" with "insulin" OR "metformin" OR "sulfonylurea (SU)" OR "thiazolidindione (TZD)" OR "dipeptidyl peptidase-4 (DPP-4) inhibitor" OR "glucagon-like peptide-1 (GLP-1) receptor agonist" OR "sodium-glucose cotransporter-2 (SGLT-2) inhibitor" issued 28 supplementary papers, which were also included in our review. When potential mechanistical explanations were useful, we also referred to other relevant review papers, selected by the same two search algorithms; as an only exception, we included a case report which filled a gap in an area of scarce evidence. The following sections summarize the data related to the risk of AF and stroke for each class of antihyperglycemic agents.

2.1. *Insulin*

In a case-control study on Taiwan registries, insulin therapy was associated with a higher risk of new-onset AF in diabetic patients than with other antihyperglycemic medications [12]. Among patients in the PREvention oF thromboembolic events—European Registry in Atrial Fibrillation (PREFER in AF) registry, insulin users, but not diabetic patients treated with non-insulin antihyperglycemic drugs, were shown to have a higher risk of stroke compared with non-diabetic individuals [13]. In a Medicare analysis on 798,592 AF patients, insulin-requiring diabetic subjects also had a higher risk of stroke than diabetic patients not requiring insulin therapy or non-diabetic individuals; use of insulin therapy was associated in this registry study with an attenuation in the efficacy of anticoagulant drugs [6]. However, the association between insulin therapy and this pro-arrhythmic status may be biased by the longer duration of type 2 diabetes usually seen in patients treated with insulin. Such subjects may have experienced years of suboptimal glycemic control on other non-insulin therapies, and may have had the time to develop significant comorbidities [12]. The real possibility exists that hyperinsulinism (either due to insulin resistance or, in this case, having an iatrogenic component) may be associated with an increased anti-fibrinolytic status, as insulin stimulates the Plasminogen Activator Inhibitor-1 (PAI-1) production in adipocytes [14].

2.2. *Metformin*

In a cohort study on 645,710 Taiwan patients, monotherapy with metformin was associated with a 19% reduction in the risk of AF compared with the use of other antihyperglycemic medications during a 13-year follow-up. Metformin users had the lowest AF incidence rates in the first two years after diagnosis, but the protective effect tended to fade afterward [15]. Possible explanations accounting for the favorable effect of metformin include its actions on adenosine monophosphate-activated kinase, and the drug-induced reduction of the oxidative stress and the myolysis in the atrial tissue [15,16]. The loss of its protective effect over time may be underlain by the progressive deterioration of β-cell function typically observed in type 2 diabetes, which may lead to a worsened glycemic control, or by the gradual remodeling of the atrial wall [15]. In the above-mentioned case-control study, also originating from Taiwan registries, biguanides, of which metformin is the main representative today, were also associated with a lower risk of developing AF [12].

Current evidence suggests that metformin also has a protective effect against ischemic stroke, even though specific outcome studies analyzing a potential cause–effect relationship between the protective role of metformin against AF development and the rate of thromboembolic events are lacking in the medical literature. The results of the United Kingdom Prospective Diabetes Study (UKPDS) suggested that intensive blood glucose control with metformin, compared with the use of sulfonylureas or insulin, significantly reduced the risk of stroke [17]. After a four-year follow-up, the administration of metformin within the antihyperglycemic therapy was associated with a 54% reduction in the risk of stroke, with the best results observed in the highest risk patients [18].

2.3. *Sulfonylureas*

Most researchers analyzing the risk of AF development have considered SU therapy as only a control to report comparative AF outcomes of other antidiabetic medications. Among the few studies making an exception, the previously mentioned Taiwan case-control study found SUs to not be associated with an increased risk of new-onset AF [12].

Research on the stroke risk associated with SU use generally precedes the publication of most studies using these drugs as an active comparator for other medications' AF risk. This class of hypoglycemiant drugs acts on the SU receptor (SUR) unit of the ATP-sensitive potassium channels. In normal conditions, these ionic channels may play a protective role against neuronal ischemia. SUs were therefore feared by some authors to inhibit this neuroprotective mechanism, and thus to increase the risk of stroke [19–21]. Initial results of clinical studies were contradictory, varying between reports of potential benefits [22], neutral effects [23], or even detrimental effects [24]. A subsequent meta-analysis of 27,705 diabetic patients from 17 trials found SUs to be associated with a higher relative risk for stroke than other antihyperglycemic drugs administered for glycemic control [20].

2.4. *Thiazolidinediones*

Thiazolidinediones are insulin sensitizers acting primarily on the peroxisome proliferator-activated receptor (PPAR)-γ and, in the case of pioglitazone, also exerting a weak agonist activity on PPAR-α. Their action on these nuclear receptors is associated with anti-inflammatory and anti-oxidant benefits, potentially due to favorable effects on Transforming Growth Factor (TGF)-β, Tumor Necrosis Factor (TNF)-α, Atrial Natriuretic Peptide (ANP), superoxide dismutase (SOD), malonyldialdehyde, nicotinamide adenine dinucleotide phosphate (NADPH) oxidase subunits, or voltage-dependent calcium channels [25]. Reports of an increased risk of hydro-saline retention, heart failure, and cardiovascular events seen with rosiglitazone [26,27] drastically limited their use in diabetic patients. As a direct effect of these reports, regulatory agencies subsequently requested proof of cardiovascular safety for the newer generations of antihyperglycemic drugs by means of dedicated trials.

These conflicting features of TZDs led to research on their association with atrial fibrillation and stroke. In an observational study on 12,605 patients with insulin-naïve type 2 diabetes, the risk of developing AF was reduced by 31% after a five-year follow-up in patients treated with TZD [28]. In another smaller observational study following the arrhythmic outcomes of catheter ablation, pioglitazone was also reported to be associated with a reduced risk of post-procedural AF [29]. A better recovery to sinus rhythm was reported in isolated cases of patients with paroxysmal AF and diabetes who received rosiglitazone [30]. The use of TZDs was associated with a lower risk of developing AF in the Taiwan case-control study that was previously mentioned [12]. A large cohort study of 108,624 diabetic, AF-free Danish patients, treated with either metformin or sulfonylureas as first-line antihyperglycemic therapy, showed a 24% risk reduction in the incidence of AF when TZDs were used as a second-line drug for glycemic control, compared with other antidiabetic drugs [31]. Post hoc analyses on the incidence of AF in the PROactive (PROspective pioglitAzone Clinical Trial In macroVascular Events) and BARI 2D (Bypass Angioplasty Revascularization Investigation 2 Diabetes) trials did not show significant differences in the number of patients developing AF [32,33]. However, neither of these two randomized studies were designed to include AF between their specific endpoints, so they did not systematically search for its existence using any ECG-monitoring device. The number of patients receiving TZDs who developed AF was lower than their counterparts in both studies [32,33]. A meta-analysis including 130,854 patients from three randomized clinical trials and four observational studies found a 30% reduction in the AF risk in patients treated with TZD, with significantly reduced incidences of both new-onset AF and recurrent AF [34]. In this meta-analysis, results were observed predominantly with pioglitazone, but not with rosiglitazone, and were driven by the data in the observational studies, as the pooled analysis of the results from the three randomized clinical trials showed no statistical differences in the AF incidence [34].

Similar to the case of metformin, no specific evidence links the potentially protective role of TZDs against AF and the effect of these drugs on the risk of cerebrovascular events. However, some data indicate a real possibility that TZDs have the ability to protect diabetic patients against stroke development. In another sub-analysis of the PROactive study, the risk for fatal or non-fatal stroke was significantly reduced with pioglitazone in type 2 diabetes patients with a history of previous stroke, but not in those without a history of cerebrovascular events [35]. In the Insulin Resistance Intervention after Stroke (IRIS) trial, performed in non-diabetic but insulin-resistant patients with a history of stroke or transient ischemic attack, pioglitazone was able to lower the risk for recurrent stroke or myocardial infarction compared with placebo therapy [36]. Finally, a meta-analysis on three randomized controlled trials, incorporating 4980 subjects with previous stroke and either insulin resistance, prediabetes, or type 2 diabetes mellitus, found the use of pioglitazone to be associated with a 32% lower risk of stroke recurrence compared with a placebo [37].

2.5. DPP-4 Inhibitors

In a cohort study on 90,880 patients with type 2 diabetes previously treated with metformin as a first-line antihyperglycemic drug, the add-on of DPP-4 inhibitors (mostly sitagliptin) as a second-line therapy was found to be associated with a lower risk of AF development than the use of other drugs (mainly SUs) as the second antidiabetic medication [38]. The use of DPP-4 inhibitors was associated with neither an increased nor a decreased risk of new-onset AF in the case-control study on Taiwan registries that was previously mentioned [12].

These positive or neutral results on AF risk raised the question of potentially protective effects of DPP-4 inhibitors against stroke. In another longitudinal observational Taiwan study on 123,050 type 2 diabetes patients that were newly initiated on oral antidiabetic drugs, the use of DPP-4 inhibitors was associated with a lower risk for ischemic stroke compared with meglitinides or insulin; however, their risk for stroke was comparable to that observed in metformin users, and higher than the risk observed in patients treated with pioglitazone [39]. None of the cardiovascular outcome trials with DPP-4 inhibitors identified a reduced risk for stroke with any of these medications [40–44]. When a meta-analysis was performed on 19 small randomized trials and the first three cardiovascular outcome trials with DPP-4 inhibitors that were published, a non-significant trend toward protection against stroke was found, but this trend disappeared when only the cardiovascular outcome trials were introduced into another pooled analysis [45]. Likewise, a meta-analysis of the five cardiovascular outcome trials with DPP-4 inhibitors available at the end of 2018 showed a neutral effect on the risk for stroke, similar to the profile of safety, but showed a lack of benefits in terms of the risk for myocardial infarction, cardiovascular death, or heart failure [46]. Similar to the case with other drugs, none of the cardiovascular outcome trials or meta-analyses with DPP-4 inhibitors published so far have differentiated between stroke events of hemorrhagic or ischemic origin, least of all between atherothrombotic or thromboembolic events.

2.6. GLP-1 Receptor Agonists

A side effect of GLP-1 receptor agonists includes a moderate increase in heart rate [47], which may be due to either an effect of the direct stimulation of the GLP-1 receptor found on sino-atrial cells, or a compensatory response to the relative lowering of blood pressure levels seen with GLP-1 receptor agonists [48,49]. Acknowledgement of this effect on the heart rate led to concerns that GLP-1 receptor agonists may be associated with a higher risk for AF, especially after a pooled analysis of the phase 2b and phase 3 trials in the Albiglutide and cardiovascular outcomes in patients with type 2 diabetes and cardiovascular disease (Harmony Outcomes) program with albiglutide showed a statistically significant increase in the AF incidence with this drug [50]. However, the cardiovascular outcome trials with lixisenatide, liraglutide, or semaglutide found no differences in the AF incidence between any of the active drugs and the placebo comparator [51–53]. As cardiovascular outcome trials are specifically designed to follow major cardiovascular events, it is plausible to think that an AF episode—even though not counting as a pre-defined endpoint—should be more recognized in such studies than in trials with metabolic outcomes, to therefore offer a better statistical accuracy. Since these three cardiovascular outcome trials included patients with pre-existing cardiovascular disease, it is also presumable that such subjects would be treated with β-blockers, thus reducing the probability of AF occurrence and reducing the number of cases below the limit of statistical significance. Subsequently, a meta-analysis of all trials available in 2017 with GLP-1 receptor agonists (including studies with albiglutide, but also with exenatide, lixisenatide, liraglutide, dulaglutide, and semaglutide) showed no increase in the risk of AF with these drugs [54].

However, aside from speculations about the risks of AF, GLP-1 receptor agonists are definitely not associated with a higher risk for stroke. All GLP-1 receptor agonists developed from the human GLP-1 backbone (liraglutide, injectable semaglutide, albiglutide, and dulaglutide) are able to lower the risk for the composite outcome of major cardiovascular events (cardiovascular death, non-fatal myocardial infarction, and non-fatal stroke) [53,55–57]. When endpoints included in the composite outcome were analyzed separately in each of these trials, liraglutide and albiglutide demonstrated non-significant differences opposite to the placebo in terms of the risk of stroke [55,56], whereas injectable semaglutide showed a significant 39% reduction [53], and dulaglutide was associated with a 24% reduction in the calculated risks for non-fatal stroke [57]. In a previously mentioned meta-analysis, including, in this case, the four cardiovascular outcome trials with GLP-1 receptor agonists available at the end of 2018, this class of drugs was associated with a 13% reduction in the risk for non-fatal stroke, even if atherothrombotic, thromboembolic, and/or hemorrhagic events were not differentiated [46].

2.7. SGLT-2 Inhibitors

SGLT-2 inhibitors exert their actions by inhibiting the active reabsorption performed by this specific co-transporter of sodium and glucose at the level of the proximal convoluted tubule. As a result, glucose, sodium, and water are lost in the final urine, lowering blood pressure and blood glucose levels, and creating a negative energy balance that induces weight loss. Based on these direct effects on multiple cardiovascular risk factors, but also on other adjunctive metabolic actions, SGLT-2 inhibitors seem able to lower the cardiovascular risk in diabetic patients. In the dedicated cardiovascular outcome trials, empagliflozin and canagliflozin were shown to reduce the progression to the composite outcome of major cardiovascular events [58,59], whereas dapagliflozin reduced the risk for the composite outcome of cardiovascular death and hospitalization for heart failure [60]. Currently, no research on the risk of AF development with any of the SGLT-2 inhibitors has been published, but a sub-analysis of the Empagliflozin Cardiovascular Outcome Event Trial in Type 2 Diabetes Mellitus Patients-Removing Excess Glucose (EMPA-REG OUTCOME) acknowledged a slightly increased incidence of stroke in the empagliflozin treatment group, even though not reaching statistical significance [61]. A subsequent meta-analysis of 57 studies using seven different approved or unapproved SGLT-2 inhibitors reported a 30% higher risk of non-fatal stroke [62]. Hypothetical explanations attribute this negative effect either to chance or to the relative increase in hematocrit, leading to a higher blood viscosity, as these agents exert an effect of osmotic diuresis [63]. However, another meta-analysis of trials with SGLT-2 inhibitors, this time including studies lasting at least 24 weeks and reporting at least one cardiovascular outcome, did not confirm an increased risk of stroke, thus assuring a reasonable level of cerebrovascular safety with this class of drugs [64]. The above-mentioned pooled analysis, including all three available cardiovascular outcome trials with SGLT-2 inhibitors, revealed no supplementary risk of stroke with SGLT-2 inhibitors compared with placebo comparators [46].

3. Conclusions

Current evidence supports the existence of a relationship between diabetes mellitus and an increased risk for atrial fibrillation and stroke. In these high-risk patients, several reports linking antidiabetic medications to modified risks for atrial fibrillation, stroke, or both, have been published in the last years. The most relevant of these results are summarized in Table 2.

Table 2. Summary of the main current evidence on the association of current antihyperglycemic drugs with risks of atrial fibrillation (AF) and stroke.

Drug	Risk for AF	Risk for Stroke
Insulin	Increased [12]	Increased [6,13]
Metformin	Reduced [12,15]	Reduced [17,18]
Sulfonylureas	Unchanged [12]	Reduced [22], unchanged [23], or increased [20,24]
Thiazolidinediones	Reduced [12,28,29,31,34] or unchanged [32,33]	Reduced [35–37]
DPP-4 inhibitors	Reduced [38] or unchanged [12]	Reduced [39] or unchanged [40–46]
GLP-1 receptor agonists	Increased with albiglutide [50], unchanged with semaglutide, liraglutide, and dulaglutide, or in meta-analyses [51–54]	Reduced in meta-analyses [46] and with semaglutide [53], unchanged with liraglutide, albiglutide, and dulaglutide [55–57]
SGLT-2 inhibitors	Data not available	Increased in some meta-analyses [62], unchanged in others [46,64]

The cause–effect relationship between the modified risk for atrial fibrillation of these drugs and cerebrovascular disease due to thromboembolic events has not yet been analyzed in studies with dedicated outcomes. However, depicting the ability of some specific antihyperglycemic therapies in reducing the risks for both atrial fibrillation and stroke as completely separate mechanisms would mean allowing the existence of slightly too much coincidental evidence. Trials searching for a potentially causal triangular relationship between antidiabetic drugs, risks for atrial fibrillation, and cerebral thromboembolism are needed to fill in a gap in evidence, and to potentially supplement the adaptation of the recommendations of current guidelines to prevent the negative outcomes of cardiovascular disease in diabetic patients as much as possible.

Author Contributions: Conceptualization, C.-M.L. and B.-M.M.; methodology, C.-M.L. and E.-D.G.; validation, C.-M.L. and B.-M.M.; formal analysis, C.-M.L., E.-D.G., A.O., and B.-M.M.; investigation, E.-D.G., C.S., R.A.S., and A.O.; resources, E.-D.G., C.S., R.A.S., and A.O.; writing—original draft preparation, C.-M.L., E.-D.G., C.S., and R.A.S.; writing—review and editing, C.-M.L. and B.-M.M.; visualization, C.-M.L.; supervision, B.-M.M.; project administration, C.-M.L. and E.-D.G.

References

1. Gæde, P.; Lund-Andersen, H.; Parving, H.-H.; Pedersen, O. Effect of a Multifactorial Intervention on Mortality in Type 2 Diabetes. *N. Engl. J. Med.* **2008**, *358*, 580–591. [CrossRef] [PubMed]
2. Rawshani, A.; Rawshani, A.; Franzén, S.; Sattar, N.; Eliasson, B.; Svensson, A.-M.; Zethelius, B.; Miftaraj, M.; McGuire, D.K.; Rosengren, A.; et al. Risk Factors, Mortality, and Cardiovascular Outcomes in Patients with Type 2 Diabetes. *N. Engl. J. Med.* **2018**, *379*, 633–644. [CrossRef] [PubMed]
3. Davies, M.; D'Alessio, D.; Fradkin, J.; Kernan, W.; Mathieu, C.; Mingrone, G.; Rossing, P.; Tsapas, A.; Wexler, D.; Buse, J. Management of hyperglycaemia in type 2 diabetes, 2018. A consensus report by the American Diabetes Association (ADA) and the European Association for the Study of Diabetes (EASD). *Diabetologia* **2018**, *61*, 2461–2498. [CrossRef] [PubMed]
4. Emerging Risk Factors Collaboration. The Emerging Risk Factors Collaboration Diabetes mellitus, fasting blood glucose concentration, and risk of vascular disease: A collaborative meta-analysis of 102 prospective studies. *Lancet* **2010**, *375*, 2215–2222. [CrossRef]

5. Proietti, R.; Russo, V.; Wu, M.A.; Maggioni, A.P.; Marfella, R. Diabetes mellitus and atrial fibrillation: Evidence of a pathophysiological, clinical and epidemiological association beyond the thromboembolic risk. *G. Ital. Cardiol. (Rome)* **2017**, *18*, 199–207.
6. Mentias, A.; Shantha, G.; Adeola, O.; Barnes, G.D.; Narasimhan, B.; Siontis, K.C.; Levine, D.A.; Sah, R.; Giudici, M.C.; Vaughan-Sarrazin, M. Role of diabetes and insulin use in the risk of stroke and acute myocardial infarction in patients with atrial fibrillation: A Medicare analysis. *Am. Heart J.* **2019**, *214*, 158–166. [CrossRef]
7. Bell, D.; Goncalves, E. Atrial fibrillation and type 2 diabetes: Prevalence, etiology, pathophysiology and effect of anti-diabetic therapies. *Diabetes Obes. Metab.* **2019**, *21*, 210–217. [CrossRef] [PubMed]
8. Bonnet, F.; Scheen, A. Impact of glucose-lowering therapies on risk of stroke in type 2 diabetes. *Diabetes Metab.* **2017**, *43*, 299–313. [CrossRef] [PubMed]
9. Chiao, Y.W.; Chen, Y.J.; Kuo, Y.H.; Lu, C.Y. Traditional Chinese Medical Care and Incidence of Stroke in Elderly Patients Treated with Antidiabetic Medications. *Int. J. Environ. Res. Public Health* **2018**, *15*, 1267. [CrossRef]
10. Naydenov, S.; Runev, N.; Manov, E.; Vasileva, D.; Rangelov, Y.; Naydenova, N. Risk Factors, Co-Morbidities and Treatment of In-Hospital Patients with Atrial Fibrillation in Bulgaria. *Medicina* **2018**, *54*, 34. [CrossRef]
11. Bandemer, S.V.; Merkel, S.; Nimako-Doffour, A.; Weber, M.M. Diabetes and atrial fibrillation: Stratification and prevention of stroke risks. *EPMA J.* **2014**, *5*, 17. [CrossRef] [PubMed]
12. Liou, Y.S.; Yang, F.Y.; Chen, H.Y.; Jong, G.P. Antihyperglycemic drugs use and new-onset atrial fibrillation: A population-based nested case control study. *PLoS ONE* **2018**, *13*, e0197245. [CrossRef] [PubMed]
13. Patti, G.; Lucerna, M.; Cavallari, I.; Ricottini, E.; Renda, G.; Pecen, L.; Romeo, F.; Le Heuzey, J.Y.; Zamorano, J.L.; Kirchhof, P.; et al. Insulin-Requiring Versus Noninsulin-Requiring Diabetes and Thromboembolic Risk in Patients with Atrial Fibrillation. *J. Am. Coll. Cardiol.* **2017**, *69*, 409–419. [CrossRef] [PubMed]
14. Asghar, O.; Alam, U.; Hayat, S.A.; Aghamohammadzadeh, R.; Heagerty, A.M.; Malik, R.A. Obesity, Diabetes and Atrial Fibrillation; Epidemiology, Mechanisms and Interventions. *Curr. Cardiol. Rev.* **2012**, *8*, 253–264. [CrossRef] [PubMed]
15. Chang, S.H.; Wu, L.S.; Chiou, M.J.; Liu, J.R.; Yu, K.H.; Kuo, C.F.; Wen, M.S.; Chen, W.J.; Yeh, Y.H.; See, L.C. Association of metformin with lower atrial fibrillation risk among patients with type 2 diabetes mellitus: A population-based dynamic cohort and in vitro studies. *Cardiovasc. Diabetol.* **2014**, *13*, 123. [CrossRef] [PubMed]
16. Homan, E.A.; Reyes, M.V.; Hickey, K.T.; Morrow, J.P. Clinical Overview of Obesity and Diabetes Mellitus as Risk Factors for Atrial Fibrillation and Sudden Cardiac Death. *Front. Physiol.* **2019**, *9*, 1847. [CrossRef] [PubMed]
17. UK Prospective Diabetes Study (UKPDS) Group. Effect of intensive blood-glucose control with metformin on complications in overweight patients with type 2 diabetes (UKPDS 34). *Lancet* **1998**, *352*, 854–865. [CrossRef]
18. Cheng, Y.Y.; Leu, H.B.; Chen, T.J.; Chen, C.L.; Kuo, C.H.; Lee, S.D.; Kao, C.L. Metformin-inclusive Therapy Reduces the Risk of Stroke in Patients with Diabetes: A 4-Year Follow-up Study. *J. Stroke Cerebrovasc. Dis.* **2014**, *23*, 99–105. [CrossRef]
19. Hatch, G.M.; Parkinson, F.E. Is There Enhanced Risk of Cerebral Ischemic Stroke by Sulfonylureas in Type 2 Diabetes? *Diabetes* **2016**, *65*, 2479–2481.
20. Liu, R.; Wang, H.; Xu, B.; Chen, W.; Turlova, E.; Dong, N.; Sun, C.; Lu, Y.; Fu, H.; Shi, R.; et al. Cerebrovascular Safety of Sulfonylureas: The Role of KATP Channels in Neuroprotection and the Risk of Stroke in Patients with Type 2 Diabetes. *Diabetes* **2016**, *65*, 2795–2809. [CrossRef]
21. Castilla-Guerra, L.; Fernandez-Moreno, M.; Leon-Jimenez, D.; Carmona-Nimo, E. Antidiabetic drugs and stroke risk Current evidence. *Eur. J. Intern. Med.* **2018**, *48*, 1–5. [CrossRef] [PubMed]
22. Kunte, H.; Schmidt, S.; Eliasziw, M.; Del Zoppo, G.J.; Simard, J.M.; Masuhr, F.; Weih, M.; Dirnagl, U. Sulfonylureas Improve Outcome in Patients with Type 2 Diabetes and Acute Ischemic Stroke. *Stroke* **2007**, *38*, 2526–2530. [CrossRef] [PubMed]
23. Weih, M.; Amberger, N.; Wegener, S.; Dirnagl, U.; Reuter, T.; Einhäupl, K. Sulfonylurea Drugs Do Not Influence Initial Stroke Severity and In-Hospital Outcome in Stroke Patients with Diabetes. *Stroke* **2001**, *32*, 2029–2032. [CrossRef] [PubMed]

24. Bannister, C.A.; Holden, S.E.; Morgan, C.L.; Halcox, J.P.; Schernthaner, G.; Mukherjee, J.; Currie, C.J.; Jenkins-Jones, S.; Halcox, J.; Bannister, C.; et al. Can people with type 2 diabetes live longer than those without? A comparison of mortality in people initiated with metformin or sulphonylurea monotherapy and matched, non-diabetic controls. *Diabetes Obes. Metab.* **2014**, *16*, 1165–1173. [CrossRef] [PubMed]
25. Goudis, C.A.; Korantzopoulos, P.; Ntalas, I.V.; Kallergis, E.M.; Liu, T.; Ketikoglou, D.G. Diabetes mellitus and atrial fibrillation: Pathophysiological mechanisms and potential upstream therapies. *Int. J. Cardiol.* **2015**, *184*, 617–622. [CrossRef] [PubMed]
26. Nesto, R.W.; Bell, D.; Bonow, R.O.; Fonseca, V.; Grundy, S.M.; Horton, E.S.; Le Winter, M.; Porte, D.; Semenkovich, C.F.; Smith, S.; et al. Thiazolidinedione Use, Fluid Retention, and Congestive Heart Failure. *Circulation* **2003**, *108*, 2941–2948. [CrossRef]
27. Wolski, K.; Nissen, S.E. Effect of Rosiglitazone on the Risk of Myocardial Infarction and Death from Cardiovascular Causes. *N. Engl. J. Med.* **2007**, *356*, 2457–2471.
28. Chao, T.F.; Leu, H.B.; Huang, C.C.; Chen, J.W.; Chan, W.L.; Lin, S.J.; Chen, S.A. Thiazolidinediones can prevent new onset atrial fibrillation in patients with non-insulin dependent diabetes. *Int. J. Cardiol.* **2012**, *156*, 199–202. [CrossRef]
29. Liu, X.; Wang, X.; Shi, H.; Tan, H.; Zhou, L.; Gu, J.; Jiang, W.; Wang, Y. Beneficial effect of pioglitazone on the outcome of catheter ablation in patients with paroxysmal atrial fibrillation and type 2 diabetes mellitus. *Europace* **2011**, *13*, 1256–1261.
30. Korantzopoulos, P.; Kokkoris, S.; Kountouris, E.; Protopsaltis, I.; Siogas, K.; Melidonis, A. Regression of paroxysmal atrial fibrillation associated with thiazolidinedione therapy. *Int. J. Cardiol.* **2008**, *125*, e51–e53. [CrossRef]
31. Pallisgaard, J.; Lindhardt, T.; Staerk, L.; Olesen, J.; Torp-Pedersen, C.; Hansen, M.; Gislason, G. Thiazolidinediones are associated with a decreased risk of atrial fibrillation compared with other antidiabetic treatment: A nationwide cohort study. *Eur. Heart J. Cardiovasc. Pharm.* **2017**, *3*, 140–146. [CrossRef] [PubMed]
32. Dormandy, J.; Charbonnel, B.; Eckland, D.; Erdmann, E.; Massi-Benedetti, M.; Moules, I.; Skene, A.; Tan, M.; Lefèbvre, P.; Murray, G.; et al. Secondary prevention of macrovascular events in patients with type 2 diabetes in the PROactive Study (PROspective pioglitAzone Clinical Trial In macroVascular Events): A randomised controlled trial. *Lancet* **2005**, *366*, 1279–1289. [CrossRef]
33. Pallisgaard, J.L.; Brooks, M.M.; Chaitman, B.R.; Boothroyd, D.B.; Perez, M.; Hlatky, M.A. Thiazolidinediones and Risk of Atrial Fibrillation among Patients with Diabetes and Coronary Disease. *Am. J. Med.* **2018**, *131*, 805–812. [CrossRef] [PubMed]
34. Zhang, Z.; Zhang, X.; Korantzopoulos, P.; Letsas, K.; Tse, G.; Gong, M.; Meng, L.; Li, G.; Liu, T. Thiazolidinedione use and atrial fibrillation in diabetic patients: A meta-analysis. *BMC Cardiovasc. Disord.* **2017**, *17*, 96. [CrossRef] [PubMed]
35. Wilcox, R.; Bousser, M.-G.; Betteridge, D.J.; Schernthaner, G.; Pirags, V.; Kupfer, S.; Dormandy, J. Effects of Pioglitazone in Patients with Type 2 Diabetes with or without Previous Stroke. *Stroke* **2007**, *38*, 865–873. [CrossRef] [PubMed]
36. Kernan, W.; Viscoli, C.; Furie, K.; Young, L.; Inzucchi, S.; Gorman, M.; Guarino, P.; Lovejoy, A.; Peduzzi, P.; Conwit, R.; et al. Pioglitazone after Ischemic Stroke or Transient Ischemic Attack. *N. Engl. J. Med.* **2016**, *374*, 1321–1331. [CrossRef]
37. Lee, M.; Saver, J.L.; Liao, H.-W.; Lin, C.-H.; Ovbiagele, B. Pioglitazone for Secondary Stroke Prevention. *Stroke* **2017**, *48*, 388–393. [CrossRef]
38. Chang, C.Y.; Yeh, Y.H.; Chan, Y.H.; Liu, J.R.; Chang, S.H.; Lee, H.F.; Wu, L.S.; Yen, K.C.; Kuo, C.T.; See, L.C. Dipeptidyl peptidase-4 inhibitor decreases the risk of atrial fibrillation in patients with type 2 diabetes: A nationwide cohort study in Taiwan. *Cardiovasc. Diabetol.* **2017**, *16*, 159. [CrossRef]
39. Ou, H.T.; Chang, K.C.; Li, C.Y.; Wu, J.S. Risks of cardiovascular diseases associated with dipeptidyl peptidase-4 inhibitors and other antidiabetic drugs in patients with type 2 diabetes: A nation-wide longitudinal study. *Cardiovasc. Diabetol.* **2016**, *15*, 41. [CrossRef]
40. Scirica, B.; Bhatt, D.; Braunwald, E.; Steg, P.; Davidson, J.; Hirshberg, B.; Ohman, P.; Frederich, R.; Wiviott, S.; Hoffman, E.; et al. Saxagliptin and Cardiovascular Outcomes in Patients with Type 2 Diabetes Mellitus. *N. Engl. J. Med.* **2013**, *369*, 1317–1326. [CrossRef]

41. White, W.; Cannon, C.; Heller, S.; Nissen, S.; Bergenstal, R.; Bakris, G.; Perez, A.; Fleck, P.; Mehta, C.; Kupfer, S.; et al. Alogliptin after Acute Coronary Syndrome in Patients with Type 2 Diabetes. *N. Engl. J. Med.* **2013**, *369*, 1327–1335. [CrossRef] [PubMed]
42. Green, J.; Bethel, M.; Armstrong, P.; Buse, J.; Engel, S.; Garg, J.; Josse, R.; Kaufman, K.; Koglin, J.; Korn, S.; et al. Effect of Sitagliptin on Cardiovascular Outcomes in Type 2 Diabetes. *N. Engl. J. Med.* **2015**, *373*, 232–242. [CrossRef] [PubMed]
43. Gantz, I.; Chen, M.; Suryawanshi, S.; Ntabadde, C.; Shah, S.; O'Neill, E.A.; Engel, S.S.; Kaufman, K.D.; Lai, E. A randomized, placebo-controlled study of the cardiovascular safety of the once-weekly DPP-4 inhibitor omarigliptin in patients with type 2 diabetes mellitus. *Cardiovasc. Diabetol.* **2017**, *16*, 112. [CrossRef] [PubMed]
44. Rosenstock, J.; Perkovic, V.; Johansen, O.; Cooper, M.; Kahn, S.; Marx, N.; Alexander, J.; Pencina, M.; Toto, R.; Wanner, C.; et al. Effect of Linagliptin vs Placebo on Major Cardiovascular Events in Adults with Type 2 Diabetes and High Cardiovascular and Renal Risk. *JAMA* **2019**, *321*, 69–79. [CrossRef] [PubMed]
45. Barkas, F.; Elisaf, M.; Tsimihodimos, V.; Milionis, H. Dipeptidyl peptidase-4 inhibitors and protection against stroke: A systematic review and meta-analysis. *Diabetes Metab.* **2017**, *43*, 1–8. [CrossRef] [PubMed]
46. Sinha, B.; Ghosal, S. Meta-analyses of the effects of DPP-4 inhibitors, SGLT2 inhibitors and GLP1 receptor analogues on cardiovascular death, myocardial infarction, stroke and hospitalization for heart failure. *Diabetes Res. Clin. Pract.* **2019**, *150*, 8–16. [CrossRef] [PubMed]
47. Sun, F.; Wu, S.; Guo, S.; Yu, K.; Yang, Z.; Li, L.; Zhang, Y.; Quan, X.; Ji, L.; Zhan, S. Impact of GLP-1 receptor agonists on blood pressure, heart rate and hypertension among patients with type 2 diabetes: A systematic review and network meta-analysis. *Diabetes Res. Clin. Pract.* **2015**, *110*, 26–37. [CrossRef] [PubMed]
48. Smits, M.M.; Muskiet, M.H.A.; Tonneijck, L.; Hoekstra, T.; Kramer, M.H.H.; Diamant, M.; Van Raalte, D.H. Exenatide acutely increases heart rate in parallel with augmented sympathetic nervous system activation in healthy overweight males. *Br. J. Clin. Pharmacol.* **2016**, *81*, 613–620. [CrossRef]
49. Lorenz, M.; Lawson, F.; Owens, D.; Raccah, D.; Roy-Duval, C.; Lehmann, A.; Perfetti, R.; Blonde, L. Differential effects of glucagon-like peptide-1 receptor agonists on heart rate. *Cardiovasc. Diabetol.* **2017**, *16*, 6. [CrossRef]
50. Fisher, M.; Petrie, M.C.; Ambery, P.D.; Donaldson, J.; Ye, J.; McMurray, J.J.V. Cardiovascular safety of albiglutide in the Harmony programme: A meta-analysis. *Lancet Diabetes Endocrinol.* **2015**, *3*, 697–703. [CrossRef]
51. Pfeffer, M.; Claggett, B.; Diaz, R.; Dickstein, K.; Gerstein, H.; Køber, L.; Lawson, F.; Ping, L.; Wei, X.; Lewis, E.; et al. Lixisenatide in Patients with Type 2 Diabetes and Acute Coronary Syndrome. *N. Engl. J. Med.* **2015**, *373*, 2247–2257. [CrossRef] [PubMed]
52. Liraglutide Effect and Action in Diabetes: Evaluation of Cardiovascular Outcome Results—Study Results—ClinicalTrials.gov. Available online: https://clinicaltrials.gov/ct2/show/results/NCT01179048 (accessed on 20 June 2019).
53. Marso, S.P.; Bain, S.C.; Consoli, A.; Eliaschewitz, F.G.; Jódar, E.; Leiter, L.A.; Lingvay, I.; Rosenstock, J.; Seufert, J.; Warren, M.L.; et al. Semaglutide and Cardiovascular Outcomes in Patients with Type 2 Diabetes. *N. Engl. J. Med.* **2016**, *375*, 1834–1844. [CrossRef] [PubMed]
54. Monami, M.; Nreu, B.; Scatena, A.; Giannini, S.; Andreozzi, F.; Sesti, G.; Mannucci, E. Glucagon-like peptide-1 receptor agonists and atrial fibrillation: A systematic review and meta-analysis of randomised controlled trials. *J. Endocrinol. Investig.* **2017**, *40*, 1251–1258. [CrossRef] [PubMed]
55. Marso, S.P.; Daniels, G.H.; Brown-Frandsen, K.; Kristensen, P.; Mann, J.F.; Nauck, M.A.; Nissen, S.E.; Pocock, S.; Poulter, N.R.; Ravn, L.S.; et al. Liraglutide and Cardiovascular Outcomes in Type 2 Diabetes. *N. Engl. J. Med.* **2016**, *375*, 311–322. [CrossRef] [PubMed]
56. Hernandez, A.; Green, J.; Janmohamed, S.; D'Agostino, R.; Granger, C.; Jones, N.; Leiter, L.; Rosenberg, A.; Sigmon, K.; Somerville, M.; et al. Albiglutide and cardiovascular outcomes in patients with type 2 diabetes and cardiovascular disease (Harmony Outcomes): A double-blind, randomised placebo-controlled trial. *Lancet* **2018**, *392*, 1519–1529. [CrossRef]
57. Gerstein, H.; Colhoun, H.; Dagenais, G.; Diaz, R.; Lakshmanan, M.; Pais, P.; Probstfield, J.; Riesmeyer, J.; Riddle, M.; Rydén, L.; et al. Dulaglutide and cardiovascular outcomes in type 2 diabetes (REWIND): A double-blind, randomised placebo-controlled trial. *Lancet* **2019**, in press. [CrossRef]

58. Zinman, B.; Wanner, C.; Lachin, J.; Fitchett, D.; Bluhmki, E.; Hantel, S.; Mattheus, M.; Devins, T.; Johansen, O.; Woerle, H.; et al. Empagliflozin, Cardiovascular Outcomes, and Mortality in Type 2 Diabetes. *N. Engl. J. Med.* **2015**, *373*, 2117–2128. [CrossRef]
59. Neal, B.; Perkovic, V.; Mahaffey, K.W.; De Zeeuw, D.; Fulcher, G.; Erondu, N.; Shaw, W.; Law, G.; Desai, M.; Matthews, D.R.; et al. Canagliflozin and Cardiovascular and Renal Events in Type 2 Diabetes. *N. Engl. J. Med.* **2017**, *377*, 644–657. [CrossRef]
60. Wiviott, S.; Raz, I.; Bonaca, M.; Mosenzon, O.; Kato, E.; Cahn, A.; Silverman, M.; Zelniker, T.; Kuder, J.; Murphy, S.; et al. Dapagliflozin and Cardiovascular Outcomes in Type 2 Diabetes. *N. Engl. J. Med.* **2019**, *380*, 347–357. [CrossRef]
61. Zinman, B.; Inzucchi, S.E.; Lachin, J.M.; Wanner, C.; Fitchett, D.; Kohler, S.; Mattheus, M.; Woerle, H.J.; Broedl, U.C.; Johansen, O.E.; et al. Empagliflozin and Cerebrovascular Events in Patients with Type 2 Diabetes Mellitus at High Cardiovascular Risk. *Stroke* **2017**, *48*, 1218–1225. [CrossRef]
62. Wu, J.; Foote, C.; Blomster, J.; Toyama, T.; Perkovic, V.; Sundström, J.; Neal, B. Effects of sodium-glucose cotransporter-2 inhibitors on cardiovascular events, death, and major safety outcomes in adults with type 2 diabetes: A systematic review and meta-analysis. *Lancet Diabetes Endocrinol.* **2016**, *4*, 411–419. [CrossRef]
63. Imprialos, K.P.; Boutari, C.; Stavropoulos, K.; Doumas, M.; Karagiannis, A.I. Stroke paradox with SGLT-2 inhibitors: A play of chance or a viscosity-mediated reality? *J. Neurol. Neurosurg. Psychiatry* **2016**, *88*, 249–253. [CrossRef] [PubMed]
64. Usman, M.S.; Siddiqi, T.J.; Memon, M.M.; Khan, M.S.; Rawasia, W.F.; Ayub, M.T.; Sreenivasan, J.; Golzar, Y. Sodium-glucose co-transporter 2 inhibitors and cardiovascular outcomes: A systematic review and meta-analysis. *Eur. J. Prev. Cardiol.* **2018**, *25*, 495–502. [CrossRef] [PubMed]

16

Outcome after Interdisciplinary Treatment for Aneurysmal Subarachnoid Hemorrhage

Benjamin Voellger [1,*], Rosita Rupa [1], Christian Arndt [2], Barbara Carl [1] and Christopher Nimsky [1]

1 Department of Neurosurgery, University Hospital Marburg, 35033 Marburg, Germany; rupar@med.uni-marburg.de (R.R.); carlb@med.uni-marburg.de (B.C.); nimsky@med.uni-marburg.de (C.N.)
2 Department of Anaesthesiology, University Hospital Marburg, 35033 Marburg, Germany; arndtc@med.uni-marburg.de
* Correspondence: voellger@med.uni-marburg.de

Abstract: *Background and Objectives:* To identify predictors of outcome after aneurysmal subarachnoid hemorrhage (aSAH) in our interdisciplinary setting. *Materials and Methods:* 176 patients who had been treated for aSAH by a team of neurosurgeons and neuroradiologists between 2009 and 2017 were analyzed retrospectively. Age, gender, clinical presentation according to the Hunt and Hess (H&H) grading on admission, overall clot burden, aneurysm localization, modality of aneurysm obliteration, early deterioration (ED), occurrence of vasospasm in transcranial Doppler ultrasonography, delayed cerebral ischemia (DCI), spasmolysis, decompressive craniectomy (DC), cerebrospinal fluid (CSF) shunt placement, deep vein thrombosis (DVT), pulmonary embolism (PE), severe cardiac events (SCE), mortality on Days 14, and 30 after admission, and outcome at one year after the hemorrhage according to the Glasgow Outcome Scale (GOS) were recorded. Chi square, Fisher's exact, Welch's t, and Wilcoxon rank sum served as statistical tests. Generalized linear models were fitted, and ordered logistic regression was performed. *Results*: SCE ($p = 0.049$) were a significant predictor of mortality at 14 days after aSAH, but not later during the first year after the hemorrhage. Clipping as opposed to coiling ($p = 0.049$) of ruptured aneurysms was a significant predictor of survival on Day 30 after aSAH, but not later during the first year after the hemorrhage, while coiling as opposed to clipping of ruptured aneurysms was significantly related to a lower frequency of DVT during hospitalization ($p = 0.024$). Aneurysms of the anterior circulation were significantly more often clipped, while aneurysms of the posterior circulation were significantly more often coiled ($p < 0.001$). Age over 70 years ($p = 0.049$), H&H grade on admission ($p = 0.022$), overall clot burden ($p = 0.035$), ED ($p = 0.009$), DCI ($p = 0.013$), DC ($p = 0.0005$), and CSF shunt placement ($p = 0.038$) proved to be predictive of long-term outcome after aSAH. *Conclusion:* Long-term results after clipping and coiling of ruptured aneurysms appear equal in an interdisciplinary setting that takes aneurysm localization, available staff, and equipment into account.

Keywords: aneurysmal subarachnoid hemorrhage; outcome; interdisciplinary setting

1. Introduction

The high-level evidence provided by the International Subarachnoid Aneurysm Trial (ISAT) [1] led to favor coiling, a technique first described by Guglielmi [2], over clipping for the obliteration of ruptured cerebral aneurysms. Nonetheless, interdisciplinary settings were tailored to the local particularities at many neurovascular centers over time, due to the indisputable weaknesses of ISAT, namely the disproportionately high number of coiled aneurysms of the anterior communicating artery, and the comparison of the results of aneurysm obliteration performed by highly specialized neuroradiologists with those performed by averagely trained neurosurgeons in ISAT. The Barrow Ruptured Aneurysm Trial (BRAT) [3] initially seemed to confirm the results of ISAT, while data from the BRAT study at six years after the hemorrhage [4] suggested that the modality of aneurysm obliteration of ruptured aneurysms of the anterior circulation would not affect long-term results as long as treatment remained in experienced hands. Furthermore, data from the BRAT study at 10 years after the hemorrhage demonstrated that rates of complete aneurysm obliteration and rates of retreatment actually favored clipping over coiling [5].

There is, however, only a limited number of publications on results after single-center interdisciplinary treatment for aSAH. Güresir et al. [6] identified intraparenchymal hemorrhage as prognostically unfavorable in 585 patients treated interdisciplinarily for aSAH. Proust et al. [7] found a decrease of verbal memory capabilities in 50 patients after clipping versus coiling of ruptured aneurysms of the anterior communicating artery, while other neuropsychological deficiencies and quality of life did not differ significantly between treatment groups. The same group [8] reported on the results of interdisciplinary treatment at six months after aSAH, according to the modified Rankin Scale (mRS) [9] in 64 patients who were 70 years of age or older at the time of bleeding; an unfavorable correlation of initially poor clinical presentation and delayed cerebral ischemia with outcome was found. Schöller et al. [10] described an initially good clinical presentation and an age of less than 70 years on admission as prognostically favorable factors. In a small series of patients with ruptured aneurysms of the posterior inferior cerebellar artery, Sejkorova et al. [11] identified an initially high Hunt and Hess (H&H) [12] grade as unfavorable for the outcome after interdisciplinary treatment. Schwartz et al. [13] found young age at the time of admission and absence of cerebral ischemia to yield a favorable prognosis in 106 cases of interdisciplinary treated ruptured cerebral aneurysms. AlMatter et al. [14] identified age, initial clinical presentation, re-rupture of the aneurysm, intraparenchymal hemorrhage, and ruptured aneurysms of the middle cerebral artery as relevant prognostic factors; they described a trend towards unfavorable outcomes after vasospasm, intraventricular hemorrhage, and rupture of large aneurysms.

In our study, we aimed to retrospectively identify predictive factors after treatment for aSAH in a single center series of 176 cases.

2. Materials and Methods

2.1. Patients

In this single center retrospective study, 176 patients admitted to our university hospital between 2009 and 2017 were included. The patients fulfilled each of the following inclusion criteria: subarachnoid hemorrhage diagnosed after cranial computed tomography (CCT) or lumbar puncture, detection of at least one cerebral aneurysm in digital subtraction angiography (DSA) or computed tomography angiography (CTA), obliteration of the ruptured aneurysm by coiling or clipping within 24 h after admission. Patients with a history of severe cognitive impairment prior to the hemorrhage, such as progressive dementia, and patients with H&H grade 5 hemorrhages who did not benefit from external ventricular drainage (EVD) insertion were not included.

Age, gender, aneurysm localization, blood distribution according to the modified Fisher scale [15], and clinical findings according to the H&H scale on admission were recorded.

Necessity of EVD insertion, modality of aneurysm obliteration, detection of cerebral vasospasm, frequencies of spasmolysis, delayed cerebral ischemia (DCI), decompressive craniectomy (DC), cerebrospinal fluid (CSF) shunt dependency, deep vein thrombosis (DVT), pulmonary embolism (PE), and severe cardiac events (SCE), i.e., incidents requiring electrical cardioversion or cardiopulmonary resuscitation, were recorded.

Survival at Days 14 and 30 after SAH was recorded. Follow-up at one year after the hemorrhage was recorded according to the Glasgow Outcome Scale (GOS) [16]. Favorable outcomes were defined as GOS 4 or 5.

2.2. Interdisciplinary Setting

Urgent EVD insertion was performed in cases with symptomatic hydrocephalus. Obliteration of the ruptured aneurysm was achieved within 24 h after admission. In all but one patient with a ruptured aneurysm of the middle cerebral artery (MCA), the aneurysm was clipped, while, in one patient with a ruptured aneurysm of the MCA, the aneurysm was coiled. In the remaining cases, an interdisciplinary decision as to the modality of aneurysm obliteration was made, and the ruptured aneurysm was treated accordingly. In cases with multiple aneurysms, sequence and modality of aneurysm obliteration were determined interdisciplinarily. All patients received neurosurgical intensive care.

2.3. Statistical Analysis

Statistical analysis was conducted using OpenOffice 4.1.3 and R 3.5.1 with R Studio 1.1.383 on a Mac OS X 10.14.4. Figures were created with R and R Studio. Chi square, Fisher's exact, Welch's t, and Wilcoxon rank sum served as statistical tests. To assess the impact of predictors on outcome variables, generalized linear models were fitted, and a proportional odds logistic regression was performed. Statistical significance was assumed with p values less than 0.05.

2.4. Ethical Approval

Upon our request in March 2018, the local ethics committee at the University Hospital Marburg considered an ethical approval unnecessary for this pseudonymized retrospective analysis.

3. Results

Mean age on admission was 56 years (range: 22–90 years). On admission, 63 patients (35.8%) were 60 years of age or older, and 9 patients (5.1%) were 80 years of age or older. One hundred six patients (60.2%) were female.

Overall, 167 of 176 patients (94.9%) presented with symptomatic hydrocephalus on admission and urgently received an EVD.

Clinical findings according to the H&H scale [12] on admission are given in Table 1. Information on blood distribution according to the modified Fisher scale in the initial CCT is provided in Table 2.

Table 1. Clinical presentation according to the Hunt and Hess (H&H) scale [12] on admission in 176 patients with aneurysmal subarachnoid hemorrhage.

Initial H&H Grade	Number of Ruptured Aneurysms Clipped (n = 108)	Number of Ruptured Aneurysms Coiled (n = 68)	Statistical Test, p-Value
1	9	9	
2	27	16	
3	26	16	
4	29	17	
5	17	10	
			Wilcoxon rank sum, $p = 0.14$

Table 2. Blood distribution in the initial cranial computerized tomography (CCT) scan according to the modified Fisher scale [15] in 176 patients with aneurysmal subarachnoid hemorrhage.

Modified Fisher Grade	Number of Ruptured Aneurysms Clipped (n = 108)	Number of Ruptured Aneurysms Coiled (n = 68)
0	2	4
1	9	6
2	4	7
3	38	18
4	55	33

Clipped and coiled aneurysms by location are tabulated in Table 3. In 42 patients (23.9%), multiple cerebral aneurysms were detected. Ruptured aneurysms of the anterior circulation were significantly more often clipped, while ruptured aneurysms of the posterior circulation were significantly more often coiled (chi square test, $p < 0.001$).

Table 3. Clipped and coiled aneurysms by location in 176 patients with aneurysmal subarachnoid hemorrhage.

Aneurysm Location	Number of Ruptured Aneurysms Clipped (n = 108)	Number of Ruptured Aneurysms Coiled (n = 68)	Statistical Test, p-Value
MCA [1]	52	1	
ACA [1]	11	4	
Acomm [1]	27	26	
ICA paraophthalmic [1]	3	4	
ICA supraophthalmic [1]	13	12	
Pcomm [1]	2	0	
SCA [2]	0	1	
PICA [2]	0	3	
Basilar artery [2]	0	13	
Vertebral artery [2]	0	4	
Ruptured aneurysms of the anterior circulation (subtotal of locations marked with superscript 1) *	108	47	
Ruptured aneurysms of the posterior circulation (subtotal of locations marked with superscript 2) *	0	21	
			chi square, $p < 0.001$

Abbreviations: MCA, middle cerebral artery; ACA, anterior cerebral artery; Acomm, anterior communicating artery; ICA, internal carotid artery; Pcomm, posterior communicating artery; SCA, superior cerebellar artery; PICA, posterior inferior cerebellar artery. Superscript 1, anterior circulation; superscript 2, posterior circulation. * Statistically significant finding.

Events of clinical significance during hospitalization are listed in Table 4. We found a significantly higher probability of DVT in patients who underwent clipping as opposed to coiling of ruptured cerebral aneurysms (Fisher's exact test, $p = 0.024$).

Table 4. Events of clinical significance during hospitalization in 176 patients with aneurysmal subarachnoid hemorrhage.

Clinical Event	Number of Ruptured Aneurysms Clipped (n = 108)	Number of Ruptured Aneurysms Coiled (n = 68)	Statistical Test, p-Value
EVD insertion = yes	102	65	Fisher's exact, $p = 1$
SCE = yes	5	7	Fisher's exact, $p = 0.218$
Vasospasm in TCD = yes	39	16	chi square, $p = 0.113$
DCI = yes	49	34	chi square, $p = 0.657$
Spasmolysis = yes	5	4	Fisher's exact, $p = 0.736$
DC performed = yes	29	13	chi square, $p = 0.322$
CSF shunt placed = yes	48	31	chi square, $p = 1$
DVT detected = yes *	8	0	Fisher's exact, $p = 0.024$
PE detected = yes	4	1	Fisher's exact, $p = 0.65$

Abbreviations: EVD, external ventricular drainage; SCE, severe cardiac event; TCD, transcranial Doppler sonography; DCI, delayed cerebral ischemia; DC, decompressive craniectomy; CSF, cerebrospinal fluid; DVT, deep vein thrombosis; PE, pulmonary embolism. * Statistically significant finding.

Information on survival during the first month after the hemorrhage is provided in Table 5. At 30 days after the hemorrhage, we found a significantly higher probability of survival in patients who underwent clipping as opposed to coiling of ruptured cerebral aneurysms (generalized linear modeling, $p = 0.0495$). Outcome according to the GOS at one year after the hemorrhage is given in Table 6. Clinical data at 14 and 30 days after the hemorrhage were available in all patients, while follow-up at one year was obtained in 133 of 176 patients (75.6%).

Table 5. Survival during the first month in 176 patients with aneurysmal subarachnoid hemorrhage.

Survival Status	Number of Ruptured Aneurysms Clipped ($n = 108$)	Number of Ruptured Aneurysms Coiled ($n = 68$)	Statistical Model, p-Value
Survived at 14 days	102	60	generalized linear modeling, $p = 0.2107$
Survived at 30 days *	101	58	generalized linear modeling, $p = 0.0495$

* Statistically significant finding.

Table 6. Outcome according to the Glasgow Outcome Scale (GOS) [16] at one year in 176 patients with aneurysmal subarachnoid hemorrhage.

GOS	Number of Ruptured Aneurysms Clipped ($n = 108$)	Number of Ruptured Aneurysms Coiled ($n = 68$)	Statistical Model, p-Value
1 at 1 year	14	11	
2 at 1 year	6	0	
3 at 1 year	25	11	
4 at 1 year	17	9	
5 at 1 year	24	16	
			proportional odds logistic regression, $p = 0.4767$

The impact of potentially predictive variables on outcome after aSAH is illustrated in Figure 1.

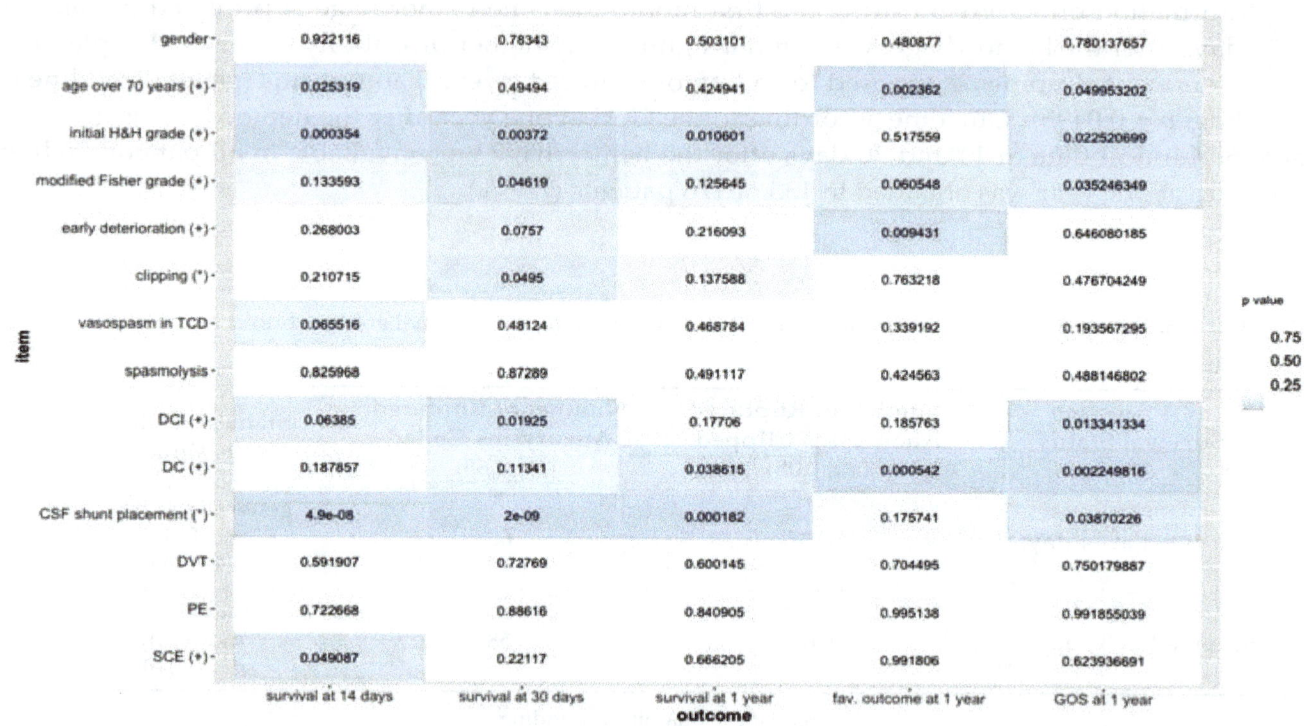

Figure 1. Statistical significance of potential predictors of outcome in 176 patients with aneurysmal subarachnoid hemorrhage as estimated from generalized linear models for dichotomous outcome variables (survival and fav. outcome) and proportional odds logistic regression for an ordinal outcome variable (GOS) after aneurysmal subarachnoid hemorrhage. Information on survival at Days 14 and 30 after the hemorrhage was available in all patients, while information on outcome at one year after the hemorrhage was obtained in 133 patients (75.6%). Abbreviations: H&H, Hunt and Hess; TCD, transcranial Doppler sonography; DCI, delayed cerebral ischemia; DC, decompressive craniectomy; CSF, cerebrospinal fluid; DVT, deep vein thrombosis; PE, pulmonary embolism; SCE, severe cardiac event; fav., favorable; GOS, Glasgow Outcome Scale; (*) true (dichotomous variables) or increasing (ordered values) values predictive of survival, favorable outcome, or high GOS score; (+) true (dichotomous variables) or increasing (ordered values) values predictive of mortality, unfavorable outcome or low GOS score.

4. Discussion

Various authors reported an initially poor H&H grade to predict an unfavorable outcome after aSAH [1,8,10,11,14]. This finding was confirmed in our study: according to our data, an initially poor H&H grade significantly predicted mortality at Days 14 and 30 after the hemorrhage, mortality at one year after the hemorrhage and a less favorable outcome according to the GOS at one year after the hemorrhage. We regularly refrain from obliterating ruptured cerebral aneurysms in patients who, prior to the onset of aSAH, have a history of severe cognitive impairment, such as progressive dementia, since we consider the potential benefit of aneurysm obliteration to these patients highly questionable.

Age as a predictor of outcome after aSAH has been reported before [10,13,14]. In our study, age of over 70 years on admission, being a cut-off age within the range of those of several other publications, was a strong predictor of mortality at 14 days after the hemorrhage, an unfavorable outcome and a less favorable outcome according to the GOS at one year after the hemorrhage. We share, however, the view of other authors that age alone should not be an objection as to the diagnosis and treatment of cerebrovascular diseases [17].

In other studies on aSAH, a high overall clot burden has been described as a predictive factor [18]. We found the extent of overall clot burden in the initial CCT, as recorded according to the modified

Fisher scale, to be significantly associated with mortality at 30 days after the hemorrhage, and with a less favorable outcome according to the GOS at one year after the hemorrhage.

Clipping as opposed to coiling of ruptured aneurysms was a significant predictor of survival at 30 days after aSAH, but not later during the first year after the hemorrhage. As far as we know, a similar finding has not been reported in other studies before. We suppose that the reduction of overall clot burden, which is part of the standard clipping procedure as opposed to the standard coiling procedure after aSAH, leads to a temporary relief from spasmogenic stimuli in the subarachnoid space, which may explain our finding.

Furthermore, our single center experience has shown that particularly in patients with poor H&H grades, clipping of a ruptured aneurysm is often accompanied by DC in the same session. By contrast, in patients with coiled aneurysms usually a clinical deterioration somewhat later in the course of the disease gives rise to DC. The earlier onset of the effect of DC may lead to temporary recovery in clinically poor patients who undergo clipping of ruptured aneurysms, which may contribute to the statistically significant effect of clipping on survival at 30 days after the hemorrhage as observed in our study.

Coiling as opposed to clipping of ruptured aneurysms was significantly correlated with a lower frequency of DVT, while the frequency of PE did not significantly depend on the modality of aneurysm obliteration in our patients. One may assume that acetylsalicylic acid (ASS) and heparin in doses with therapeutic effects, as regularly administered after aneurysm coiling, help to prevent DVT, while larger patient cohorts need to be analyzed to prove a potential impact of ASS and heparin on the frequency of PE after aSAH.

The fact that aneurysms of the anterior circulation were significantly more often clipped, while aneurysms of the posterior circulation were significantly more often coiled, is primarily attributable to particularities of our interdisciplinary approach.

ED has been reported to predict an unfavorable outcome after aSAH [19], which was confirmed in our study: ED was significantly related to an unfavorable outcome at 12 months after the hemorrhage.

Other authors have reported SCE as well as elevated Troponin levels, electrocardiographic or echocardiographic abnormalities, to be linked to unfavorable outcomes after aSAH [20–22]. In our patients, SCE were a significant predictor of mortality at 14 days after the hemorrhage, but not later during the first year after the hemorrhage. This finding may become relevant when clinical decisions have to be consented with the patient's next of kin: in patients with aSAH, a severely unstable cardiovascular situation during hospitalization after the hemorrhage occasionally tempts family members to fear lack of recovery and to demand intensive care not to be extended. Our study may provide a rationale to continue curative treatment in these cases.

We found that DCI was a significant predictor of mortality on Day 30 and of a less favorable overall outcome according to the GOS at one year after the hemorrhage, which is a finding other authors have reported before [14].

In our study, DC was a significant predictor of mortality, of an unfavorable outcome (i.e., GOS < 4) and of a less favorable outcome (i.e., a lower GOS) at one year after the hemorrhage. We found, however, that more than two out of three patients who required DC survived the first year after the hemorrhage. It therefore seems well warranted to indicate DC generously in patients who deteriorate due to malignant brain swelling after aSAH.

In our study, CSF shunt placement was a significant predictor of survival on days 14 and 30, and at one year after aSAH as well as of a less favorable outcome according to the GOS at one year after aSAH. This finding should be interpreted cautiously: of 97 patients who did not receive a CSF shunt, 14 (respectively, 17 and 21) patients were deceased at 14 (respectively, 30 and 365) days after the hemorrhage, while, of 79 patients who received a CSF shunt, 0 (respectively, 0 and 4) patients were deceased at 14 (respectively, 30 and 365) days after the hemorrhage. This observation is in accordance with the clinical experience that most patients with initially poor H&H grades simply do not survive long enough to receive a CSF shunt after aSAH.

Limitations of Our Study

When interpreting our results, it should be kept in mind that this work is a single center retrospective study with an incomplete follow-up of 75.6% at one year after the hemorrhage. These facts set limitations to any generalized conclusion one would want to derive from our data. Our patients were treated at a university hospital in a country with an overall high standard of medical care.

5. Conclusions

SCE were predictive of mortality at 14 days after aSAH but not later during the first year after the hemorrhage.

Clipping as opposed to coiling of ruptured aneurysms was a significant predictor of survival at 30 days but not later during the first year after aSAH, while coiling as opposed to clipping of ruptured aneurysms was significantly related to a lower frequency of DVT during hospitalization.

Age over 70 years, H&H grade on admission, overall clot burden, ED, DCI, DC, and CSF shunt placement proved to be predictive of long-term outcome after aSAH.

Long-term results after clipping and coiling of ruptured aneurysms appear equal in an interdisciplinary setting that takes aneurysm localization, available staff, and equipment into account.

Author Contributions: Conceptualization: B.V. and C.N.; methodology: B.V. and C.N.; validation: B.V.; formal analysis: B.V. and R.R.; investigation: R.R.; resources: C.N.; data curation: B.V. and R.R.; writing—original draft preparation: B.V.; writing—review and editing: C.N., B.C., R.R., and C.A.; visualization: B.V.; and supervision: C.N.

Acknowledgments: We are very grateful to med. Maximilian Schulze, Department of Neuroradiology, University Hospital Marburg, for the careful analysis of CCT scans in order to detect radiographic signs of DCI in our patients.

References

1. Molyneux, A.J.; Kerr, R.S.C.; Yu, L.M.; Clarke, M.; Sneade, M.; Yarnold, J.A.; Sandercock, P.; International Subarachnoid Aneurysm Trial (ISAT) Collaborative Group. International subarachnoid aneurysm trial (ISAT) of neurosurgical clipping versus endovascular coiling in 2143 patients with ruptured intracranial aneurysms: A randomised comparison of effects on survival, dependency, seizures, rebleeding, subgroups, and aneurysm occlusion. *Lancet* **2005**, *366*, 809–817.
2. Guglielmi, G.; Viñuela, F.; Dion, J.; Duckwiler, G. Electrothrombosis of saccular aneurysms via endovascular approach. Part 2: Preliminar clinical experience. *J. Neurosurg.* **1991**, *75*, 8–14. [CrossRef]
3. McDougall, C.G.; Spetzler, R.F.; Zabramski, J.M.; Partovi, S.; Hills, N.K.; Nakaji, P.; Albuquerque, F.C. The Barrow ruptured Aneurysm Trial. *J. Neurosurg.* **2012**, *116*, 135–144. [CrossRef] [PubMed]
4. Spetzler, R.F.; McDougall, C.G.; Zabramski, J.M.; Albuquerque, F.C.; Hills, N.K.; Russin, J.J.; Partovi, S.; Nakaji, P.; Wallace, R.C. The Barrow Ruptured Aneurysm Trial: 6-year results. *J. Neurosurg.* **2015**, *123*, 609–617. [CrossRef] [PubMed]
5. Spetzler, R.F.; McDougall, C.G.; Zabramski, J.M.; Albuquerque, F.C.; Hills, N.K.; Nakaji, P.; Karis, J.P.; Wallace, R.C. Ten-year analysis of saccular aneurysms in the Barrow Ruptured Aneurysm Trial. *J. Neurosurg.* **2019**, *8*, 1–6. [CrossRef] [PubMed]
6. Güresir, E.; Beck, J.; Vatter, H.; Setzer, M.; Gerlach, R.; Seifert, V.; Raabe, A. Subarachnoid hemorrhage and intracerebral hematoma: Incidence, prognostic factors, and outcome. *Neurosurgery* **2008**, *63*, 1088–1093. [CrossRef] [PubMed]
7. Proust, F.; Martinaud, O.; Gérardin, E.; Derrey, S.; Lesvèque, S.; Bioux, S.; Tollard, E.; Clavier, E.; Langlois, O.; Godefroy, O.; et al. Quality of life and brain damage after microsurgical clip occlusion or endovascular coil embolization for ruptured anterior communicating artery aneurysms: Neuropsychological assessment. *J. Neurosurg.* **2009**, *110*, 19–29. [CrossRef] [PubMed]
8. Proust, F.; Gérardin, E.; Derrey, S.; Lesvèque, S.; Ramos, S.; Langlois, O.; Tollard, E.; Bénichou, J.; Chassagne, P.; Clavier, E. Interdisciplinary treatment of ruptured cerebral aneurysms in elderly patients. *J. Neurosurg.* **2010**, *112*, 1200–1207. [CrossRef] [PubMed]

9. van Swieten, J.C.; Koudstaal, P.J.; Visser, M.C.; Schouten, H.J.; van Gijn, J. Intraobserver agreement for the assessment of handicap in stroke patients. *Stroke* **1988**, *19*, 604–607. [CrossRef]
10. Schöller, K.; Massmann, M.; Markl, G.; Kunz, M.; Fesl, G.; Brückmann, H.; Pfefferkorn, T.; Tonn, J.C. Aneurysmal subarachnoid hemorrhage in elderly patients: Long-term outcome and prognostic factors in an interdisciplinary treatment approach. *J. Neurol.* **2013**, *260*, 1052–1060. [CrossRef]
11. Sejkorova, A.; Cihlar, F.; Hejcl, A.; Lodin, J.; Vachata, P.; Sames, M. Microsurgery and endovascular treatment of posterior inferior cerebellar artery aneurysms. *Neurosurg. Rev.* **2016**, *39*, 159–168. [CrossRef] [PubMed]
12. Hunt, W.E.; Hess, R.M. Surgical risk as related to time of intervention in the repair of intracranial aneurysms. *J. Neurosurg.* **1968**, *28*, 14–20. [CrossRef] [PubMed]
13. Schwartz, C.; Pfefferkorn, T.; Ebrahimi, C.; Ottomeyer, C.; Fesl, G.; Bender, A.; Straube, A.; Pfister, H.W.; Heck, S.; Tonn, J.C.; et al. Long-term neurological outcome and quality of life after World Federation of Neurological Societies Grades IV and V aneurysmal subarachnoid hemorrhage in an interdisciplinary treatment concept. *Neurosurgery* **2017**, *80*, 967–974. [CrossRef] [PubMed]
14. AlMatter, M.; Aguilar Pereza, M.; Bhogal, P.; Hellstern, V.; Ganslandt, O.; Henkes, H. Results of interdisciplinary management of 693 patients with aneurysmal subarachnoid hemorrhage: Clinical outcome and relevant prognostic factors. *Clin. Neurol. Neurosurg.* **2018**, *167*, 106–111. [CrossRef] [PubMed]
15. Frontera, J.A.; Claassen, J.; Schmidt, J.M.; Wartenberg, K.E.; Temes, R.; Connolly, E.S., Jr.; MacDonald, R.L.; Mayer, S.A. Prediction of symptomatic vasospasm after subarachnoid hemorrhage: The modified Fisher scale. *Neurosurgery* **2006**, *59*, 21–27. [CrossRef] [PubMed]
16. Jennett, B.; Bond, M. Assessment of Outcome after severe brain damage. *Lancet* **1975**, *1*, 480–484. [CrossRef]
17. Subic, A.; Cermakova, P.; Norrving, B.; Winblad, B.; von Euler, M.; Kramberger, M.B.; Eriksdotter, M.; Garcia-Ptacek, S. Management of acute ischaemic stroke in patients with dementia. *J. Intern. Med.* **2017**, *281*, 348–364. [CrossRef]
18. Claassen, J.; Bernardini, G.L.; Kreiter, K.; Bates, J.; Du, Y.E.; Copeland, D.; Connolly, E.S.; Mayer, S.A. Effect of cisternal and ventricular blood on risk of delayed cerebral ischemia after subarachnoid hemorrhage: The Fisher scale revisited. *Stroke* **2001**, *32*, 2012–2020. [CrossRef]
19. Ransom, E.R.; Mocco, J.; Komotar, R.J.; Sahni, D.; Chang, J.; Hahn, D.K.; Kim, G.H.; Schmidt, J.M.; Sciacca, R.R.; Mayer, S.A.; et al. External ventricular drainage response in poor grade aneurysmal subarachnoid hemorrhage: Effect on preoperative grading and prognosis. *Neurocrit. Care* **2007**, *6*, 174–180. [CrossRef]
20. van der Bilt, I.; Hasan, D.; van den Brink, R.; Cramer, M.J.; van der Jagt, M.; van Kooten, F.; Meertens, J.; van den Berg, M.; Groen, R.; Ten Cate, F.; et al. Cardiac dysfunction after aneurysmal subarachnoid hemorrhage: Relationship with outcome. *Neurology* **2014**, *82*, 351–358. [CrossRef]
21. Norberg, E.; Odenstedt-Herges, H.; Rydenhag, B.; Oras, J. Impact of acute cardiac complications after subarachnoid hemorrhage on long-term mortality and cardiovascular events. *Neurocrit. Care* **2018**, *29*, 404–412. [CrossRef] [PubMed]
22. Zaroff, J.G.; Leong, J.; Kim, H.; Young, W.L.; Cullen, S.P.; Rao, V.A.; Sorel, M.; Quesenberry, C.P., Jr.; Sidney, S. Cardiovascular predictors of long-term outcomes after non-traumatic subarachnoid hemorrhage. *Neurocrit. Care* **2012**, *17*, 374–381. [CrossRef] [PubMed]

17

Subclinical and Asymptomatic Atrial Fibrillation: Current Evidence and Unsolved Questions in Clinical Practice

Andrea Ballatore [1], Mario Matta [2], Andrea Saglietto [1], Paolo Desalvo [1], Pier Paolo Bocchino [1], Fiorenzo Gaita [3], Gaetano Maria De Ferrari [1] and Matteo Anselmino [1,*]

1 Division of Cardiology, "Città della Salute e della Scienza di Torino" Hospital, Department of Medical Sciences, University of Turin, 10126 Turin, Italy
2 Division of Cardiology, Electrophysiology Lab, Sant'Andrea Hospital, 13100 Vercelli, Italy
3 Cardiology Department, Clinica Pinna Pintor, 10129 Turin, Italy
* Correspondence: matteo.anselmino@unito.it

Abstract: Atrial Fibrillation (AF) may be diagnosed due to symptoms, or it may be found as an incidental electrocardiogram (ECG) finding, or by implanted devices recordings in asymptomatic patients. While anticoagulation, according to individual risk profile, has proven definitely beneficial in terms of prognosis, rhythm control strategies only demonstrated consistent benefits in terms of quality of life. In fact, evidence collected by observational data showed significant benefits in terms of mortality, stroke incidence, and prevention of cognitive impairment for patients referred to AF catheter ablation compared to those medically treated, however randomized trials failed to confirm such results. The aims of this review are to summarize current evidence regarding the treatment specifically of subclinical and asymptomatic AF, to discuss potential benefits of rhythm control therapy, and to highlight unclear areas.

Keywords: subclinical atrial fibrillation; stroke; ischemic cerebral events; catheter ablation; screening; cognitive impairment

---

1. Introduction

Atrial fibrillation (AF), the most common sustained arrhythmia [1], is associated with an increased risk of thromboembolic events such as transient ischemic attack (TIA), ischemic stroke with overt neurological sequelae [2], or micro-embolic events resulting in subclinical brain lesions (revealed by neuroimaging techniques). On the other hand, AF is independently associated with a higher risk of developing dementia [3], with up to a 30% increased risk regardless of clinical cerebrovascular events [4]. Therefore, given the high prevalence of AF in the general population and its considerable impact on both life expectancy and quality of life, correct and prompt management of the arrhythmia is mandatory. However, early diagnosis can be difficult in the case of an asymptomatic presentation, defined as sustained AF episodes in patients not presenting palpitations, dyspnea, fatigue, or other AF related symptoms [5]. The exact percentage of asymptomatic presentations among patients with AF has not been clearly established. Different studies provide estimates between 10% and 40%, according to the characteristics of the population in exam [6–10]. A higher prevalence has been reported in patients with persistent AF, males, elderlies, and in the presence of relevant comorbidities [7]. However, subclinical AF can also be diagnosed in patients with fewer risk factors [10] as paroxysmal AF, for example, at the early phase of arrhythmia development and progression. Moreover, variability in terminology among studies, as later discussed, increases uncertainty related to the description of asymptomatic AF.

In the present review, we shed light on several aspects of this clinical entity, highlighting doubtful elements for which further research is needed: first, we discuss the complex pathophysiological links between AF, dementia, and stroke, focusing on the clinical impact of asymptomatic AF, which has been demonstrated not to be a benign condition. Subsequently, we address the issue of screening for AF, which is of great interest from both a clinical and population medicine point of view. Finally, we discuss management of the patient with asymptomatic and subclinical AF, considering clinical recommendations, anticoagulation, antiarrhythmic drugs (AAD) therapy, and catheter ablation.

2. Definitions

Despite being a widely discussed topic, terminology in literature is often inconsistent and the terms "asymptomatic AF", "subclinical AF", "silent AF", and "atrial high rate episodes (AHRE)" are used to identify different entities (Table 1). Different studies define "asymptomatic AF" as AF diagnosed incidentally [11] or by ECG in patients reporting no symptoms, or, alternatively, with European Heart Rhythm Association (EHRA) score 1 [6–10,12]. Other studies [6,7,10] consider silent AF and asymptomatic AF as synonyms. The STROKESTOP trial names AF "silent AF" when the diagnosis is established through screening [13]. However, in other experiences [14–16] assessing the benefit of AF screening, the arrhythmia diagnosed through a screening program is simply referred to as AF. Conversely, AHRE are defined, with variable temporal cutoffs according to different studies, as atrial tachycardia episodes recorded by the intra-atrial electrode of implanted devices. However, when an intra-atrial electrogram is available, as in the subgroup of patients of the ARTESiA trial [17], the arrhythmia episode has been defined as "subclinical AF" and not as AHRE. Instead, the ASSERT trial refers to AHRE as subclinical AF [18]: in this study the devices were able to detect atrial arrhythmias, but it remains unclear whether the electrograms were finally analyzed to define the episodes or not. These studies, in fact, consider both asymptomatic and symptomatic AF as "clinical" only when diagnosed by surface ECG. For the purpose of this review we consider device detected atrial tachycardia without electrogram documentation as AHRE; subclinical AF refers to AF either diagnosed through screening programs, incidental findings during routine ECG, or after implanted device electrograms analysis; finally, we define asymptomatic AF in patients with a clearly established AF diagnosis, undergoing a defined clinical management and who remain asymptomatic based on physician's evaluation. According to these definitions, subclinical and asymptomatic AF are a continuum in the diagnostic process and subsequent management of AF: in fact, once the diagnosis has been confirmed and treatment has begun, subclinical AF should be referred to as clinical asymptomatic AF.

Table 1. Details on the terminology used in available literature.

<table>
<tr><th>Authors (Study Year)</th><th>AHRE/Subclinical/Asymptomatic AF Diagnostic Method</th><th>Terminology Used in the Study</th><th>Terminology Used in This Review</th></tr>
<tr><td colspan="4">Implanted device monitoring</td></tr>
<tr><td>Glotzer et al. (2003) [19]</td><td>AHRE: atrial rate ≥ 220 bpm lasting at least 5 min (detected by pacemaker)</td><td>AHRE</td><td rowspan="5">AHRE</td></tr>
<tr><td>Glotzer et al. (2006) [20]</td><td>AHRE: atrial rate > 175 bpm lasting at least 20 s</td><td>Device-detected atrial tachycardia (AT)/AF burden (AHRE)</td></tr>
<tr><td>Hohnloser et al. (2006) [21]</td><td>AHRE: atrial rate ≥ 190 bpm lasting at least 6 min (detected by pacemaker or ICD)</td><td>Asymptomatic AF/AHRE</td></tr>
<tr><td>Ip et al. (2009) [22]</td><td>AHRE: atrial rate ≥ 220 beat/min lasting at least 5 min,</td><td>AHRE</td></tr>
<tr><td>Kirchhof et al. (2017) [23]</td><td>AHRE: atrial rate ≥ 180 bpm lasting at least 6 min</td><td>AHRE</td></tr>
<tr><td>Lopes et al. (2017) [17]</td><td>One episode of device-detected subclinical AF lasting at least 6 min. Subclinical AF requires at least one episode of electrogram confirmation</td><td>Subclinical AF</td><td>Subclinical AF</td></tr>
</table>

Table 1. *Cont.*

Authors (Study Year)	AHRE/Subclinical/Asymptomatic AF Diagnostic Method	Terminology Used in the Study	Terminology Used in This Review
	Non-Invasive ECG monitoring		
Flaker et al. (2005) [12]	AF diagnosed with ECG or rhythm strip. Symptoms evaluated by a questionnaire	Asymptomatic AF	Asymptomatic AF
Rienstra et al. (2014) [10]	Recurrent persistent AF without symptoms according to a questionnaire	Asymptomatic AF/Silent AF	
Boriani et al. (2015) [7]	ECG diagnosed AF and EHRA score I	Asymptomatic AF/Silent AF	
Freeman et al. (2015) [9]	Electrocardiographically documented AF and EHRA score I	Asymptomatic AF	
Bakhai et al. (2016) [6]	ECG diagnosed AF and EHRA score I	Asymptomatic AF/Silent AF	
Siontis et al. (2016) [11]	AF detected incidentally (routine physical examination, preoperative evaluation, emergency department or clinic visit for unrelated problem)	Asymptomatic AF	Subclinical AF
Jaakkola et al. (2017) [15]	ECG diagnosis in a screening program	AF	
Halcox et al. (2017) [16]	Device detected AF in a screening program	AF	
Friberg et al. (2013) [13]	Device detected AF in a screening program and confirmed by Holter for uncertain cases	Silent AF	

AF: atrial fibrillation; AHRE: atrial high rate episodes; ICD: implantable cardioverter-defibrillator.

3. Pathophysiological Links between AF, Dementia, and Stroke

AF confers an increased risk of cognitive decline and dementia development independently from stroke occurrence. Indeed, this has been recently demonstrated in a large cohort study conducted on 262,611 patients registered in the Korea National Health Insurance Service—Senior, 60 years of age or older and no history of valvular heart disease, stroke, dementia, and AF before enrolment [24]. After adjustment, in the incident AF population the risk of developing dementia was increased after censoring for stroke (HR, 1.27; 95% CI 1.18–1.37). Interestingly, anticoagulation therapy was associated with a lower risk of developing dementia (HR, 0.61; 95% 0.54–0.68). These results are consistent, in fact, with a recent meta-analysis showing a 30% increased risk of AF patients to develop dementia regardless of cerebrovascular events [4].

The association between AF and cognitive impairment in patients without clinical stroke has been linked to several possible mechanisms: micro-embolic events occurring in cerebral circulation may lead to silent cerebral ischemia (SCI), visible by neuroimaging techniques as magnetic resonance imaging (MRI). The correlation between SCIs and cognitive impairment has been demonstrated by ad hoc questionnaires and tests designed to examine cognitive function, both in retrospective [25] and prospective studies [26]. Additionally, a computational analysis showed that AF directly affects cerebral hemodynamic, resulting in hypoperfusions and hypertensive events, possibly associated with non-embolic SCI and microbleedings in the deep cerebral circle [27,28]. Dementia and cognitive decline, however, can also be caused by clinical strokes, a well-known and feared complication of AF. Several questions on the relation between AF and stroke are actually still unsolved: the classical mechanism, based on the Virchow's triad [29], by which AF causes strokes is thrombus formation in the left atrium (typically in the left atrial appendage), and its subsequent embolism in a cerebral vessel. Nevertheless, studies conducted in patients with implanted devices and who suffered a thromboembolic event showed that, in a large portion of patients, no AF events occurred the months before [30,31].

The link between fibrosis and AF is rather complex, since AF causes atrial remodeling and fibrosis itself causes and sustains AF. Animal experimental models demonstrated that sustained AF induces several structural changes in atrial myocytes, including glycogen accumulation, sarcomeres reduction, mitochondrial modification, collagen deposition, and fibrosis [32]. Late gadolinium enhancement MRI studies demonstrated that more severe atrial remodeling with extensive fibrosis is associated with more advanced disease and a higher risk of AF recurrences after catheter ablation [33]. Voltage map during invasive procedures demonstrated that the magnitude of atrial fibrosis is greater in persistent [34] in comparison to paroxysmal AF, and it predicts ablation success [35]. Finally, AF can be a marker of other atrial abnormalities including atrial dilation, left atrial appendage dysfunction, endothelial disease; all these features may cause thromboembolic stroke without an AF episode occurring prior to the cerebrovascular event. Indeed, an "atrial cardiomyopathy" exists, according to which extensive atrial disease can be, at least partially, the cause rather than the consequence of AF [36,37]. Therefore, it has been proposed [30] that AF can cause atrial remodeling and be the manifestation of an atrial disease that increases per se the risk of stroke and thrombi formation, independently from the heart's rhythm.

Actually, the association between dementia and the different clinical presentation of AF has not been thoroughly analyzed. In fact, no published studies directly analyzed cognitive impairment in patients with asymptomatic AF. Several studies evaluated the relation between subclinical AF and the risk of stroke, focusing on subclinical atrial tachyarrhythmia detected by implanted devices. Indeed, it has been thoroughly demonstrated that evaluation of pacemakers recordings is a reliable method to detect AF [38]. The TRENDS trial [39], in fact, evaluated stroke and systemic thromboembolic events in patients with at least one stroke risk factor (defined by the CHADS2 score) by assessing pacemaker or defibrillator recordings. The study was meant to detect a difference in stroke rate among patients with a high, low burden, or no events of atrial arrhythmias/tachycardia (AHRE). Unfortunately, the study failed to show any significant differences, likely due to underpowering as the event rate was lower than expected. An ancillary analysis of the MOST study, instead, demonstrated that AHRE in patients with sinus node dysfunction conferred an increased risk of stroke, death, and to develop clinical AF [19]. Of note, patients with previously diagnosed supraventricular arrhythmia were not excluded, and a large portion of patients with AHRE presented symptoms. Nevertheless, the authors concluded that symptoms were poorly correlated with and were not reliable markers of AHRE. Analogous results were found in the ASSERT trial, which demonstrated that AHRE in patients without a history of AF confer a greater risk of developing clinical AF and are associated with a higher rate of stroke and systemic thromboembolic events [18].

Finally, also AF burden needs consideration: as thoroughly explained by Kennedy [40], AF burden defines the overall amount of AF duration among each patient, providing additional insight on the magnitude of AF episodes. Many clinical conditions (such as, genetics, obesity, hypertension, diabetes, heart failure, older age [40]) affect AF burden and have an important role in AF morbidity. Indeed, it is now clear that prompt correction of comorbidities and cardiovascular risk factors reduces AF burden [41,42] and is, therefore, recommended in all patients suffering from AF [43,44]. Several arrhythmic entities, including AHRE, detected by non-invasive ECG monitoring and implanted devices, are markers of AF and contribute to define the AF burden [40]: however, despite the association between persistent AF and worse prognosis [45–47], current guidelines suggest to base the decision of anticoagulation therapy for stroke prevention on patient's risk factors (quantified by CHA2DS2-VASc score) and not on AF burden. In fact, an AF burden cutoff identifying an increased risk of stroke or mortality has not yet been established, and its quest is at the heart of many studies.

4. Asymptomatic AF and Its Impact on Prognosis

Whether asymptomatic presentation of AF confers a worse prognosis than symptomatic AF is still debated (Table 2). A prospective observational study conducted by Boriani et al. on 3119 patients with AF (the EORP-AF Registry) demonstrated that patients with asymptomatic AF, in comparison to symptomatic patients, have a worse prognosis and an increased risk of mortality at 1 year. At multivariate analysis, however, EHRA score I was not independently associated with a worse prognosis. Therefore, increased mortality was likely mainly driven by the differences in patients' comorbidities and global risk rather than to the different AF presentation [7]. Another study reported that both patients with subclinical AF and atypical presentations of AF (fatigue, shortness of breath, chest pain, light-headedness, syncope, decreased exercise tolerance without palpitations) are at higher risk of cerebrovascular events (CVE) in comparison with patients with typical AF symptoms (palpitations). Moreover, the risk of cardiovascular and global mortality was greater in asymptomatic patients after adjustment for confounding factors (CHA2DS2-VASc score and age) [11]. A sub-study conducted on the PREFER in AF Registry showed that ischemic stroke and TIA occurred with similar frequency in symptomatic and asymptomatic patients [6]. These results confirm, in fact, those of a retrospective analysis of the AFFIRM trial that revealed no differences in outcomes after adjustment for baseline characteristics between patients with asymptomatic and symptomatic AF [12]. Conversely, in a sub-analysis of the RACE study, asymptomatic AF was associated with improved prognosis (lower hospitalization due to heart failure and antiarrhythmic drugs adverse effect rate) in comparison with symptomatic patients, but no differences were found on the risk of thromboembolic events [10]. However, these trials were not designed to evaluate the prognostic implications of different subtypes of AF, and AF presentation was not considered when deciding treatment throughout follow up.

Table 2. Summary of studies on the clinical relevance of asymptomatic and subclinical atrial fibrillation (AF).

Authors (Study Year)	AHRE/Subclinical/Asymptomatic AF Diagnostic Method	Stroke and TE Incidence (%) *	Mortality (%) *	Correlation with Stroke or Mortality
		Implanted device monitoring		
Glotzer et al. (2003) [19]	AHRE: atrial rate ≥ 220 bpm lasting at least 5 min (detected by pacemaker)	AHRE: 33/160 (20.6) No AHRE: 16/152 (10.5)	AHRE: 28/160 (17.5) No AHRE: 16/152 (10.5)	Yes (for total mortality, stroke, and AF development)
Glotzer et al. (2009) [39]	AHRE: atrial rate > 175 bpm lasting at least 20 s. Patients were stratified according to 30 days window monitoring in: zero, low, and high AHRE burden	Annualized TE incidence rate: zero AHRE burden 1.1%; Low AHRE burden 1.1%; High AHRE burden 2.4%	NA	No
Healey et al. (2012) [18]	AHRE: atrial rate ≥ 190 bpm lasting at least 6 min (detected by pacemaker or ICD)	AHRE in the previous 3 months: 11/261 (4.2) No AHRE in the previous 3 months: 40/2319 (1.7)	From vascular causes AHRE in the previous 3 months: 19/261 (7.3) No AHRE in the previous 3 months: 153/2319 (6.6)	Yes
		Non-Invasive ECG monitoring		
Flaker et al. (2005) [12]	AF diagnosed with ECG or rhythm strip. Symptoms evaluated by a questionnaire	Asymptomatic AF: 21 Symptomatic AF: 136	Asymptomatic AF: 60 (19) Symptomatic AF: 606 (27)	No (in comparison with symptomatic patients)
Rienstra et al. (2014) [10]	Recurrent persistent AF without symptoms according to a questionnaire	Asymptomatic AF: 8/157 Symptomatic AF: 28/365	Asymptomatic AF: 9/157 Symptomatic AF: 26/365 (death from cardiovascular causes)	No †
Boriani et al. (2015) [7]	ECG diagnosed AF and EHRA score I	EHRA I: 10/962 (1.0%) EHRA II–IV: 15/1344 (1.1%)	EHRA I: 102/1086 (9.4%) EHRA II–IV: 65/1556 (4.2%)	Yes (for mortality compared to symptomatic patients)
Freeman et al. (2015) [9]	Electrocardiographically documented AF and EHRA score I	EHRA I: 99/3682 EHRA II–IV: 168/5918	EHRA I: 311/3682 EHRA II–IV: 561/5918	No ‡
Bakhai et al. (2016) [6]	ECG diagnosed AF and EHRA score I	EHRA I: ischemic stroke 8/489 (1.6) TIA 7/488 (1.4) arterial embolism 2/488 (0.4) EHRA II–IV: ischemic stroke 44/5514 (0.8) TIA 73/5510 (1.3) arterial embolism 11/5514 (0.2)	NA	No (only EHRA score IV was associated with a higher events occurrence)

Table 2. *Cont.*

Authors (Study Year)	AHRE/Subclinical/Asymptomatic AF Diagnostic Method	Stroke and TE Incidence (%) *	Mortality (%) *	Correlation with Stroke or Mortality
Siontis et al. (2016) [11]	AF detected incidentally (routine physical examination, preoperative evaluation, emergency department, or clinic visit for unrelated problem)	HR compared to typical AF: Subclinical AF 2.60 (95% C.I. 1.10–6.11) Atypical AF 3.12 (95% C.I. 1.27–7.66)	HR compared to typical AF: Subclinical AF 4.01 (95% C.I. 2.32–6.91) Atypical AF 3.19 (95% C.I. 1.78–5.71)	Yes (compared to typical AF)

AF: atrial fibrillation; AHRE: atrial high rate episodes; NA: not applicable; TIA: transient ischemic attack; TE: thromboembolism * If not otherwise indicated. † In this study asymptomatic AF compared to symptomatic presentation conferred a lower risk of heart failure and severe antiarrhythmic drugs adverse effects. ‡ In this study AF symptoms and decreased quality of life were associated with higher risk of hospitalization.

Bearing in mind that the first manifestation of AF can be an ischemic stroke with severe consequences (as death, dementia, and lower quality of life), that AF is first diagnosed in 11%–24% of patients with recent ischemic stroke or TIA [48,49], and that AF-associated strokes have a high risk of recurrences, interest in the screening for subclinical AF has grown during the recent years.

5. Screening for Atrial Fibrillation

A screening program to early detect subclinical AF entails several questions: what is the appropriate method for the screening? Who should be screened? Is a screening program cost-effective? Current European guidelines for the management of AF suggest opportunistic screening in patients older than 65 years by pulse check or single-lead ECG portable devices (Class of recommendation I). In patients with an implanted device it is recommended to evaluate the occurrence of AHRE on a regular basis: if AHRE are detected, AF must be searched by further electrocardiographic monitoring prior to starting treatment. In patients with cryptogenic ischemic stroke or TIA an initial ECG followed by electrocardiographic monitoring for 72 h is recommended (Class of recommendation I), and a long term strategy should be considered (Class of recommendation IIa) [5]. The AHA/ACC/HRS guidelines, instead, do not provide definite recommendations for screening [50]. In addition, a statement appears suggesting that ECG based screening does not improve detection rate of asymptomatic AF in comparison with a pulse palpation based approach, and there are currently no evidence to support the benefits of an ECG based screening [51,52].

Several methods have been proposed for AF screening in populations with risk factors: pulse palpation has been described as an effective method to detect subclinical AF [14]. However, pulse characteristics are seldom evaluated in primary care settings and adequately trained patients' compliance in self-monitoring is low in the long term [15]. Handheld ECG is a reliable and effective method for AF screening in at risk populations, with a fourfold increase in AF diagnosis over 12 months according to the REHEARSE-AF study [16]. This study showed that stroke and TIA incidence was not statistically different in screened and unscreened patients. However, clinical events were not considered as a primary outcome, and the study was not designed and powered to detect a significant difference in these events. The ongoing STROKESTOP trial aims at evaluating the efficacy and cost effectiveness in reducing stroke incidence of an AF screening program based on single lead discontinuous ambulatory ECG monitoring in a 75–76 years old population from two regions in Sweden [13]. An analysis of the ongoing investigation demonstrated that this strategy increased AF detection fourfold, as AF has been first diagnosed in 3% of the screened-population; 93% of patients with new detection of AF have initiated oral anticoagulation (OAC) therapy [53]. Awaiting for the conclusion of the trial and its final results, a simulation study based on the study design and available data of this trial, concluded that screening for AF with an ECG recorder is cost effective with a reduction of eight strokes, and an increase of 11 life-years and 12 quality-adjusted life years (QALYs) per 1000 screened patients [54].

In patients who suffered a cryptogenic stroke and in whom standard 24 h ECG monitoring failed to detect AF, two randomized trials, instead, demonstrated the benefits of further prolonging rhythm monitoring. The CRYSTAL-AF trial [55,56] randomized 441 patients, 40 years of age or older, who suffered a cryptogenic stroke or TIA, without history of AF and no other indications to anticoagulant therapy, to implant a cardiac monitoring device or standard care: the AF detection rate was higher in the long term monitoring strategy group both at 6 and 12 months (HR 6.4; 95% CI 1.9–21.7; HR 7.3; 95% CI 2.6–20.8, respectively). The EMBRACE trial [57] compared standard care and 30-days non-invasive ECG monitoring to detect AF in patients over 55 years old, with cryptogenic stroke or TIA within the 6 months prior to randomization. By 90 days after the randomization AF lasting 30 s was detected in significantly more patients in the intervention group (absolute difference 12.9%, 95% CI 8.0–17.6), with a number needed to screen of eight. Moreover, in the AHA/ACC/HRS focused update of AF guidelines recommendation for the use of implantable device for AF detection after cryptogenic stroke has been implemented, according to which a more extensive and thorough long-term cardiac monitoring needs to be considered [44].

6. Management of Subclinical and Asymptomatic AF

6.1. Clinical Approach to the Patient with Asymptomatic Atrial Fibrillation

Clinical approach to a patient with asymptomatic AF is indeed complex and needs to take into account several aspects of the arrhythmia and presence of comorbidities. First, it must be taken into consideration that asymptomatic AF patients are not always truly asymptomatic, since they may undergo progressive involuntary lifestyle restriction or suffer unrecognized anxiety or depression; moreover, a large portion of AF patients may already present cerebral ischemic lesions (about four out of 10 according to results of the prospective observational SWISS-AF study [58]) which have been demonstrated to affect cognitive functions [26,58]. To assess definitively whether a patient is truly asymptomatic, cardioversion should be performed, and symptoms and quality of life evaluated after sinus rhythm restoration; subsequently, in those who felt improvement after sinus rhythm restoration, a rhythm control strategy should be pursued. It has been demonstrated that catheter ablation for AF significantly improves quality of life and symptoms [59,60]: however subanalysis of these studies demonstrated that, once the patients were divided according to symptoms intensity, the observed benefit was mostly driven by patients with more severe symptoms, whereas those who at baseline were barely symptomatic had little or no improvement after ablation. Therefore, patients' symptoms (not only typical AF symptoms such as palpitations, but also fatigue and dyspnea) and exercise tolerance should be thoroughly examined and a quality of life questionnaire administered; comorbidities should be evaluated, since they can be a cause of symptoms experienced by the patient, and promptly treated. Control of cardiovascular risk factors, hypertension, smoke habit, sedentary life, and obesity should be also encouraged and recommended, as they worsen symptoms and play a role in disease progression [44]. Finally, a regular cardiological follow-up is recommended, including clinical examination for heart failure signs and echocardiographic control of ejection fraction; the latter, in fact, is a crucial aspect to promptly recognize and address patients with a reduced ejection fraction to rhythm control strategy by catheter ablation in order to prevent further heart failure progression [5] and reduce mortality, as suggested by the recent CASTLE-AF findings [61].

Treatment strategies for prevention of cognitive decline are, instead, debated [62]: in addition to physical exercise and optimal control of cardiovascular risk factors, appropriate anticoagulation therapy is recommended; non-vitamin K antagonist oral anticoagulants (NOAC) should be preferred because of the higher safety profile. Moreover, a rhythm control strategy, including catheter ablation, is indicated; nevertheless, it should be borne in mind that the benefit of restoring sinus rhythm may be partially offset by subclinical cerebral lesions occurring during the procedure [63,64].

6.2. Anticoagulation Therapy

The cornerstone of AF therapy for prevention of stroke and systemic thromboembolic events is OAC therapy. The 2016 ESC guidelines recommend to initiate OAC therapy upon evaluation of the individual stroke risk based on the number of CHA2DS2-VASc risk factors; in the absence of contraindications, OAC therapy is recommended when the CHA2DS2-VASc score is ≥2 in male patients or ≥3 in female patients and it should be considered with CHA2DS2-VASc scores 1 or 2 respectively. Whereas vitamin K antagonists are the only recommended anticoagulants for valvular AF patients, i.e., patients with mechanical heart valve or moderate to severe mitral stenosis, NOAC should be preferred in non-valvular AF patients [5]. The net benefit of CHA2DS2-VASc-guided OAC therapy in preventing stroke occurrence and recurrence in AF patients has been thoroughly demonstrated [65,66]. A large meta-analysis showed the superiority of NOAC over VKA with respect to safety and efficacy [67].

As far as OAC therapy in subclinical AF or AHRE is concerned, there is actually no direct evidence that early initiation of OAC treatment in this setting can improve hard clinical endpoints without significantly increasing bleeding risk [51]. It has been proposed that intermittent OAC might provide a better balance between stroke prevention and bleeding risk than uninterrupted OAC therapy. Nevertheless, the IMPACT trial, which evaluated intermittent versus OAC initiated upon standard physician's indication after detection of AHRE at implanted defibrillator follow-up sessions, failed to show clinical benefit regarding the composite outcome of stroke, systemic embolism, and bleeding events (HR 1.06; 95% CI 0.75–1.51; p value: 0.732) [68]. In this perspective, two ongoing clinical trials are designed to assess the feasibility of continuous OAC therapy in patients with subclinical AF or AHRE recorded by implanted devices (Table 3). The randomized, double-blind, multicenter NOAH-AFNET 6 study, including older patients (>65 years old) with at least one additional CHA2DS2-VASc risk factor but without clinical AF nor any other indication to OAC therapy, will evaluate the efficacy of edoxaban compared to aspirin or no antithrombotic therapy in preventing stroke, cardiovascular death, and systemic embolism after AHRE detection by implanted devices' recordings; the primary safety endpoint will be major bleeding [23]. The ARTESiA trial is a prospective, multicenter, double-blind, randomized controlled trial, which enrolls patients with risk factors for stroke and subclinical AF detected by implanted devices; patients will be randomized to either apixaban or aspirin with a primary composite endpoint of stroke, TIA, and systemic thromboembolic events during an estimated follow-up of 3 years [17].

Table 3. Details of ongoing trials.

Name of Study	Number of Patients	Study Arms	Primary Endpoints	Secondary Endpoints
STROKESTOP (NCT01593553)	7173 (in screening) 14,381 (controls not screened)	Intervention group: ECG screening for AF using intermittent ECG recorder. Control group: standard of care	Composite of ischemic and hemorrhagic stroke, systemic embolism, major bleeding requiring hospitalization, and all-cause mortality	Each single component of the composite primary outcome; dementia; cardiovascular mortality; hospitalization due to cardiovascular disease; cost-effectiveness; OAC initiation and compliance; AF detection; pulmonary embolism and deep vein thrombosis
NOAH-AFNET 6 (NCT02618577)	2686 (3400 estimated) patients (≥65 years old and ≥1 additional CHA2DS2-VASc factor) with AHRE documented by implanted devices	Intervention group: Edoxaban (standard AF dosing) Control group: ASA or placebo	Composite of stroke, systemic embolism and cardiovascular death (measured as time from randomization to event occurrence)	MACE (cardiac death, MI, acute coronary syndrome), all-cause death, major bleeding events, quality of life changes at 12 and 24 months, patient satisfaction at 12 and 24 months, cost effectiveness and health resource utilization, autonomy status changes in patients affected by stroke during study participation, cognitive function at 12 and 24 months
ARTESiA (NCT01938248)	≈4000 patients with subclinical AF at high risk for stroke (estimated)	Intervention group: Apixaban (standard AF dosing) Control group: ASA (81 mg/die)	Efficacy outcome: composite of stroke (including TIA) and systemic embolism. Safety outcome: major bleeding	Ischemic stroke; MI; vascular death; total death; composite of stroke, MI, systemic embolism and total death; composite of stroke, MI, systemic embolism, total death, and major bleeding.

Table 3. *Cont.*

Name of Study	Number of Patients	Study Arms	Primary Endpoints	Secondary Endpoints
EAST (NCT01288352)	2789 patients with new AF (<1 year) and risk factors for stroke	Intervention group: guidelines-based therapy andearly rhythm control therapy (AAD or PVI) Control group: usual care	First coprimary outcome: composite of cardiovascular death, stroke (including TIA), acute coronary syndrome, and worsening of heart failure. Second coprimary outcome: nights in hospital per year	Cardiovascular death, stroke, worsening of heart failure, acute coronary syndrome, time to recurrent AF, cardiovascular hospitalizations, all-cause hospitalizations, left ventricular function, quality of life, cognitive function
OCEAN (NCT02168829)	1572 patients free from AF for at least 1 year after catheter ablation for non-valvular AF (estimated)	Active Comparator: rivaroxaban 15 mg/die Active Comparator: ASA 75–160 mg/die	Composite of clinically overt stroke, systemic embolism, and covert stroke detected by brain MRI	Each single component of the composite primary outcome; major bleeding, clinically relevant non-major bleeding, minor bleeding and their composite; overt intracranial hemorrhage; microbleedings as detected by MRI; TIA; all-cause mortality; net clinical benefit; occurrence of nonprimary end point MRI changes; correlation of AF burden/recurrence to occurrence of clinical or covert stroke; neuropsychological testing; quality of life
OAT (NCT01959425)	100 patients free from AF for at least 3 months after catheter ablation and at high risk for stroke (estimated)	Intervention group: OAC discontinuation Control group: OAC continuation	Composite of any major thromboembolic event and major hemorrhagic complication	Bleeding; hospitalization; mortality; quality of Life; AF recurrence; repeat ablation
SWISS-AF (NCT02105844)	2415 AF patients	NA	Stroke or systemic embolism	Hospitalization for heart failure

AAD: antiarrhythmic drugs; AF: atrial fibrillation; AHRE: atrial high rate episodes; ASA: acetylsalicylic acid; MACE: major adverse cardiovascular events; MI: myocardial infarction; MRI: magnetic resonance imaging; NA: not applicable; OAC: oral anticoagulant; PVI: pulmonary veins isolation; TIA: transient ischemic attack.

6.3. Anti-Arrhythmic Drug Management

A rhythm control approach in the subset of patients with subclinical and asymptomatic AF is perhaps even more controversial than the previously discussed OAC therapy. The AFFIRM [69,70] and RACE [71] trials demonstrated no advantage on mortality and stroke in pursuing a rhythm control over a rate control strategy in AF patients. Nevertheless, the CASTLE-AF [61] study showed a clear benefit in cardiovascular death and hospitalizations for worsening heart failure in patients with heart failure and paroxysmal or persistent AF treated by catheter ablation. According to current European guidelines, rhythm control therapy is recommended in symptomatic patients presenting with recent onset AF in order to improve quality of life [5].

Some considerations are needed in this regard. First, a subanalysis of the AFFIRM [72] study showed that maintaining sinus rhythm confers half the risk of death compared to AF persistence. AAD, however, were associated with increased mortality after adjustment for sinus rhythm restoration, therefore the authors concluded that the beneficial effects of AAD in maintaining sinus rhythm were offset by their adverse effects, resulting in no net survival advantage. Similarly, an observational study [73] comparing stroke and TIA incidence in patients treated with either rate or rhythm control strategy (n = 41.193 and 16.325 respectively) showed that rhythm control strategy was associated with a lower risk of stroke and TIA during a mean follow-up of 2.8 years at multivariate analysis (HR 0.80; 95% CI 0.74–0.87). After stratification for CHADS2 score, absolute stroke and TIA incidences were reduced only in patients with CHADS2 score ≥ 2.

6.4. Catheter Ablation

The aforementioned studies compared only AAD with rate control therapy, but AF catheter ablation has now become an effective and widespread option for rhythm control: indeed, ESC guidelines do recommend catheter ablation as a first-line alternative to AAD in symptomatic patients with paroxysmal AF. A large meta-analysis [74] including 1481 patients with AF and 11 randomized controlled trials compared the efficacy and safety of catheter ablation versus AAD therapy ($n = 785$ and 696 respectively): catheter ablation was associated with lower AF recurrences (RR, 0.40; 95% CI 0.31−0.52; p value = 0.00001) both as first- and second-line approaches (RR, 0.52; 95% CI, 0.30−0.91; p value = 0.02 and RR, 0.37; 95% CI, 0.29−0.48; p value < 0.00001, respectively), but there was a significant increase of adverse events incidence (RR, 2.04; 95% CI, 1.10–3.77; p value = 0.02). However, after stratification by date, no difference in safety endpoints was found considering only the results of the studies conducted after 2009 (RR, 1.51; 95% CI, 0.55–4,15; p value = 0.42). This finding may be due to increased experience and improved technology in catheter ablation, leading to lower complications and adverse events.

Since catheter ablation proved more effective than AAD therapy in maintaining sinus rhythm [74], it has been hypothesized that indication to this procedure could reflect into better long-term prognosis. However, the recent CABANA trial [75], which was supposed to shed light on this clinical dilemma, failed to demonstrate a statistically significant superiority of catheter ablation over both rhythm and rate control pharmacological therapy for a composite primary endpoint including death, disabling stroke, serious bleeding, or cardiac arrest (HR, 0.86; 95% CI 0.65–1.15; p value = 0.30). A detailed analysis of the results, however, shows that the study was characterized by a greater than expected cross-over between treatment groups, with 301 (27.5%) patients assigned to medical therapy switching to catheter ablation. Indeed, in the 12-month per-protocol analysis of the results, patients who had undergone catheter ablation presented a reduced risk of meeting the primary endpoint than those managed pharmacologically (HR 0.73; 95% CI 0.54–0.99).

Several other investigations, albeit limited by their unrandomized nature, provided evidence in favor of catheter ablation. One study comparing patients with similar CHADS2 scores showed that catheter ablation confers a risk of ischemic stroke similar to that of the population without AF, but the details on OAC treatment were lacking [76]. A multicenter study conducted by Hunter et al. [77] compared patients undergoing AF ablation with a cohort treated with medical therapy and an AF-free cohort representing the general population; of note, in the medical therapy cohort CHADS2 score was higher than in catheter ablation group (1.6 ± 1.2 and 0.7 ± 0.9 respectively). After a mean follow-up of 3.1 years, catheter ablation was associated with a lower risk of stroke and death in comparison with medical therapy, presenting a stroke rate comparable to the general population. Moreover, freedom from AF was a protective factor against stroke at multivariate analysis (HR 0.33; 95% CI 0.17–0.67). Discontinuation of OAC therapy occurred in 64% of patients who underwent pulmonary veins (isolation (85% of these were on single antiplatelet agent therapy) and it was more frequent in patients without AF recurrences in comparison to patients with AF recurrences, despite a small difference in CHADS2 score between the two groups (0.7 ± 0.9 vs. 0.9 ± 0.9, respectively). These findings confirm those of another observational study [78] which reported no statistically significant difference between patients who stopped or continued OAC after AF ablation. Along with history of stroke, and unlike OAC interruption, except in intermediate risk patients, recurrent AF was a predictor of thromboembolic events, whereas OAC continuation was associated with an increased risk of bleeding. Another multicenter observational study [79] recruiting 1500 AF patients compared rate control and OAC therapy with catheter ablation associated with either OAC continuation or discontinuation after the procedure: no differences were found as for thromboembolic events incidence (2.2% in rate control strategy and OAC, 1% in catheter ablation with OAC, 1.4% catheter ablation and OAC discontinuation, p value = 0.45), whereas OAC discontinuation after catheter ablation conferred a lower risk of hemorrhagic events (2.4% in rate control strategy and OAC, 1.8% in catheter ablation with OAC, and no events in catheter ablation and OAC discontinuation, p value < 0.001).

Based on the aforementioned studies, preservation of sinus rhythm, achieved by AAD therapy or catheter ablation, holds the potential to confer an improved clinical outcome in the general population. Among patients with fewer risk factors and lower event rates than those with heart failure, a longer follow-up and greater sample sizes are possibly needed to identify a statistically significant benefit in hard clinical end-points. Indeed, maintenance of sinus rhythm can prevent atrial structural remodeling process accompanying the arrhythmia, hampering disease progression. In this perspective, the currently ongoing EAST [80] trial will assess if rhythm control therapy in the early phase following AF diagnosis can improve prognosis in comparison with a more conservative approach; the trial primary endpoint is a composite of cardiovascular death, stroke, worsening heart failure and myocardial infarction; cognitive function will be evaluated as a secondary outcome as in the STROKESTOP, NOAH-AFNET 6, and OCEAN studies. Additionally, two ongoing trials will shed light on another quandary in clinical management of AF patients: the open, multicenter, randomized OCEAN trial [81] will compare rivaroxaban and acetylsalicylic acid efficacy in reducing stroke, systemic embolism and subclinical brain lesions incidence among high-risk patients free from AF for at least 1 year after pulmonary veins isolation after a 3 years follow-up period. In the OAT trial (NCT01959425) patients without AF recurrences three months after catheter ablation will be randomized to suspend or continue OAC. Should these trials meet their outcomes, a rhythm control strategy with catheter ablation in an early phase of the disease would be recommended aiming to interrupt disease progression and prevent AF-related complications. Moreover, it would be possible to consider catheter ablation in asymptomatic patients as well; as a matter of fact, as thoroughly explained by Kalman et al. [82], subclinical AF can become symptomatic with arrhythmia progression, therefore it may prove useful to treat the arrhythmia in this early "window of opportunity" in order to prevent symptoms onset and atrial remodeling. Finally, patients' compliance to OAC therapy for AF diagnosed after a single ECG in the absence of any symptoms is of great concern in clinical practice; in this scenario catheter ablation may be a valid tool potentially providing the expected benefits (Figure 1).

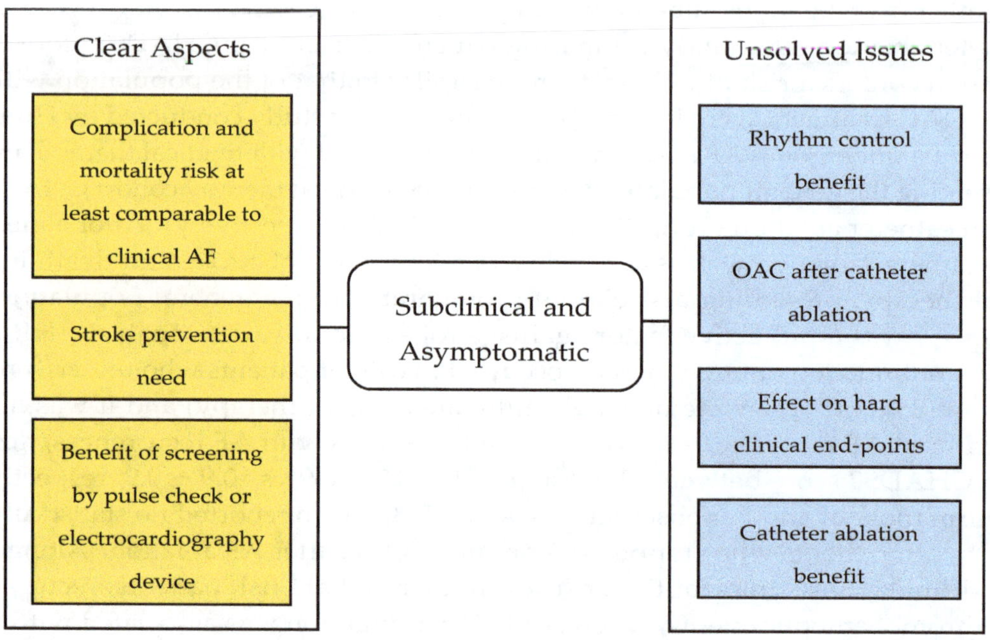

Figure 1. Current certainties and doubts on the management of subclinical and asymptomatic AF.

7. Conclusions

The treatment of asymptomatic AF patients should be personalized, evaluating individual risk factors and comorbidities as well as patient's own preference. High risk individuals with heart failure, should be promptly treated, and catheter ablation should be offered due to the strong evidence supporting AF ablation in this setting. As for patients with early-diagnosed asymptomatic AF and no comorbidities, ongoing clinical trials will assess the benefits of catheter ablation and pharmacological rhythm control therapy, but currently there is not enough evidence to clearly support this approach.

Author Contributions: M.A., G.M.D.F., F.G., A.B., M.M. participated in the conception of the research; A.B. and M.M. drafted the manuscript; M.A., G.M.D.F., F.G., A.S., P.D., P.P.B. helped draft and critically revised the manuscript.

References

1. Andrade, J.; Khairy, P.; Dobrev, D.; Nattel, S. The clinical profile and pathophysiology of atrial fibrillation: Relationships among clinical features, epidemiology, and mechanisms. *Circ. Res.* **2014**. [CrossRef] [PubMed]
2. Wolf, P.A.; Abbott, R.D.; Kannel, W.B. Atrial fibrillation as an independent risk factor for stroke: The Framingham Study. *Stroke* **1991**, *22*, 983–988. [CrossRef] [PubMed]
3. Kalantarian, S.; Stern, T.A.; Mansour, M.; Ruskin, J.N. Cognitive Impairment Associated With Atrial Fibrillation: A Meta-analysis. *Ann. Intern. Med.* **2013**, *158*, 338. [CrossRef] [PubMed]
4. Saglietto, A.; Matta, M.; Gaita, F.; Jacobs, V.; Bunch, T.J.; Anselmino, M. Stroke-independent contribution of atrial fibrillation to dementia: A meta-analysis. *Open Heart* **2019**, *6*, e000984. [CrossRef] [PubMed]
5. Kirchhof, P.; Benussi, S.; Kotecha, D.; Ahlsson, A.; Atar, D.; Casadei, B.; Castella, M.; Diener, H.C.; Heidbuchel, H.; Hendriks, J.; et al. 2016 ESC Guidelines for the management of atrial fibrillation developed in collaboration with EACTS. *Eur. J. Cardiothorac. Surg.* **2016**, *50*, e1–e88. [CrossRef] [PubMed]
6. Bakhai, A.; Darius, H.; De Caterina, R.; Smart, A.; Le Heuzey, J.Y.; Schilling, R.J.; Zamorano, J.L.; Shah, M.; Bramlage, P.; Kirchhof, P. Characteristics and outcomes of atrial fibrillation patients with or without specific symptoms: Results from the PREFER in AF registry. *Eur. Heart J. Qual. Care Clin. Outcomes* **2016**, *2*, 299–305. [CrossRef]
7. Boriani, G.; Laroche, C.; Diemberger, I.; Fantecchi, E.; Popescu, M.I.; Rasmussen, L.H.; Sinagra, G.; Petrescu, L.; Tavazzi, L.; Maggioni, A.P.; et al. Asymptomatic Atrial Fibrillation: Clinical Correlates, Management, and Outcomes in the EORP-AF Pilot General Registry. *Am. J. Med.* **2015**, *128*, 509–518. [CrossRef]
8. Lévy, S.; Maarek, M.; Coumel, P.; Guize, L.; Lekieffre, J.; Medvedowsky, J.L.; Sebaoun, A. Characterization of different subsets of atrial fibrillation in general practice in France: The ALFA study. The College of French Cardiologists. *Circulation* **1999**, *99*, 3028–3035. [CrossRef]
9. Freeman, J.V.; Simon, D.N.; Go, A.S.; Spertus, J.; Fonarow, G.C.; Gersh, B.J.; Hylek, E.M.; Kowey, P.R.; Mahaffey, K.W.; Thomas, L.E.; et al. Association between Atrial Fibrillation Symptoms, Quality of Life, and Patient Outcomes: Results from the Outcomes Registry for Better Informed Treatment of Atrial Fibrillation (ORBIT-AF). *Circ. Cardiovasc. Qual. Outcomes* **2015**, *8*, 393–402. [CrossRef]
10. Rienstra, M.; Vermond, R.A.; Crijns, H.J.G.M.; Tijssen, J.G.P.; Van Gelder, I.C. Asymptomatic persistent atrial fibrillation and outcome: Results of the RACE study. *Heart Rhythm* **2014**, *11*, 939–945. [CrossRef]
11. Siontis, K.C.; Gersh, B.J.; Killian, J.M.; Noseworthy, P.A.; McCabe, P.; Weston, S.A.; Roger, V.L.; Chamberlain, A.M. Typical, atypical, and asymptomatic presentations of new-onset atrial fibrillation in the community: Characteristics and prognostic implications. *Heart Rhythm* **2016**, *13*, 1418–1424. [CrossRef] [PubMed]
12. Flaker, G.C.; Belew, K.; Beckman, K.; Vidaillet, H.; Kron, J.; Safford, R.; Mickel, M.; Barrell, P.; AFFIRM Investigators. Asymptomatic atrial fibrillation: Demographic features and prognostic information from the Atrial Fibrillation Follow-up Investigation of Rhythm Management (AFFIRM) study. *Am. Heart J.* **2005**, *149*, 657–663. [CrossRef] [PubMed]
13. Friberg, L.; Engdahl, J.; Frykman, V.; Svennberg, E.; Levin, L.Å.; Rosenqvist, M. Population screening of 75- and 76-year-old men and women for silent atrial fibrillation (STROKESTOP). *Europace* **2013**, *15*, 135–140. [CrossRef] [PubMed]
14. Fitzmaurice, D.A.; Hobbs, F.D.R.; Jowett, S.; Mant, J.; Murray, E.T.; Holder, R.; Raftery, J.P.; Bryan, S.; Davies, M.; Lip, G.Y.; et al. Screening versus routine practice in detection of atrial fibrillation in patients aged 65 or over: Cluster randomised controlled trial. *Br. Med. J.* **2007**, *335*, 383–386. [CrossRef] [PubMed]
15. Jaakkola, J.; Virtanen, R.; Vasankari, T.; Salminen, M.; Airaksinen, K.E.J. Self-detection of atrial fibrillation in an aged population: Three-year follow-up of the LietoAF intervention study. *BMC Geriatr.* **2017**, *17*, 218. [CrossRef] [PubMed]

16. Halcox, J.P.J.; Wareham, K.; Cardew, A.; Gilmore, M.; Barry, J.P.; Phillips, C.; Gravenor, M.B. Assessment of Remote Heart Rhythm Sampling Using the AliveCor Heart Monitor to Screen for Atrial Fibrillation. *Circulation* **2017**, *136*, 1784–1794. [CrossRef] [PubMed]
17. Lopes, R.D.; Alings, M.; Connolly, S.J.; Beresh, H.; Granger, C.B.; Mazuecos, J.B.; Boriani, G.; Nielsen, J.C.; Conen, D.; Hohnloser, S.H.; et al. Rationale and design of the Apixaban for the Reduction of Thrombo-Embolism in Patients With Device-Detected Sub-Clinical Atrial Fibrillation (ARTESiA) trial. *Am. Heart J.* **2017**, *189*, 137–145. [CrossRef]
18. Healey, J.S.; Connolly, S.J.; Gold, M.R.; Israel, C.W.; Van Gelder, I.C.; Capucci, A.; Lau, C.P.; Fain, E.; Yang, S.; Bailleul, C.; et al. Subclinical Atrial Fibrillation and the Risk of Stroke. *N. Engl. J. Med.* **2012**, *366*, 120–129. [CrossRef]
19. Glotzer, T.V.; Hellkamp, A.S.; Zimmerman, J.; Sweeney, M.O.; Yee, R.; Marinchak, R.; Cook, J.; Paraschos, A.; Love, J.; Radoslovich, G.; et al. Atrial High Rate Episodes Detected by Pacemaker Diagnostics Predict Death and Stroke. *Circulation* **2003**, *107*, 1614–1619. [CrossRef]
20. Glotzer, T.V.; Daoud, E.G.; Wyse, D.G.; Singer, D.E.; Holbrook, R.; Pruett, K.; Smith, K.; Hilker, C.E. Rationale and design of a prospective study of the clinical significance of atrial arrhythmias detected by implanted device diagnostics: The TRENDS study. *J. Interv. Card. Electrophysiol.* **2006**, *15*, 9–14. [CrossRef]
21. Hohnloser, S.H.; Capucci, A.; Fain, E.; Gold, M.R.; van Gelder, I.C.; Healey, J.; Israel, C.W.; Lau, C.P.; Morillo, C.; Connolly, S.J.; et al. ASymptomatic atrial fibrillation and Stroke Evaluation in pacemaker patients and the atrial fibrillation Reduction atrial pacing Trial (ASSERT). *Am. Heart J.* **2006**, *152*, 442–447. [CrossRef]
22. Ip, J.; Waldo, A.L.; Lip, G.Y.H.; Rothwell, P.M.; Martin, D.T.; Bersohn, M.M.; Choucair, W.K.; Akar, J.G.; Wathen, M.S.; Rohani, P.; et al. Multicenter randomized study of anticoagulation guided by remote rhythm monitoring in patients with implantable cardioverter-defibrillator and CRT-D devices: Rationale, design, and clinical characteristics of the initially enrolled cohort. The IMPACT study. *Am. Heart J.* **2009**, *158*, 364–370. [CrossRef]
23. Kirchhof, P.; Blank, B.F.; Calvert, M.; Camm, A.J.; Chlouverakis, G.; Diener, H.-C.; Goette, A.; Huening, A.; Lip, G.Y.H.; Simantirakis, E.; et al. Probing oral anticoagulation in patients with atrial high rate episodes: Rationale and design of the Non–vitamin K antagonist Oral anticoagulants in patients with Atrial High rate episodes (NOAH–AFNET 6) trial. *Am. Heart J.* **2017**, *190*, 12–18. [CrossRef]
24. Kim, D.; Yang, P.-S.; Yu, H.T.; Kim, T.-H.; Jang, E.; Sung, J.-H.; Pak, H.N.; Lee, M.Y.; Lee, M.H.; Lip, G.Y.H.; et al. Risk of dementia in stroke-free patients diagnosed with atrial fibrillation: Data from a population-based cohort. *Eur. Heart J.* **2019**, *40*, 2313–2323. [CrossRef]
25. Chen, L.Y.; Lopez, F.L.; Gottesman, R.F.; Huxley, R.R.; Agarwal, S.K.; Loehr, L.; Mosley, T.; Alonso, A. Atrial Fibrillation and Cognitive Decline–The Role of Subclinical Cerebral Infarcts. *Stroke* **2014**, *45*, 2568–2574. [CrossRef]
26. Gaita, F.; Corsinovi, L.; Anselmino, M.; Raimondo, C.; Pianelli, M.; Toso, E.; Bergamasco, L.; Boffano, C.; Valentini, M.C.; Cesarani, F.; et al. Prevalence of silent cerebral ischemia in paroxysmal and persistent atrial fibrillation and correlation with cognitive function. *J. Am. Coll. Cardiol.* **2013**, *62*, 1990–1997. [CrossRef]
27. Scarsoglio, S.; Saglietto, A.; Anselmino, M.; Gaita, F.; Ridolfi, L. Alteration of cerebrovascular haemodynamic patterns due to atrial fibrillation: An in silico investigation. *J. R. Soc. Interface* **2017**, *14*, 20170180. [CrossRef]
28. Anselmino, M.; Scarsoglio, S.; Saglietto, A.; Gaita, F.; Ridolfi, L. Transient cerebral hypoperfusion and hypertensive events during atrial fibrillation: A plausible mechanism for cognitive impairment. *Sci. Rep.* **2016**, *6*, 28635. [CrossRef]
29. Watson, T.; Shantsila, E.; Lip, G.Y. Mechanisms of thrombogenesis in atrial fibrillation: Virchow's triad revisited. *Lancet* **2009**, *373*, 155–166. [CrossRef]
30. Brambatti, M.; Connolly, S.J.; Gold, M.R.; Morillo, C.A.; Capucci, A.; Muto, C.; Lau, C.P.; Van Gelder, I.C.; Hohnloser, S.H.; Carlson, M.; et al. Temporal Relationship Between Subclinical Atrial Fibrillation and Embolic Events. *Circulation* **2014**, *129*, 2094–2099. [CrossRef]
31. Daoud, E.G.; Glotzer, T.V.; Wyse, D.G.; Ezekowitz, M.D.; Hilker, C.; Koehler, J.; Ziegler, P.D.; TRENDS Investigators. Temporal relationship of atrial tachyarrhythmias, cerebrovascular events, and systemic emboli based on stored device data: A subgroup analysis of TRENDS. *Heart Rhythm* **2011**, *8*, 1416–1423. [CrossRef]
32. Ausma, J.; Wijffels, M.; Thoné, F.; Wouters, L.; Allessie, M.; Borgers, M. Structural changes of atrial myocardium due to sustained atrial fibrillation in the goat. *Circulation* **1997**, *96*, 3157–3163. [CrossRef]
33. Marrouche, N.F.; Wilber, D.; Hindricks, G.; Jais, P.; Akoum, N.; Marchlinski, F.; Kholmovski, E.; Burgon, N.;

Hu, N.; Mont, L.; et al. Association of Atrial Tissue Fibrosis Identified by Delayed Enhancement MRI and Atrial Fibrillation Catheter Ablation. *JAMA* **2014**, *311*, 498. [CrossRef]

34. Rolf, S.; Kircher, S.; Arya, A.; Eitel, C.; Sommer, P.; Richter, S.; Gaspar, T.; Bollmann, A.; Altmann, D.; Piedra, C.; et al. Tailored Atrial Substrate Modification Based on Low-Voltage Areas in Catheter Ablation of Atrial Fibrillation. *Circ. Arrhythmia Electrophysiol.* **2014**, *7*, 825–833. [CrossRef]
35. Verma, A.; Wazni, O.M.; Marrouche, N.F.; Martin, D.O.; Kilicaslan, F.; Minor, S.; Schweikert, R.A.; Saliba, W.; Cummings, J.; Burkhardt, J.D.; et al. Pre-existent left atrial scarring in patients undergoing pulmonary vein antrum isolation. *J. Am. Coll. Cardiol.* **2005**, *45*, 285–292. [CrossRef]
36. Kottkamp, H. Human atrial fibrillation substrate: Towards a specific fibrotic atrial cardiomyopathy. *Eur. Heart J.* **2013**, *34*, 2731–2738. [CrossRef]
37. Kottkamp, H. Fibrotic Atrial Cardiomyopathy: A Specific Disease/Syndrome Supplying Substrates for Atrial Fibrillation, Atrial Tachycardia, Sinus Node Disease, AV Node Disease, and Thromboembolic Complications. *J. Cardiovasc. Electrophysiol.* **2012**, *23*, 797–799. [CrossRef]
38. Pollak, W.M.; Simmons, J.D.; Interian, A.; Atapattu, S.A.; Castellanos, A.; Myerburg, R.J.; Mitrani, R.D. Clinical utility of intraatrial pacemaker stored electrograms to diagnose atrial fibrillation and flutter. *Pacing Clin. Electrophysiol.* **2001**, *24*, 424–429. [CrossRef]
39. Glotzer, T.V.; Daoud, E.G.; Wyse, D.G.; Singer, D.E.; Ezekowitz, M.D.; Hilker, C.; Miller, C.; Qi, D.; Ziegler, P.D. The Relationship Between Daily Atrial Tachyarrhythmia Burden from Implantable Device Diagnostics and Stroke Risk. *Circ. Arrhythmia Electrophysiol.* **2009**, *2*, 474–480. [CrossRef]
40. Kennedy, H.L. Silent Atrial Fibrillation: Definition, Clarification, and Unanswered Issues. *Ann. Noninvasive Electrocardiol.* **2015**, *20*, 518–525. [CrossRef]
41. Abed, H.S.; Wittert, G.A.; Leong, D.P.; Shirazi, M.G.; Bahrami, B.; Middeldorp, M.E.; Lorimer, M.F.; Lau, D.H.; Antic, N.A.; Brooks, A.G.; et al. Effect of weight reduction and cardiometabolic risk factor management on symptom burden and severity in patients with atrial fibrillation: A randomized clinical trial. *JAMA J. Am. Med. Assoc.* **2013**, *310*, 2050–2060. [CrossRef]
42. Malmo, V.; Nes, B.M.; Amundsen, B.H.; Tjonna, A.E.; Stoylen, A.; Rossvoll, O.; Wisloff, U.; Loennechen, J.P. Aerobic interval training reduces the burden of Atrial fibrillation in the short term: A randomized trial. *Circulation* **2016**, *133*, 466–473. [CrossRef]
43. Chen, L.Y.; Chung, M.K.; Allen, L.A.; Ezekowitz, M.; Furie, K.L.; McCabe, P.; Noseworthy, P.A.; Perez, M.V.; Turakhia, M.P.; American Heart Association Council on Clinical Cardiology; et al. Atrial Fibrillation Burden: Moving Beyond Atrial Fibrillation as a Binary Entity: A Scientific Statement From the American Heart Association. *Circulation* **2018**, *137*, e623–e644. [CrossRef]
44. January, C.T.; Wann, L.S.; Calkins, H.; Chen, L.Y.; Cigarroa, J.E.; Cleveland, J.C.; Ellinor, P.T.; Ezekowitz, M.D.; Field, M.E.; Furie, K.L.; et al. 2019 AHA/ACC/HRS Focused Update of the 2014 AHA/ACC/HRS Guideline for the Management of Patients With Atrial Fibrillation: A Report of the American College of Cardiology/American Heart Association Task Force on Clinical Practice Guidelines and the Heart, R. *Circulation* **2019**, *140*, 125–151. [CrossRef]
45. Al-Khatib, S.M.; Thomas, L.; Wallentin, L.; Lopes, R.D.; Gersh, B.; Garcia, D.; Ezekowitz, J.; Alings, M.; Yang, H.; Alexander, J.H. Outcomes of apixaban vs. warfarin by type and duration of atrial fibrillation: Results from the ARISTOTLE trial. *Eur. Heart J.* **2013**, *34*, 2464–2471. [CrossRef]
46. Link, M.S.; Giugliano, R.P.; Ruff, C.T.; Scirica, B.M.; Huikuri, H.; Oto, A.; Crompton, A.E.; Murphy, S.A.; Lanz, H.; Mercuri, M.F. Stroke and Mortality Risk in Patients with Various Patterns of Atrial Fibrillation: Results from the ENGAGE AF-TIMI 48 Trial (Effective Anticoagulation with Factor Xa Next Generation in Atrial Fibrillation-Thrombolysis in Myocardial Infarction 48). *Circ. Arrhythmia Electrophysiol.* **2017**, *10*, 1–7. [CrossRef]
47. Steinberg, B.A.; Hellkamp, A.S.; Lokhnygina, Y.; Patel, M.R.; Breithardt, G.; Hankey, G.J.; Becker, R.C.; Singer, D.E.; Halperin, J.L.; Hacke, W.; et al. Higher risk of death and stroke in patients with persistent vs. paroxysmal atrial fibrillation: Results from the ROCKET-AF Trial. *Eur. Heart J.* **2015**, *36*, 288–296. [CrossRef]
48. Sposato, L.A.; Cipriano, L.E.; Saposnik, G.; Vargas, E.R.; Riccio, P.M.; Hachinski, V. Diagnosis of atrial fibrillation after stroke and transient ischaemic attack: A systematic review and meta-analysis. *Lancet Neurol.* **2015**, *14*, 377–387. [CrossRef]
49. Kishore, A.; Vail, A.; Majid, A.; Dawson, J.; Lees, K.R.; Tyrrell, P.J.; Smith, C.J. Detection of Atrial Fibrillation After Ischemic Stroke or Transient Ischemic Attack. *Stroke* **2014**, *45*, 520–526. [CrossRef]
50. January, C.T.; Wann, L.S.; Alpert, J.S.; Calkins, H.; Cigarroa, J.E.; Cleveland, J.C.; Conti, J.B.; Ellinor, P.T.;

Ezekowitz, M.D.; Field, M.E.; et al. 2014 AHA/ACC/HRS Guideline for the Management of Patients with Atrial Fibrillation. *Circulation* **2014**, *130*, 1–2. [CrossRef]

51. Jonas, D.E.; Kahwati, L.C.; Yun, J.D.Y.; Middleton, J.C.; Coker-Schwimmer, M.; Asher, G.N. Screening for Atrial Fibrillation with Electrocardiography. *JAMA* **2018**, *320*, 485. [CrossRef]
52. Curry, S.J.; Krist, A.H.; Owens, D.K.; Barry, M.J.; Caughey, A.B.; Davidson, K.W.; Doubeni, C.A.; Epling, J.W., Jr.; Kemper, A.R.; Kubik, M.; et al. Screening for Atrial Fibrillation with Electrocardiography. *JAMA* **2018**, *320*, 478. [CrossRef]
53. Svennberg, E.; Engdahl, J.; Al-Khalili, F.; Friberg, L.; Frykman, V.; Rosenqvist, M. Mass Screening for Untreated Atrial Fibrillation. *Circulation* **2015**, *131*, 2176–2184. [CrossRef]
54. Aronsson, M.; Svennberg, E.; Rosenqvist, M.; Engdahl, J.; Al-Khalili, F.; Friberg, L.; Frykman-Kull, V.; Levin, L.Å. Cost-effectiveness of mass screening for untreated atrial fibrillation using intermittent ECG recording. *Europace* **2015**, *17*, 1023–1029. [CrossRef]
55. Sinha, A.-M.; Diener, H.-C.; Morillo, C.A.; Sanna, T.; Bernstein, R.A.; Di Lazzaro, V.; Passman, R.; Beckers, F.; Brachmann, J. Cryptogenic Stroke and underlying Atrial Fibrillation (CRYSTAL AF): Design and rationale. *Am. Heart J.* **2010**, *160*, 36–41. [CrossRef]
56. Sanna, T.; Diener, H.-C.; Passman, R.S.; Di Lazzaro, V.; Bernstein, R.A.; Morillo, C.A.; Rymer, M.M.; Thijs, V.; Rogers, T.; Beckers, F.; et al. Cryptogenic Stroke and Underlying Atrial Fibrillation. *N. Engl. J. Med.* **2014**, *370*, 2478–2486. [CrossRef]
57. Gladstone, D.J.; Spring, M.; Dorian, P.; Panzov, V.; Thorpe, K.E.; Hall, J.; Vaid, H.; O'Donnell, M.; Laupacis, A.; Côté, R.; et al. Atrial Fibrillation in Patients with Cryptogenic Stroke. *N. Engl. J. Med.* **2014**, *370*, 2467–2477. [CrossRef]
58. Conen, D.; Rodondi, N.; Müller, A.; Beer, J.H.; Ammann, P.; Moschovitis, G.; Auricchio, A.; Hayoz, D.; Kobza, R.; Shah, D.; et al. Relationships of Overt and Silent Brain Lesions with Cognitive Function in Patients With Atrial Fibrillation. *J. Am. Coll. Cardiol.* **2019**, *73*, 989–999. [CrossRef]
59. Mark, D.B.; Anstrom, K.J.; Sheng, S.; Piccini, J.P.; Baloch, K.N.; Monahan, K.H.; Monahan, K.H.; Daniels, M.R.; Bahnson, T.D.; Poole, J.E.; et al. Effect of Catheter Ablation vs Medical Therapy on Quality of Life Among Patients With Atrial Fibrillation. *JAMA* **2019**, *321*, 1275. [CrossRef]
60. Wokhlu, A.; Monahan, K.H.; Hodge, D.O.; Asirvatham, S.J.; Friedman, P.A.; Munger, T.M.; Bradley, D.J.; Bluhm, C.M.; Haroldson, J.M.; Packer, D.L. Long-Term Quality of Life After Ablation of Atrial Fibrillation. *J. Am. Coll. Cardiol.* **2010**, *55*, 2308–2316. [CrossRef]
61. Marrouche, N.F.; Brachmann, J.; Andresen, D.; Siebels, J.; Boersma, L.; Jordaens, L.; Merkely, B.; Pokushalov, E.; Sanders, P.; Proff, J.; et al. Catheter Ablation for Atrial Fibrillation with Heart Failure. *N. Engl. J. Med.* **2018**, *378*, 417–427. [CrossRef]
62. Dagres, N.; Chao, T.-F.; Fenelon, G.; Aguinaga, L.; Benhayon, D.; Benjamin, E.J.; Bunch, T.J.; Chen, L.Y.; Chen, S.A.; Darrieux, F.; et al. European Heart Rhythm Association (EHRA)/Heart Rhythm Society (HRS)/Asia Pacific Heart Rhythm Society (APHRS)/Latin American Heart Rhythm Society (LAHRS) expert consensus on arrhythmias and cognitive function: What is the best practice? *Europace* **2018**, *20*, 1399–1421. [CrossRef]
63. Herm, J.; Fiebach, J.B.; Koch, L.; Kopp, U.A.; Kunze, C.; Wollboldt, C.; Brunecker, P.; Schultheiss, H.P.; Schirdewan, A.; Endres, M.; et al. Neuropsychological effects of MRI-detected brain lesions after left atrial catheter ablation for atrial fibrillation: Long-term results of the MACPAF study. *Circ. Arrhythmia Electrophysiol.* **2013**, *6*, 843–850. [CrossRef]
64. Medi, C.; Evered, L.; Silbert, B.; Teh, A.; Halloran, K.; Morton, J.; Kistler, P.; Kalman, J. Subtle post-procedural cognitive dysfunction after atrial fibrillation ablation. *J. Am. Coll. Cardiol.* **2013**, *62*, 531–539. [CrossRef]
65. Allan, V.; Banerjee, A.; Shah, A.D.; Patel, R.; Denaxas, S.; Casas, J.-P.; Hemingway, H. Net clinical benefit of warfarin in individuals with atrial fibrillation across stroke risk and across primary and secondary care. *Heart* **2017**, *103*, 210–218. [CrossRef]
66. Friberg, L.; Rosenqvist, M.; Lip, G.Y.H. Net clinical benefit of warfarin in patients with atrial fibrillation: A report from the swedish atrial fibrillation cohort study. *Circulation* **2012**, *125*, 2298–2307. [CrossRef]
67. Ruff, C.T.; Giugliano, R.P.; Braunwald, E.; Hoffman, E.B.; Deenadayalu, N.; Ezekowitz, M.D.; Camm, A.J.; Weitz, J.I.; Lewis, B.S.; Parkhomenko, A.; et al. Comparison of the efficacy and safety of new oral anticoagulants with warfarin in patients with atrial fibrillation: A meta-analysis of randomised trials. *Lancet* **2014**, *383*, 955–962. [CrossRef]
68. Martin, D.T.; Bersohn, M.M.; Lwaldo, A.; Wathen, M.S.; Choucair, W.K.; Lip, G.Y.; Ip, J.; Holcomb, R.;

Akar, J.G.; Halperin, J.L.; et al. Randomized trial of atrial arrhythmia monitoring to guide anticoagulation in patients with implanted defibrillator and cardiac resynchronization devices. *Eur. Heart J.* **2015**, *36*, 1660–1668. [CrossRef]

69. Greene, H.L. Baseline characteristics of patients with atrial fibrillation: The AFFIRM study. *Am. Heart J.* **2002**, *143*, 991–1001. [CrossRef]
70. Investigators TAFFI of RM (AFFIRM). A Comparison of Rate Control and Rhythm Control in Patients with Atrial Fibrillation. *N. Engl. J. Med.* **2002**, *347*, 1825–1833. [CrossRef]
71. Van Gelder, I.C.; Hagens, V.E.; Bosker, H.A.; Kingma, J.H.; Kamp, O.; Kingma, T.; Said, S.A.; Darmanata, J.I.; Timmermans, A.J.; Tijssen, J.G.; et al. A Comparison of Rate Control and Rhythm Control in Patients with Recurrent Persistent Atrial Fibrillation. *N. Engl. J. Med.* **2002**, *347*, 1834–1840. [CrossRef]
72. Epstein, A.E. Relationships Between Sinus Rhythm, Treatment, and Survival in the Atrial Fibrillation Follow-Up Investigation of Rhythm Management (AFFIRM) Study. *Circulation* **2004**, *109*, 1509–1513. [CrossRef]
73. Tsadok, M.A.; Jackevicius, C.A.; Essebag, V.; Eisenberg, M.J.; Rahme, E.; Humphries, K.H.; Tu, J.V.; Behlouli, H.; Pilote, L. Rhythm Versus Rate Control Therapy and Subsequent Stroke or Transient Ischemic Attack in Patients with Atrial Fibrillation. *Circulation* **2012**, *126*, 2680–2687. [CrossRef]
74. Khan, A.R.; Khan, S.; Sheikh, M.A.; Khuder, S.; Grubb, B.; Moukarbel, G.V. Catheter ablation and antiarrhythmic drug therapy as first- or second-line therapy in the management of atrial fibrillation: Systematic review and meta-analysis. *Circ. Arrhythmia Electrophysiol.* **2014**, *7*, 853–860. [CrossRef]
75. Packer, D.L.; Mark, D.B.; Robb, R.A.; Monahan, K.H.; Bahnson, T.D.; Poole, J.E.; Noseworthy, P.A.; Rosenberg, Y.D.; Jeffries, N.; Mitchell, L.B.; et al. Effect of Catheter Ablation vs Antiarrhythmic Drug Therapy on Mortality, Stroke, Bleeding, and Cardiac Arrest Among Patients with Atrial Fibrillation. *JAMA* **2019**, *321*, 1261–1274. [CrossRef]
76. Bunch, T.J.; May, H.T.; Bair, T.L.; Weiss, J.P.; Crandall, B.G.; Osborn, J.S.; Mallender, C.; Anderson, J.L.; Muhlestein, B.J.; Lappe, D.L.; et al. Atrial fibrillation ablation patients have long-term stroke rates similar to patients without atrial fibrillation regardless of CHADS2 score. *Heart Rhythm* **2013**, *10*, 1272–1277. [CrossRef]
77. Hunter, R.J.; McCready, J.; Diab, I.; Page, S.P.; Finlay, M.; Richmond, L.; French, A.; Earley, M.J.; Sporton, S.; Jones, M.; et al. Maintenance of sinus rhythm with an ablation strategy in patients with atrial fibrillation is associated with a lower risk of stroke and death. *Heart* **2012**, *98*, 48–53. [CrossRef]
78. Karasoy, D.; Gislason, G.H.; Hansen, J.; Johannessen, A.; K'ber, L.; Hvidtfeldt, M.; Özcan, C.; Torp-Pedersen, C.; Hansen, M.L. Oral anticoagulation therapy after radiofrequency ablation of atrial fibrillation and the risk of thromboembolism and serious bleeding: Long-term follow-up in nationwide cohort of Denmark. *Eur. Heart J.* **2015**, *36*, 307–314. [CrossRef]
79. Gallo, C.; Battaglia, A.; Anselmino, M.; Bianchi, F.; Grossi, S.; Nangeroni, G.; Toso, E.; Gaido, L.; Scaglione, M.; Ferraris, F.; et al. Long-term events following atrial fibrillation rate control or transcatheter ablation. *J. Cardiovasc. Med.* **2016**, *17*, 187–193. [CrossRef]
80. Kirchhof, P.; Breithardt, G.; Camm, A.J.; Crijns, H.J.; Kuck, K.-H.; Vardas, P.; Wegscheider, K. Improving outcomes in patients with atrial fibrillation: Rationale and design of the Early treatment of Atrial fibrillation for Stroke prevention Trial. *Am. Heart J.* **2013**, *166*, 442–448. [CrossRef]
81. Verma, A.; Ha, A.C.T.; Kirchhof, P.; Hindricks, G.; Healey, J.S.; Hill, M.D.; Sharma, M.; Wyse, D.G.; Champagne, J.; Essebag, V.; et al. The Optimal Anti-Coagulation for Enhanced-Risk Patients Post–Catheter Ablation for Atrial Fibrillation (OCEAN) trial. *Am. Heart J.* **2018**, *197*, 124–132. [CrossRef]
82. Kalman, J.M.; Sanders, P.; Rosso, R.; Calkins, H. Should We Perform Catheter Ablation for Asymptomatic Atrial Fibrillation? *Circulation* **2017**, *136*, 490–499. [CrossRef]

18

Thromboembolic Events Following Atrial Fibrillation Cardioversion and Ablation: What's the Culprit?

Francesco De Sensi [1,*], Gennaro Miracapillo [1], Luigi Addonisio [1], Marco Breschi [1], Alberto Cresti [1], Pasquale Baratta [1], Francesco Paneni [2] and Ugo Limbruno [1]

1 Cardiology Department, Misericordia Hospital, 58100 Grosseto, Italy
2 Center for Molecular Cardiology, University Hospital, 8057 Zürich, Switzerland
* Correspondence: desensi_francesco@libero.it

Abstract: Stroke is a rare but possible complication after atrial fibrillation (AF) ablation. However, its etiopathogenesis is far from being completely characterized. Here we report a case of stroke, with recurrent peripheral embolism after AF ablation procedure. In our patient, an in situ femoral vein thrombosis and iatrogenic atrial septal defect were simultaneously detected. A comprehensive review of multiple pathophysiological mechanisms of stroke in this context is provided. The case underlines the importance of a global evaluation of patients undergoing AF ablation.

Keywords: atrial fibrillation ablation; stroke; iatrogenic interatrial septum defect; paradoxical embolism; anticoagulant interruption

1. Case Report

A gentleman, 76 years old, was scheduled for catheter ablation of atrial fibrillation (AF) and atypical left atrial flutter in the context of symptomatic left ventricular dysfunction. He reported fatigue and exertional dyspnea, and presented persistent AF on EKG. He had a weight of 68 kg, and a height of 170 cm (BMI = 23 kg/m^2), with high estimated thromboembolic risk (CHA_2DS_2VASc = 4). He was previously prescribed with anticoagulation (Dabigatran 110 mg bid), beta-blocker (bisoprolol 5 mg od), ACE-inhibitor (ramipril 5 mg od), diuretic (furosemide 50 mg) therapy. A 2D-echocardiogram documented left ventricle dilation (LVEDD (end diastolic diameter): 61 mm) with systolic dysfunction (EF (ejection fraction): 38%). A 2D-transesophageal echocardiogram (TEE) showed absence of images referable to atrial and auricular thrombosis. Single-lobe left appendage displayed reduced function with velocity peaks of 25 cm/sec. The left atrial area was 28 cm^2. No relevant atherosclerotic plaques were found in the thoracic aorta. Written informed consent was obtained and the patient underwent radiofrequency electrical pulmonary veins isolation plus roof and mitral isthmus ablation lines during systemic intraprocedural heparinization (activation clotting time (ACT)-target: 300–350 s). Electrical cardioversion was also performed due to presence of persistent AF. The total procedural time was 180 min. Dabigatran was temporarily interrupted for 36 h across the procedure and the patient was discharged the next day. After one week he was admitted to the emergency department for sudden dyspnea, being hospitalized for acute heart failure. At admission the EKG showed sinus tachycardia, while chest X-ray depicted bilateral alveolar edema. During hospitalization, after achieving hemodynamic stabilization, the patient suffered aphasia and space-time disorientation with near loss of consciousness. The Angio-CT (computational tomography) showed hypodense lesions in the left cortico-subcortical temporo-occipital area and in the left cerebellar hemisphere as showed in Figure 1. Carotid and vertebral arteries were free from hemodynamic atherosclerotic plaques. Symptoms completely disappeared after two days and at the 24 h CT scan control, the lesions were stable, in the absence of hemorrhagic transformation. After a few days, the patient complained left limb pain and an acute distal embolism was diagnosed. A new transthoracic echocardiogram revealed a further deterioration of left ventricular ejection fraction (EF: 30%) with no evidence of intraventricular thrombosis and a clearly discernable interatrial septal defect with left-to-right shunt, this was likely attributable to the trans-septal puncture performed during the ablation (Figure 2). Ultrasonography of the groin region documented in situ not compressible left femoral vein thrombosis (Figure 3). Non fractioned heparin infusion was administered with complete resolution of both the arterial embolic occlusion and venous thrombosis. After a few days, oral anticoagulation with apixaban was initiated and the patient was discharged. At the six months follow-up, he presented with mild cognitive impairment, which persisted overtime till the last visit.

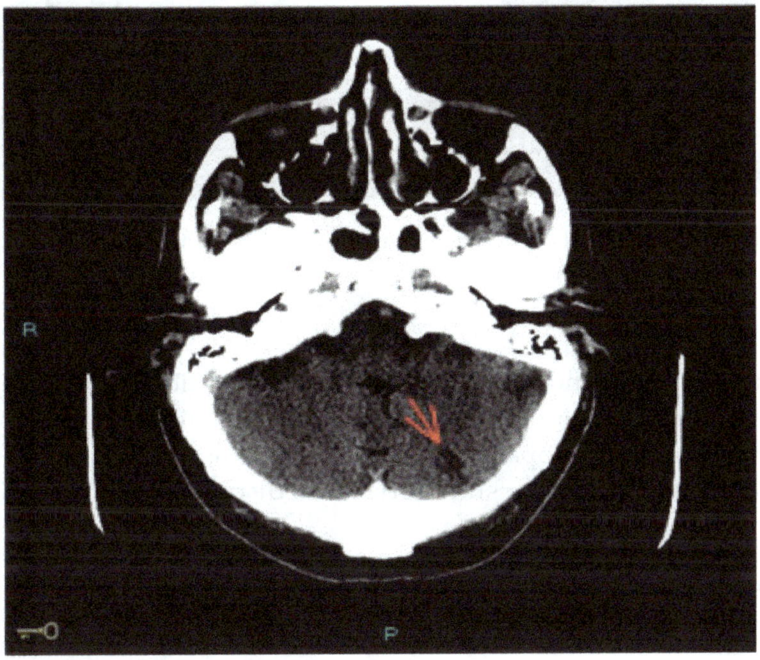

Figure 1. Angio-CT (computational tomography) brain scan. The exam showed an acute ischemic lesion in the left cortico-subcortical temporo-occipital area and in the left cerebellar hemisphere (last one marked with red arrow).

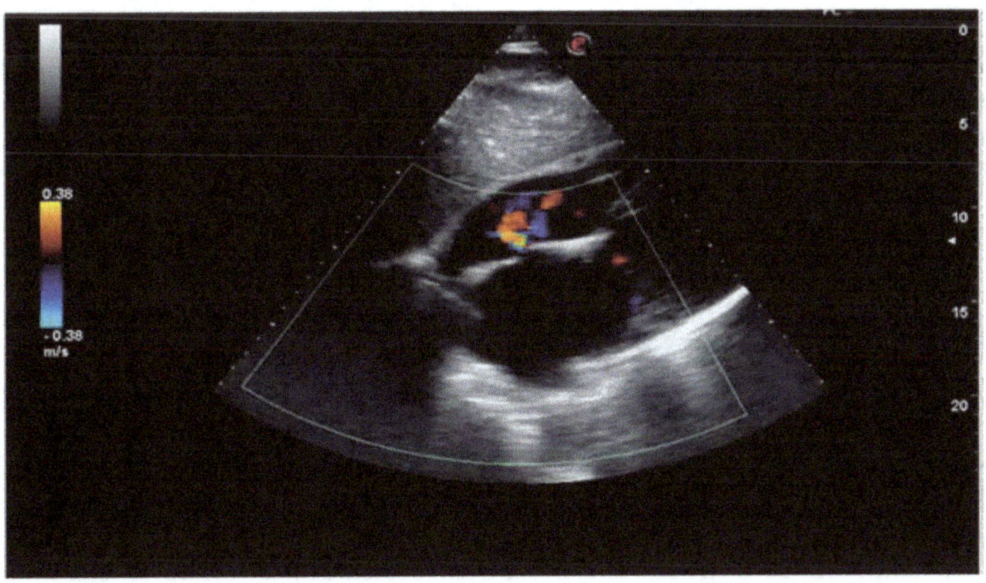

Figure 2. Transthoracic echocardiogram (subxiphoid view). The exam showed a clearly discernable interatrial septal defect with left-to-right shunt identified, at rest, with color doppler.

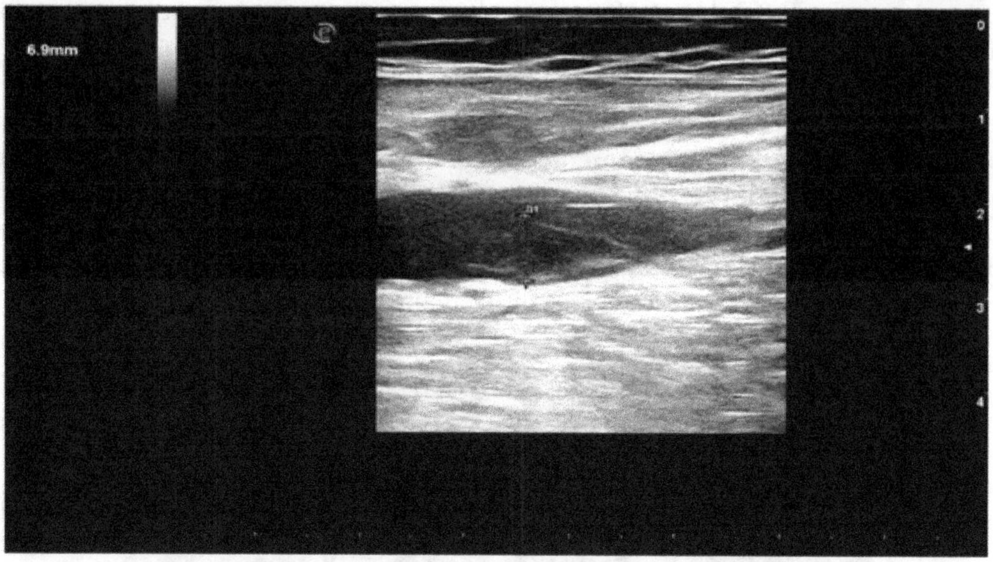

Figure 3. Ultrasonographic femoral scan. The exam showed in situ thrombosis of the left femoral vein which was not compressible with the probe.

2. Case Discussion

The case illustrates an uncommon complication after atrial fibrillation (AF) ablation manifested with recurrent embolic events: A stroke and a leg embolism. Although stroke is a well-known described complication after AF ablation, the etiopathogenetic mechanisms underlying this complication are yet to be completely characterized. Here, we summarize and discuss all the potential factors involved in this undesirable complication.

2.1. Radiofrequency Lesion Set and Ablation "Per Se"

Evidence from non-randomized studies has shown that AF catheter ablation may reduce stroke risk, when successful. Among 361,913 patients with AF of the Swedish Patient Registry, catheter ablation was associated with a lower risk of stroke (HR = 0.69) and mortality (HR = 0.50). These results were even more significant in patients with CHA_2DS_2-VASc score ≥2 (HR = 0.39) [1]. Especially in patients with CHA2DS2-VASc score of ≥2 (83% of 3953 patients) Saliba and colleagues found a reduction in stroke rate in the ablation group compared to the non-ablated group (HR = 0.61) [2]. On this ground, Hunter et al. demonstrated, in an international multicenter registry of 1273 patients, that freedom from AF was associated with stroke-free survival (HR = 0.30) [3]. However, when discussing the possibility of a catheter ablation procedure for AF treatment, physicians should clearly make their patients aware about a periprocedural stroke risk which is approximately 0.5–1% [4]. Thromboembolic risk is directly related to the amount of radiofrequency lesions applied in the left atrial cavity. In fact, radiofrequency produces colliquative necrosis, thus leading to endothelial dysfunction and activation of the Virchow triad. Hence, during ablation, tissue involvement is directly related to an increased embolic risk [5]. An approach adding linear or complex lesion sets to pulmonary vein isolation (PVI) did not demonstrate an increase in freedom from AF recurrences, thus the standard endpoint during the first procedure should be PVI alone [6]. In our case, extensive left atrial ablation was performed with PVI plus tracing of two ablation lines along the roof and the mitral isthmus. Such ablation strategy was due to the presence of atypical left atrial flutter as well as of persistent atrial fibrillation. Although stroke is considered an uncommon complication after AF ablation, a growing body of evidence is consistently reporting asymptomatic or subclinical ischemic lesions in up to 41% of patients [7,8]. An elegant Italian study by Gaita and colleagues analyzed postprocedural brain magnetic resonance imaging (MRI) of 232 consecutive patients with paroxysmal or persistent atrial fibrillation who underwent radiofrequency left atrial catheter ablation. Techniques used were PVI or PVI plus linear lesions plus atrial defragmentation. A clinical cerebrovascular accident occurred in only 1 patient. However, brain MRI returned positive for new embolic lesions in 33 patients. Cardioversion (CV) during the procedure was associated with an increased risk of 2.75 (95 confidence interval, 1.29–5.89; $p = 0.009$) [9]. Our patient underwent electrical CV during the ablation due to the presence of persistent AF at the beginning of the procedure. It has been recognized that CV is related to thromboembolic events "per se", independently by the ablation procedure. In patients undergoing TEE-guided cardioversion, patients on direct oral anticoagulants (DOACs), such as dabigatran and apixaban, experienced low incidence of thromboembolic events during follow-ups (0.6% and 1.1%, respectively), similar to warfarin, with a favorable trend of bleeding safety profile [10,11]. The highest risk period after CV is the following week, which would be a suitable timeline for our patient considering the stroke and the peripheral embolism.

Finally, it seems that techniques other than radiofrequency, such as cryoballoon based one-shot ablation and duty-cycled phased radiofrequency ablation (PVAC) are not free from silent cerebral embolisms, suggesting other mechanisms (like air embolism) could play a pivotal role in the physiopathology of these subclinical findings [12–14].

2.2. Management of Anticoagulant Therapy in the Periprocedural Period

Ablation was performed in January 2017. The patient had been prescribed Dabigatran 6 months before. We decided to perform TEE due to the patient's high thromboembolic risk ($CHA_2DS_2VASc = 4$). Indeed, despite optimal oral anticoagulation with DOACs, left atrial (LA) thrombus was detected in the left appendage (LAA) in >3.6% of AF patients undergoing catheter ablation in the real world. In this setting higher CHA_2DS_2VASc ($p = 0.02$), but not the type of DOAC, significantly predicted the presence of LA thrombus [15].

Dabigatran has been available in Italy since 2014. At the time of ablation there were no clear guidelines on appropriate periprocedural ablation management of such a new kind of drug. On the contrary, evidence available on uninterrupted warfarin showed reduction in bleeding and thromboembolic complications [16]. Since we used all the available tools in order to reduce bleeding complications (i.e., ultrasound guided femoral veins puncture, intracardiac echocardiography, contact force sensing catheters) [17,18], we felt confident to minimize dabigatran interruption. In fact, the last assumption was in the morning of the day before, and first retake was in the evening of the day of the procedure (36 h, total interruption time). Despite this short interruption and the use of heparinization during the procedure (target activation clotting time ACT = 300–350 s), we should consider this anticoagulation break as a putative factor implicated in the patient's recurrent embolic events. Indeed, the 2017 expert consensus statement on AF Ablation provide a Class I recommendation for performing the procedure with uninterrupted dabigatran (Class I, LOE A) or rivaroxaban (Class I, LOE B-R), and a 2A recommendation for the other Xa inhibitors for which specific clinical studies had not been performed at the time [5]. These recommendations derived from the results of the RE-CIRCUIT trial which was a head-to-head comparison between uninterrupted dabigatran and uninterrupted warfarin in patients undergoing AF ablation. The incidence of major bleeding was significantly lower with dabigatran than with warfarin (5 patients (1.6%) vs 22 patients (6.9%)). No strokes/TIA (transient ischemic attack) occurred in the dabigatran arm, while there was one TIA in the warfarin group. Idarucizumab, the specific reversal agent, was never used during the study [19]. Two years before, Cappato and colleagues published the results of the VENTURE-AF trial, comparing uninterrupted rivaroxaban vs uninterrupted warfarin. Complications (a major bleeding event, one ischemic stroke, and one vascular death) occurred only in the warfarin group [20]. More recently consistent evidences were provided also for apixaban and edoxaban. The AEIOU trial, published in 2018, randomized 300 patients undergoing AF ablation to uninterrupted versus minimally interrupted (holding 1 dose) periprocedural apixaban. A retrospective cohort of patients treated with uninterrupted warfarin at the same centers was matched to the apixaban-treated subjects for comparison. There were no stroke or SE events observed in all groups. The rates of clinically significant, major bleeding were similar for all apixaban patients compared with the matched warfarin group [21]. Finally, in 2019 Hohnloser et al. published results from the ELIMINATE-AF trial, which confirmed the safety and efficacy of uninterrupted edoxaban vs vitamin K antagonists (VKAs) in the same setting. Among 553 patients undergoing AF ablation, brain magnetic resonance imaging was performed in 177 subjects to assess silent cerebral infarcts. There was one ischaemic and one haemorrhagic stroke, both in patients on edoxaban. Cerebral microemboli were detected in 13.8% (16) of patients who received edoxaban and 9.6% (5) of patients in the VKA group ($p =$ ns) [22]. Based on these clinical trials, it is now clear that a strategy of performing AF ablation on patients receiving uninterrupted anticoagulation can be performed safely and will minimize the risk of thromboembolic events. Finally, international guidelines state in the absence of controlled trial data, anticoagulation management after AF ablation should follow general recommendations (i.e., on the basis of CHA_2DS_2-VASc score), regardless of the presumed rhythm outcome [23].

2.3. *Iatrogenic Interatrial Septal Defect, In Situ Thrombosis and Paradoxical Embolism*

The diagnosis in our patient, of simultaneous iatrogenic interatrial septal defect (IASD) and in-situ thrombosis, is rather unique. These are two well characterized phenomena that have rarely been discovered together in this setting. Real incidence of IASD after AF ablation is under debate. Older studies, using transesophageal echocardiography (TEE), reported up to 19% rate during follow-up [24–27].

More recently, other rates have been described (5.6% following a first procedure and 2.2% following a second procedure) [28].

The risk of persistent IASD is in part related to the tools, technologies, and approaches used for catheter ablation. For example, the incidence of IASD at 1-year follow-up following cryoballoon ablation procedure for PVI is significantly higher in front of radiofrequency procedures [29–31]. After a single-puncture, using the robotic navigation system, an IASD was detected in 38 of 40 (95%) patients one day after the ablation. At 6-months follow up, the IASDs were closed only in 30 of 39 (78.9%) patients. The authors also addressed that persistent IASDs are not associated with an increased rate of paradoxical embolism or with relevant shunting [32].

On the other side, the real incidence of in situ asymptomatic femoral thrombosis after AF ablation is unknown. Asymptomatic deep venous thrombosis (DVT) formation, following sheath placement for electrophysiological studies (EPS) in general, were detected in up to 16–44% of patients. In contrast, symptomatic DVTs are much lower (0.5–0.8%) [33]. In 2004, Chen and colleagues reported a significant incidence (17.6%) of non-occlusive DVT after multiple sheath placements for EPS. Nonetheless, in the study, all venous thrombi were non-occlusive and asymptomatic. None of the femoral veins developed occlusive DVT [34]. Although there are weak supporting data, it is reasonable to conclude that limiting the number and the size of femoral vein sheaths on the same side can minimize thrombosis risk. Despite the fact that there are no large prospective or randomized trials, prophylactic heparin administration during the procedure may be considered on an individual basis for right chamber ablations, particularly for longer procedures, or in high-risk patients [35]. Large emboli migrated from leg veins can lodge in the right ventricle [36], whereas smaller emboli are likely to pass unimpeded to the pulmonary arteries. The occurrence of pulmonary embolism following EP procedures has previously been reported, especially in patients with a thrombophilic state [37]. Moreover, two cases of floating atrial thrombi following EP studies were successfully treated with thrombolysis in asymptomatic patients [38].

To the best of our knowledge, there are no reported cases of paradoxical embolism following AF ablation where in situ thrombosis and iatrogenic atrial septal defect are detected simultaneously. Indeed, DVT developed despite fully systemic heparinization during the procedure and minimal oral anticoagulation interruption.

3. Conclusions

In conclusion, we report a case of stroke and peripheral embolism after atrial fibrillation ablation procedure. In our patient an in situ femoral vein thrombosis and iatrogenic atrial septal defect were simultaneously detected. We highlighted and discussed each etiopathogenetic mechanism underlying this clinical condition. The case encourages a critical clinical and instrumental evaluation in the management of such undesirable complications.

Author Contributions: Conceptualization, F.D.S. and A.C.; methodology, F.D.S. and L.A. and A.C.; software, M.B.; validation, F.P., U.L. and G.M.; formal analysis, F.P. and U.L.; investigation, G.M. and L.A.; data curation, A.C. and P.B.; writing—original draft preparation, F.D.S. and P.B. and F.P.; writing—review & editing, F.D.S. and F.P. and G.M.; supervision, U.L.

Acknowledgments: The authors would like to thank all the nurses working in the Electrophysiology Lab of Misericordia Hospital, Grosseto, Italy.

References

1. Friberg, L.; Tabrizi, F.; Englund, A. Catheter ablation for atrial fibrillation is associated with lower incidence of stroke and death: Data from Swedish health registries. *Eur. Heart J.* **2016**, *37*, 2478–2487. [CrossRef] [PubMed]
2. Saliba, W.; Schliamser, J.E.; Lavi, I.; Barnett-Griness, O.; Gronich, N.; Rennert, G. Catheter ablation of atrial fibrillation is associated with reduced risk of stroke and mortality: A propensity score-matched analysis. *Heart Rhythm* **2017**, *14*, 635–642. [CrossRef] [PubMed]
3. Hunter, R.J.; McCready, J., Diab, I.; Page, S.P.; Finlay, M.; Richmond, L.; French, A.; Sporton, S.; Lee, G.; Chow, A.; et al. Maintenance of sinus rhythm with an ablation strategy in patients with atrial fibrillation is associated with a lower risk of stroke and death. *Heart* **2012**, *98*, 48–53. [CrossRef] [PubMed]
4. Haeusler, K.G.; Kirchhof, P.; Endres, M. Left atrial catheter ablation and ischemic stroke. *Stroke* **2012**, *43*, 265–270. [CrossRef] [PubMed]
5. Calkins, H.; Hindricks, G.; Cappato, R.; Kim, Y.H.; Saad, E.B.; Aguinaga, L.; Akar, J.G.; Badhwar, V.; Brugada, J.; Camm, J.; et al. 2017 HRS/EHRA/ECAS/APHRS/SOLAECE expert consensus statement on catheter and surgical ablation of atrial fibrillation. *Europace* **2018**, *20*, e1–e160. [CrossRef] [PubMed]
6. Verma, A.; Jiang, C.Y.; Betts, T.R.; Chen, J.; Deisenhofer, I.; Mantovan, R.; Macle, L.; Morillo, C.A.; Haverkamp, W.; Weerasooriya, R.; et al. STAR AF II Investigators. Approaches to catheter ablation for persistent atrial fibrillation. *N. Engl. J. Med.* **2015**, *372*, 1812–1822. [CrossRef]
7. Rillig, A.; Meyerfeldt, U.; Tilz, R.R.; Talazko, J.; Arya, A.; Zvereva, V.; Birkemeyer, R.; Miljak, T.; Hajredini, B.; Wohlmuth, P.; et al. Incidence and long-term follow-up of silent cerebral lesions after pulmonary vein isolation using a remote robotic navigation system as compared with manual ablation. *Circ. Arrhythm. Electrophysiol.* **2012**, *5*, 15–21. [CrossRef]
8. Herm, J.; Fiebach, J.B.; Koch, L.; Kopp, U.A.; Kunze, C.; Wollboldt, C.; Brunecker, P.; Schultheiss, H.P.; Schirdewan, A.; Endres, M.; et al. Neuropsychological effects of MRI- detected brain lesions after left atrial catheter ablation for atrial fibrillation: Long-term results of the MACPAF study. *Circ. Arrhythmia Electrophysiol.* **2013**, *6*, 843–850. [CrossRef]
9. Gaita, F.; Caponi, D.; Pianelli, M.; Scaglione, M.; Toso, E.; Cesarani, F.; Boffano, C.; Gandini, G.; Valentini, M.C.; de Ponti, R.; et al. Radiofrequency catheter ablation of atrial fibrillation: A cause of silent thromboembolism? Magnetic resonance imaging assessment of cerebral thromboembolism in patients undergoing ablation of atrial fibrillation. *Circulation* **2010**, *122*, 1667–1673. [CrossRef]
10. Russo, V.; Rago, A.; Papa, A.A.; D'Onofrio, A.; Golino, P.; Nigro, G. Efficacy and safety of dabigatran in patients with atrial fibrillation scheduled for transoesophageal echocardiogram-guided direct electrical current cardioversion: A prospective propensity score-matched cohort study. *J. Thromb. Thrombolysis* **2018**, *45*, 206–212. [CrossRef]
11. Rago, A.; Papa, A.A.; Cassese, A.; Arena, G.; Magliocca, M.C.G.; D'Onofrio, A.; Golino, P.; Nigro, G.; Russo, V. Clinical Performance of Apixaban vs. Vitamin K Antagonists in Patients with Atrial Fibrillation Undergoing

Direct Electrical Current Cardioversion: A Prospective Propensity Score-Matched Cohort Study. *Am. J. Cardiovasc. Drugs* **2019**, *19*, 421–427. [CrossRef] [PubMed]

12. McCready, J.; Chow, A.W.; Lowe, M.D.; Segal, O.R.; Ahsan, S.; de Bono, J.; Dhaliwal, M.; Mfuko, C.; Ng, A.; Rowland, E.R.; et al. Safety and efficacy of multipolar pulmonary vein ablation catheter vs. irrigated radiofrequency ablation for paroxysmal atrial fibrillation: A randomized multicentre trial. *Europace* **2014**, *16*, 1145–1153. [CrossRef] [PubMed]
13. Wieczorek, M.; Lukat, M.; Hoeltgen, R.; Condie, C.; Hilje, T.; Missler, U.; Hirsch, J.; Scharf, C. Investigation into causes of abnormal cerebral MRI findings following PVAC duty-cycled, phased RF ablation of atrial fibrillation. *J. Cardiovasc. Electrophysiol.* **2013**, *24*, 121–128. [CrossRef] [PubMed]
14. Miyazaki, S.; Kajiyama, T.; Yamao, K.; Hada, M.; Yamaguchi, M.; Nakamura, H.; Hachiya, H.; Tada, H.; Hirao, K.; Iesaka, Y. Silent cerebral events/lesions after second-generation cryoballoon ablation: How can we reduce the risk of silent strokes? *Heart Rhythm* **2019**, *16*, 41–48. [CrossRef] [PubMed]
15. Bertaglia, E.; Anselmino, M.; Zorzi, A.; Russo, V.; Toso, E.; Peruzza, F.; Rapacciuolo, A.; Migliore, F.; Gaita, F.; Cucchini, U.; et al. NOACs and atrial fibrillation: Incidence and predictors of left atrial thrombus in the real world. *Int. J. Cardiol.* **2017**, *249*, 179–183. [CrossRef] [PubMed]
16. Hussein, A.A.; Martin, D.O.; Saliba, W.; Patel, D.; Karim, S.; Batal, O.; Banna, M.; Williams-Andrews, M.; Sherman, M.; Kanj, M.; et al. Radiofrequency ablation of atrial fibrillation under therapeutic international normalized ratio: A safe and efficacious periprocedural anticoagulation strategy. *Heart Rhythm* **2009**, *6*, 1425–1429. [CrossRef]
17. De Sensi, F.; Miracapillo, G.; Addonisio, L.; Breschi, M.; Paneni, F. A call for safety during electrophysiological procedures: US in, why not US out? *Europace* **2017**, *19*, 2048. [CrossRef] [PubMed]
18. De Sensi, F.; Miracapillo, G.; Addonisio, L.; Breschi, M.; Scalese, M.; Cresti, A.; Paneni, F.; Limbruno, U. Predictors of Successful Ultrasound Guided Femoral Vein Cannulation in Electrophysiological Procedures. *J. Atr. Fibrillation.* **2018**, *11*, 2083. [CrossRef]
19. Calkins, H.; Willems, S.; Gerstenfeld, E.P.; Verma, A.; Schilling, R.; Hohnloser, S.H.; Okumura, K.; Serota, H.; Nordaby, M.; Guiver, K.; et al. RE-CIRCUIT Investigators. Uninterrupted Dabigatran versus Warfarin for Ablation in Atrial Fibrillation. *N. Engl. J. Med.* **2017**, *376*, 1627–1636. [CrossRef]
20. Cappato, R.; Marchlinski, F.E.; Hohnloser, S.H.; Naccarelli, G.V.; Xiang, J.; Wilber, D.J.; Ma, C.S.; Hess, S.; Wells, D.S.; Juang, G.; et al. VENTURE-AF Investigators. Uninterrupted rivaroxaban vs. uninterrupted vitamin K antagonists for catheter ablation in non-valvular atrial fibrillation. *Eur. Heart J.* **2015**, *36*, 1805–1811. [CrossRef]
21. Reynolds, M.R.; Allison, J.S.; Natale, A.; Weisberg, I.L.; Ellenbogen, K.A.; Richards, M.; Hsieh, W.H.; Sutherland, J.; Cannon, C.P. A Prospective Randomized Trial of Apixaban Dosing During Atrial Fibrillation Ablation: The AEIOU Trial. *JACC Clin. Electrophysiol.* **2018**, *4*, 580–588. [CrossRef] [PubMed]
22. Hohnloser, S.H.; Camm, J.; Cappato, R.; Diener, H.C.; Heidbüchel, H.; Mont, L.; Morillo, C.A.; Abozguia, K.; Grimaldi, M.; Rauer, H.; et al. Uninterrupted edoxaban vs. vitamin K antagonists for ablation of atrial fibrillation: The ELIMINATE-AF trial. *Eur. Heart J.* **2019**, *11*. [CrossRef] [PubMed]
23. Kirchhof, P.; Benussi, S.; Kotecha, D.; Ahlsson, A.; Atar, D.; Casadei, B.; Castella, M.; Diener, H.C.; Heidbuchel, H.; Hendriks, J.; et al. ESC Scientific Document Group. 2016 ESC Guidelines for the management of atrial fibrillation developed in collaboration with EACTS. *Eur. Heart J.* **2016**, *37*, 2893–2962. [CrossRef] [PubMed]
24. Hammerstingl, C.; Lickfett, L.; Jeong, K.; Troatz, C.; Wedekind, J.A.; Tiemann, K.; Lüderitz, B.; Lewalter, T. ; Lüderitz, B.; Lewalter, T. Persistence of iatrogenic atrial septal defect after pulmonary vein isolation—An under- estimated risk? *Am. Heart J.* **2006**, *152*, 362–365. [CrossRef] [PubMed]
25. Rillig, A.; Meyerfeldt, U.; Birkemeyer, R.; Treusch, F.; Kunze, M.; Jung, W. Persistent iatrogenic atrial septal defect after pulmonary vein isolation: Incidence and clinical implications. *J. Interv. Card. Electrophysiol.* **2008**, *22*, 177–181. [CrossRef] [PubMed]
26. Fitchet, A.; Turkie, W.; Fitzpatrick, A.P. Transeptal approach to ablation of left-sided arrhythmias does not lead to persisting interatrial shunt: A transesophageal echocardiographic study. *Pacing Clin. Electrophysiol.* **1998**, *21*, 2070–2072. [CrossRef] [PubMed]
27. Obel, O.; Mansour, M.; Picard, M.; Ruskin, J.; Keane, D. Persistence of septal defects after transeptal puncture for pulmonary vein isolation procedures. *Pacing Clin. Electrophysiol.* **2004**, *27*, 1411–1414. [CrossRef]
28. Anselmino, M.; Scaglione, M.; Battaglia, A.; Muccioli, S.; Sardi, D.; Azzaro, G.; Garberoglio, L.; Miceli, S.;

Gaita, F. Iatrogenic atrial septal defects following atrial fibrillation transcatheter ablation: A relevant entity? *Europace* **2014**, *16*, 1562–1568. [CrossRef]

29. Mugnai, G.; Sieira, J.; Ciconte, G.; Hervas, M.S.; Irfan, G.; Saitoh, Y.; Hünük, B.; Ströker, E.; Velagic, V.; Wauters, K.; et al. One Year Incidence of Atrial Septal Defect after PV Isolation: A Comparison Between Conventional Radiofrequency and Cryoballoon Ablation. *Pacing Clin. Electrophysiol.* **2015**, *38*, 1049–1057. [CrossRef]
30. Sieira, J.; Chierchia, G.B.; di Giovanni, G.; Conte, G.; de Asmundis, C.; Sarkozy, A.; Droogmans, S.; Baltogiannis, G.; Saitoh, Y.; Ciconte, G. One-year incidence of iatrogenic atrial septal defect after cryoballoon ablation for atrial fibrillation. *J. Cardiovasc. Electrophysiol.* **2014**, *25*, 11–15. [CrossRef]
31. Cronin, E.M.; Collier, P.; Wazni, O.M.; Griffin, B.P.; Jaber, W.A.; Saliba, W.I. Persistence of atrial septal defect after cryoballoon ablation of atrial fibrillation. *J. Am. Coll. Cardiol.* **2013**, *62*, 1491–1492. [CrossRef] [PubMed]
32. Rillig, A.; Meyerfeldt, U.; Kunze, M.; Birkemeyer, R.; Miljak, T.; Jäckle, S.; Hajredini, B.; Treusch, F.; Jung, W. Persistent iatrogenic atrial septal defect after a single-puncture, double-transseptal approach for pulmonary vein isolation using a remote robotic navigation system: Results from a prospective study. *Europace* **2010**, *12*, 331–336. [CrossRef] [PubMed]
33. Davutoglu, V.; Kervancioglu, S.; Dinckal, H.; Soydinc, S.; Turkmen, S.; Akdemir, I.; Aksoy, M. High incidence of occult femoral vein thrombosis related to multiple venous sheaths during electrophysiology study. *Heart* **2004**, *90*, 1061–1062. [CrossRef] [PubMed]
34. Chen, J.Y.; Chang, K.C.; Lin, Y.C.; Chou, H.T.; Hung, J.S. Safety and outcomes of short-term multiple femoral venous sheath placement in cardiac electrophysiological study and radiofrequency catheter ablation. *Jpn. Heart J.* **2004**, *45*, 257–264. [CrossRef] [PubMed]
35. Blanc, J.J.; Almendral, J.; Brignole, M.; Fatemi, M.; Gjesdal, K.; Gonzalez-Torrecilla, E.; Wolpert, C. Consensus document on antithrombotic therapy in the setting of electrophysiological procedures. *Europace* **2008**, *10*, 513–527. [CrossRef] [PubMed]
36. De Sensi, F.; Cresti, A.; Addonisio, L. Migration of femoral vein thrombus to the right ventricle: An undesiderable complication in patients undergoing electrophysiological procedures. *Europace* **2017**, *19*, 1131. [CrossRef] [PubMed]
37. Nasrin, S.; Aaysha Cader, F.; Salahuddin, M.; Nazrin, T.; Iqbal, J.; Jannat, M.; Shafi, P. Pulmonary embolism as a complication of an electrophysiological study: A case report. *J. Med. Case Rep.* **2016**, *10*, 89. [CrossRef]
38. Alizadeh, A.; Rad, M.A.; Emkanjoo, Z.; Saravi, M.; Sadeghi, G.; Sadr-Ameli, M.A. Free floating right atrial thrombus in two asymptomatic patients after electrophysiological study: Role of routine echocardiography after ablation. *Europace* **2010**, *12*, 587–588. [CrossRef]

19

Physicians' Perceptions of their Patients' Attitude and Knowledge of Long-Term Oral Anticoagulant Therapy in Bulgaria

Nikolay Runev [1], Tatjana Potpara [2], Stefan Naydenov [1,*], Anita Vladimirova [3], Gergana Georgieva [3] and Emil Manov [1]

1 Department of Internal Diseases, Medical University of Sofia, 1431 Sofia, Bulgaria
2 Faculty of Medicine, University of Belgrade, 11000 Belgrade, Serbia
3 Boehringer Ingelheim RCV GmbH & Co KG Bulgarian Branch, 1505 Sofia, Bulgaria
* Correspondence: snaydenov@gmail.com

Abstract: *Background and Objectives*: Oral anticoagulation (OAC) is widely used in daily clinical practice worldwide for various indications. We aimed to explore the perception of Bulgarian clinicians about their patients' attitude and knowledge of long-term OAC, prescribed for atrial fibrillation (AF) and/or known deep venous thrombosis (DVT)/pulmonary embolism (PE). *Materials and Methods*: We performed a cross-sectional study that involved 226 specialists: 187 (82.7%) cardiologists, 23 (10.2%) neurologists, and 16 (7.1%) vascular surgeons. They filled in a questionnaire, specially designed for our study, answering various questions regarding OAC treatment in their daily clinical practice. *Results*: The mean prescription rate of OACs in AF patients was 80.3% and in DVT/PE—88.6%. One hundred and eighty-seven (82.7%) of the participants stated they see their patients on OAC at least once per month. According to more than one-third of the inquired clinicians, the patients did not understand well enough the provided information concerning net clinical benefit of OAC treatment. About 68% of the clinicians declared that their patients would prefer a "mutual" approach, discussing with the physician the OAC options and taking together the final decision, whereas according to 43 (19.0%), the patients preferred the physician to take a decision for them. Patients' OAC treatment had been interrupted at least once within the last year due to a physician's decision by 178 (78.8%) of the participants and the most common reason was elective surgery. The most influential factors for a patient's choice of OAC were the need of a specific diet to be kept, intake frequency, and possible adverse reactions. *Conclusions*: Our results suggest that a clinician's continuous medical education, shared decision-making, and appropriate local strategies for improved awareness of AF/DVT/PE patients are key factors for improvement of OAC management.

Keywords: atrial; fibrillation; venous; thrombosis; anticoagulation; perception

---

1. Introduction

Oral anticoagulation (OAC) is widely used in contemporary clinical practice for preventive and therapeutic indications [1–3]. Until recently, the OAC treatment choice was restricted to the vitamin K antagonists (VKAs) and patients' preferences were less commonly encountered [2–4]. Even after the introduction of new direct oral anticoagulants (DOACs) to clinical use and the large volume of data from clinical trials comparing VKAs' and DOACs' efficacy and safety, the patients' awareness of the treatment choices, benefits, and risks with long-term OAC remains unclear [3–7]. Moreover, their role in the decision-making process is frequently neglected thus affecting the treatment adherence and persistence [5,7].

To date, there are no large-scale, population-based studies or national registries in Bulgaria evaluating the prescription rate of OACs and/or the prevalence of atrial fibrillation (AF), deep venous thrombosis (DVT)/pulmonary embolism (PE)—some of the most common diseases requiring OAC. A single center cross-sectional study, including 1027 patients, hospitalized for different diseases in the largest Bulgarian internal clinic showed that ~62% of all patients suffered at least one episode of AF [8]. Of these patients, ~14% had undergone ischemic stroke and OAC was prescribed to ~86% [8].

These data gave us grounds to perform the present study, aiming to explore the practicing clinicians' perceptions of their patients' attitude and knowledge of long-term OAC.

2. Materials and Methods

A cross-sectional questionnaire-based study involved 226 clinical specialists from 20 cities in Bulgaria. Of these, 187 (82.7%) were cardiologists, 23 (10.2%) neurologists, and 16 (7.1%) vascular surgeons. For the purposes of the study, a structured questionnaire with 12 questions was formulated, as shown in Appendix A.

The study was conducted from 1 July to 30 September 2017. The inclusion criteria were: (1) clinical experience for at least 5 years, and (2) regular prescription of OAC for atrial fibrillation (AF) and/or deep venous thrombosis (DVT)/pulmonary embolism (PE). The regular OAC prescription was defined as at least two prescriptions per week of a VKA or a DOAC. Exclusion criteria: (1) clinicians with other clinical specialties, (2) prescription of anticoagulants for indications other than those in the inclusion criteria, and (3) inability to fill in the study questionnaire for any reason.

As this is a non-trial activity (NTA) for health care providers (no involvement of patients at all in the study), an internal approval only has been done according to Boehringer Ingelheim requirements and standards (NTA tracking no. 170432).

Statistical Analysis

Categorical variables were shown as counts and percentages, and continuous variables as mean values and standard deviation (SD). Where normal distribution was not confirmed using the Shapiro–Wilk test, the median value and interquartile range (IQR) were used for variables with skewed distribution. Categorical variables were compared using the independent samples Chi-square test. Analysis of variance (ANOVA) was used for comparison of parametric data and the Mann–Whitney U test for non-parametric data. A two-sided p-value of <0.05 was considered statistically significant. The statistical analysis was performed by SPSS statistical package, version 19.0 (SPSS Inc., Chicago, IL, USA).

3. Results

The answers of the questions 1 to 7 are provided in Tables 1 and 2. The vast majority of 226 participating physicians (210, 92.9%) reported that they treated patients with AF. The highest average monthly number of patients with AF was seen by cardiologists (46, 60.5%), whereas those with known DVT/PE by vascular surgeons (21, 60.0%). The physicians stated they had assigned an OAC to 80.3% of their AF patients for stroke prevention and to 88.6% of the patients with known DVT/PE for secondary prevention. One hundred and eighty-seven (82.7%) of the participants in our study declared they see their patients on OAC at least once per month, 28 (12.4%)—at least twice and 11 (4.9%)—three or more times per month (without significant difference between the specialties), as shown in Table 1.

According to 168 physicians (74.3%), the patients were satisfied with the provided general information about OAC treatment before its initiation, 42 (18.6%) answered their patients were very satisfied, and 16 (7.1%)—the patients were neither satisfied nor unsatisfied (no statistically significant difference between cardiologists, neurologists, and vascular surgeons). However, only 64.2% of the surveyed physicians answered that their patients understand well enough the discussed information about OAC, as shown in Table 1.

Table 1. Questions 1 to 7 and the clinicians' answers.

Question and Answers	All N (%)	Cardiologists N (%)	Neurologists N (%)	Vascular Surgeons N (%)	p Value
1. What is the average monthly number of patients with the following diagnoses in your practice?					
AF	76 (100%)	46 (60.5%)	16 (21.1%)	14 (18.4%)	$p < 0.001$
Known DVT/PE	35 (100%)	10 (28.6%)	4 (11.4%)	21 (60.0%)	$p < 0.001$
2. What is the approximate proportion of your patients with: AF treated with OAC for stroke prevention (%) or known deep vein thrombosis (DVT) with or without pulmonary embolism (PE) on OAC (%)?					
AF	61 (80.3%)	41 (67.2%)	11 (18.0%)	9 (14.8%)	$p < 0.001$
Known DVT/PE	31 (88.6%)	8 (25.8%)	2 (6.5%)	21 (67.7%)	$p < 0.001$
3. How often do you see your patients on OAC per month?					
At least once	187 (82.7%)	155 (82.9%)	19 (82.6%)	13 (81.3%)	NS
At least twice	28 (12.4%)	23 (12.3%)	3 (13.0%)	2 (12.5%)	NS
3 or more times	11 (4.9%)	9 (4.8%)	1 (4.3%)	1 (6.3%)	NS
4. In your opinion, how satisfied are your patients with the information about the OAC treatment they receive before its initiation?					
Satisfied	168 (74.3%)	139 (74.3%)	17 (73.9%)	12 (75.0%)	NS
Very satisfied	42 (18.6%)	35 (18.7%)	4 (17.4%)	3 (18.75%)	NS
Neither satisfied nor unsatisfied	16 (7.1%)	13 (7.0%)	2 (8.7%)	1 (6.25%)	NS
5. How do you rate your patients' understanding of the provided information about OAC?					
Very good	101 (44.7%)	84 (44.9%)	10 (43.5%)	7 (43.8%)	NS
Good	44 (19.5%)	36 (19.3%)	5 (21.7%)	3 (18.8%)	NS
Inadequate	81 (35.8%)	67 (35.8%)	8 (34.8%)	6 (37.5%)	NS

AF—atrial fibrillation, DVT—deep venous thrombosis, PE—pulmonary embolism, OAC—oral anticoagulation, NS—non-significant; the p value refers to the inter-physicians' answers.

Table 2. Questions 6 and 7, and the clinicians' answers.

6. In your opinion, to what extent would your patients like to be involved in the choice of OAC?					
They prefer to discuss with the physician, then make the decision together.	153 (67.7%)	135 (72.2%)	8 (34.8%)	10 (62.5%)	$p = 0.02$
They prefer to discuss with the physician, then make the decision by themselves.	30 (13.3%)	25 (13.4%)	2 (8.7%)	3 (18.75%)	$p < 0.001$
They prefer the physician to make the decision.	43 (19.0%)	27 (14.4%)	13 (56.5%)	3 (18.75%)	$p < 0.001$
7. Did you have to stop the current OAC in any of your patients within the past 12 months due to a planned surgery and/or emergency?					
Yes, I had to stop OAC	178 (78.8%)	151 (80.7%)	14 (60.9%)	13 (81.3%)	$p < 0.001$
Due to a planned surgery	167 (93.8%)	146 (96.7%)	8 (57.1%)	13 (100%)	$p = 0.02$
Because of an emergency	11 (6.2%)	5 (3.3%)	6 (42.9%)	0	$p < 0.01$

OAC—oral anticoagulation; the p value refers to the inter-physicians' answers.

In terms of the patients' role in the decision-making process concerning OAC, 153 (67.7%) of the participants stated that their patients preferred to discuss with the physician all possible treatment options (advantages and disadvantages) and then make a decision together (equal role of both sides), 43 (19.0%)—the patients preferred the physician to take a decision for them (with or without prior discussion, whereas 30 (13.3%) reported the patients would make their therapeutic choice alone irrespective of the physician's opinion during the discussion, as shown in Table 2.

Patients' OAC therapy had been interrupted at least once within the last 12 months due to a physician's decision by 178 (78.8%). This occurred significantly more often with cardiologists and vascular surgeons and more rarely with neurologists. The most common reasons for interruption of OAC was the elective surgery—reported by 167 (93.8%), followed by an emergency—by 11 (6.2%) physicians, as shown in Table 2.

The physicians' answers of the question "In your opinion, how do your patients rate the importance of treatment outcomes and attributes of OAC?" are shown in Figure 1.

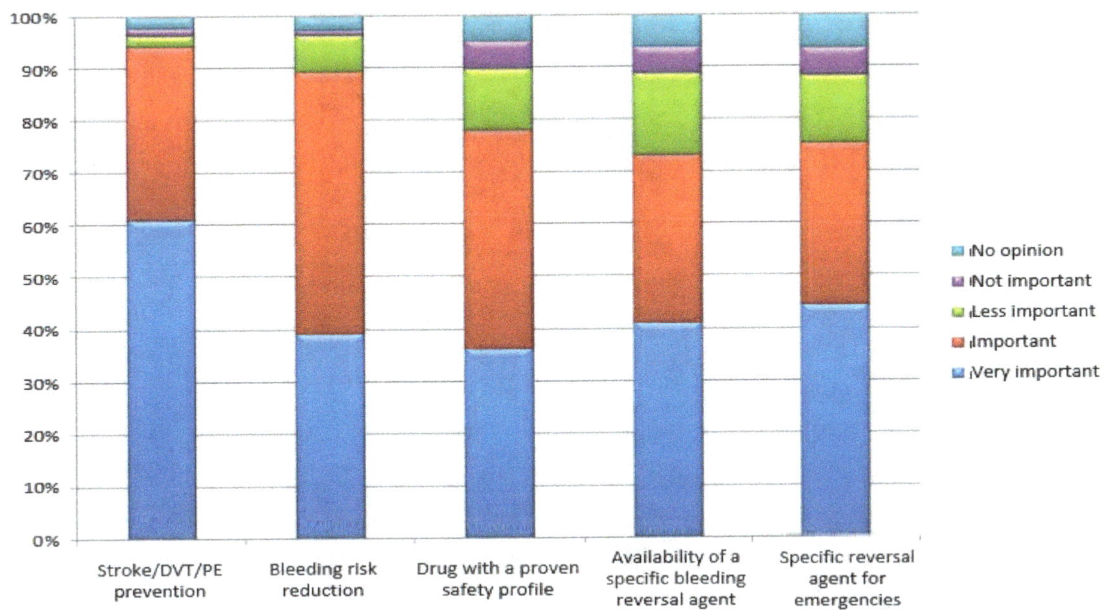

Figure 1. Some basic characteristics of the OAC treatment according to the patients (the information was provided by their physicians); DVT—deep venous thrombosis; PE—pulmonary embolism.

The responders were asked to rank up to three factors (out of a total of six) which their patients would consider the most important in their choice of OAC. The drug's efficacy was most commonly rated as the third important factor, whereas the need a specific diet to be kept, intake frequency, and possible adverse reactions were considered the most influential factors by the majority of the physicians, as shown in Figure 2.

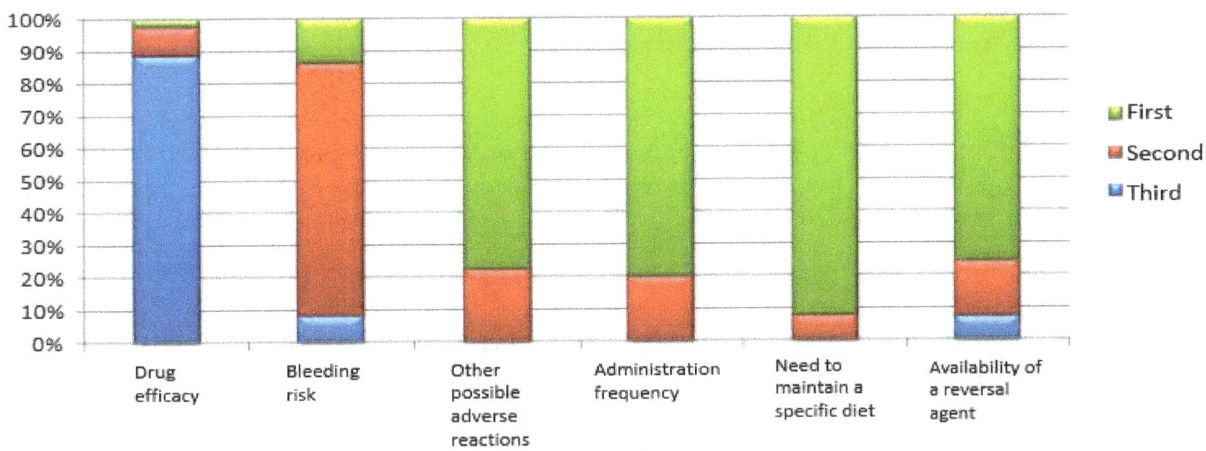

Figure 2. Rankings of factors of the surveyed physicians based on their responses to the question "If you had to discuss with your patients the OAC to be prescribed, which three factors they would consider the most important in your opinion?" (absolute number; relative share).

The physicians were asked to rate five complications by importance and then to report how they evaluate their patients' opinion about those complications. There was a close similarity between physicians' answers and their opinions about what would the patients say when they chose an OAC. The complication the physicians rated the highest was stroke/DVT/PE, followed by bleeding, and then surgical emergencies, as shown in Figure 3a,b.

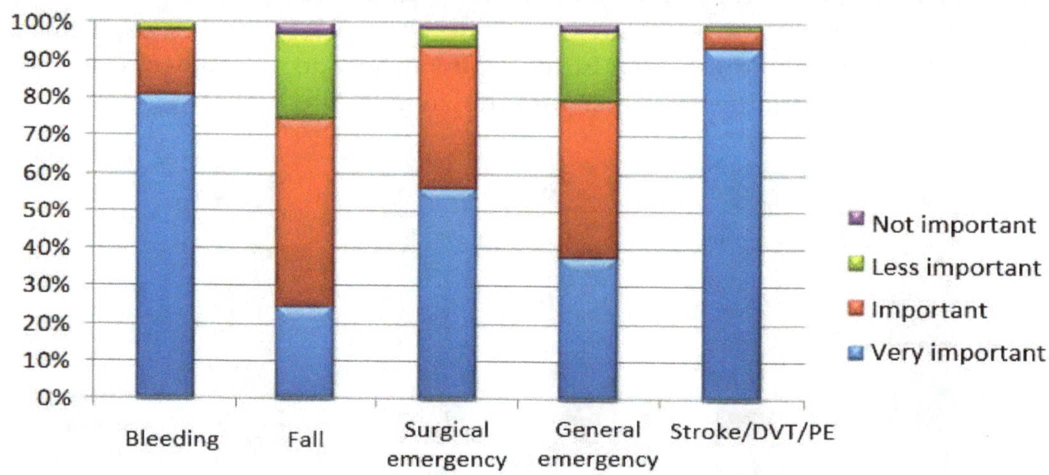

(a)

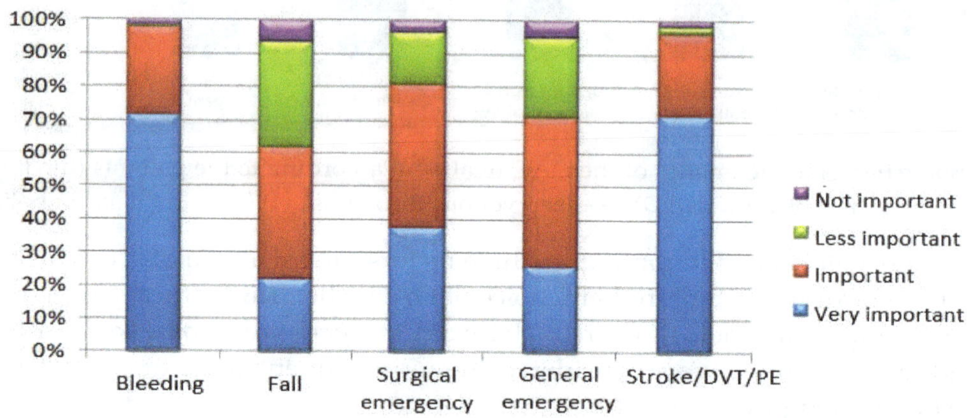

(b)

Figure 3. (**a**) Importance of five basic complications according to the physicians, when choosing an OAC. (**b**) Importance of five basic complications according to the patients, when choosing an OAC (the information was provided by their physicians); DVT—deep venous thrombosis; PE—pulmonary embolism.

Most commonly, the information about the assigned OAC was provided to patients by the prescribing physician (223 physicians, 98.7%), followed by the printed leaflet inserted into the drug package (164, 72.6%), internet and online forums (125, 55.3%), friends/family (80, 35.4%), other patients (79, 35.0%), another physician (68, 30.1%), other materials supplied together with the drugs (47, 20.8%), and nurse/pharmacist (21, 9.3%), as shown in Figure 4.

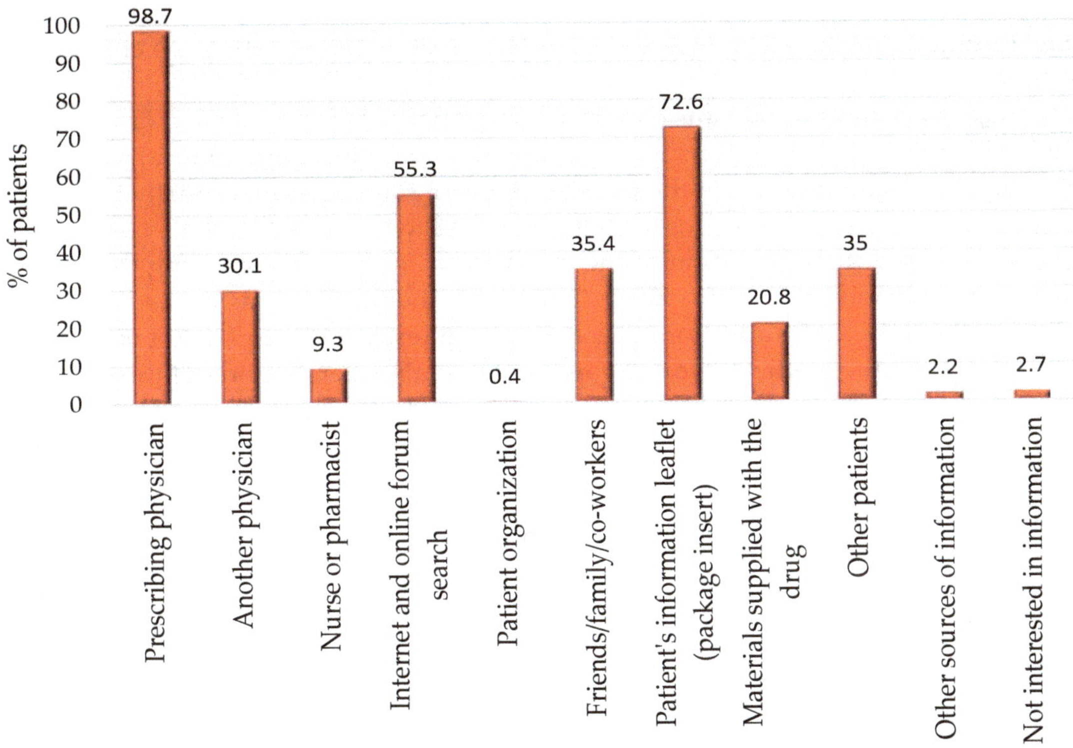

Figure 4. Sources of information from the surveyed physicians based on their responses to the question "What sources, in your opinion, do patients use to get information about the OAC they are taking?".

4. Discussion

This is a cross-sectional questionnaire-based study, conducted among 226 physicians in 20 towns of Bulgaria, the vast majority of which 82.7% were cardiologists, 10.2% were neurologists, and 7.1% were vascular surgeons. They answered specific questions in order to evaluate the attitude, knowledge, and preferences of their patients with AF and/or DVT/PE concerning the long-term OAC treatment.

The prescription rate of oral anticoagulants in our study was relatively high compared the published data of other authors—80.3% of the physicians dealing with AF (mostly cardiologists) stated their patients had been treated with an OAC (VKA or DOAC) for prevention of embolic events [1–4]. Atrial fibrillation was the most common indication for prescription of OAC [7–14]. This could be explained by the high prevalence of this arrhythmia in the general population (25% long-life risk for at least one episode of AF in people aged >40 years) and probably by the significantly improved awareness of the cardiologists and other health specialists for the last two decades about the cardio-embolic risk of AF [11,12,15–17]. In developed countries, 65% to 80% of the patients diagnosed with AF and a $CHADS_2$ or CHA_2DS_2VASc risk score higher than 2, receive long-term oral anticoagulation [2,3,15]. Data from the USA IMS Health's National Disease and Therapeutic Index revealed that OAC prescription rates in AF patients with high thromboembolic risk varied from 20% to 80% [2]. Interestingly, ~15% of all AF patients in these studies did not receive any antithrombotic treatment because of various concomitant conditions (active bleeding, patient refusal, severe comorbid illnesses, pregnancy, etc.) [3,16–19]. In our study, the percentage of non-anticoagulated AF patients was around 20%. In contrast to other studies, we found similar (~67%) prescription rates of OAC (VKA or DOAC) for AF (most often by cardiologists) and DVT/PE (by vascular surgeons). Other authors reported a higher use of oral anticoagulants for DVT and/or PE, than in the case of AF—85–88% versus 60–80%, respectively [1–5]. It should be pointed out, the level of education and patients' knowledge had a direct influence on the OAC management for embolic stroke prevention in AF [9,18–21].

Most of the physicians (~83%) of all specialties enrolled in our study stated they had visits with their patients on OAC therapy at least once per month. According to the guidelines, patients on DOACs should be seen at least once per year and if their kidney function was impaired (creatinine clearance <60 mL/min), the annual frequency of clinical visits could be calculated dividing the creatinine clearance by 10 [1,2].

The vast majority of our participants considered their patients were satisfied or very satisfied with the provided information about OACs. Since no patients were included in our study we could not discuss if the physician's opinion about the patient's level of satisfaction was really true. According to other studies, patients' satisfaction varies widely from 42% to 97% [18,22,23].

The patient's proper understanding of the provided information regarding the OAC treatment could influence the decision-making process, adherence to therapy, and the immediate and long-term prognosis, respectively [1,3]. In addition, there was frequently a discrepancy between the level of patient satisfaction from the medical information and the real understanding of this information [4,5]. According to only 64.2% of the inquired physicians in our study, their patients understood well enough the discussed information. In the study of Nadar et al., conducted in the United Kingdom, between 18% and 45% of all patients (depending on the ethnic group) had difficulties with the proper understanding about any aspect of the antithrombotic treatment [16].

Regarding the decision-making process, about 68% of our participants stated their patients would prefer a "mutual" approach, discussing with the physician the treatment options and taking together the final decision. Only 13% of the physicians answered the patients would prefer to decide themselves irrespective of the physician's opinion. These data were supported by other studies, which confirmed that shared decision-making would improve patients' adherence and persistence to OAC treatment [13,24,25].

An alarming finding of our study was that at least ~79% of all patients had stopped their OAC therapy at least once per year. These results were similar to other published data [2,5]. Our participants reported elective surgery as the most frequent cause for treatment cessation. According to other studies, gastrointestinal procedures and surgery with biopsy were the most frequent reason for temporary OAC discontinuation [1,3]. These findings were important from a clinical point of view—previous studies had shown that major thromboembolic complications, especially ischemic stroke, occurred in approximately 1% of the patients who underwent temporary discontinuation of OAC before an invasive procedure [2,3].

Intriguing answers were given by the participants concerning the most important characteristics of OAC medication according to their patients—the highest role of stroke/DVT/PE prevention, followed by the availability of a reversal agent in case of bleeding or emergencies. Obviously, the presence of a specific inhibitor of the OAC action make the patients more confident and trustworthy during a discussion of their anticoagulation management. This is particularly relevant for Dabigatran use in daily clinical practice [23].

In our study the most important factors for a patient's choice about OAC therapy were the necessity to keep a specific diet, the intake frequency, and the possible adverse reactions. They were reported as "first three factors" exerting influence on the therapeutic decision by the majority of the participants. Surprisingly, the efficacy of the OAC drugs was classified most frequently as the third important factor by many of them. This finding could be related to patients' misperception of OAC risks and benefits, which might be overcome by a well-structured patient education program [13]. However, in our study, the physicians' answers and their opinions about the patients' judgment of the complications, concerning the choice of OAC, were very similar—the highest importance was attributed to stroke/DVT/PE, followed by bleeding and surgical emergencies. Perhaps, the communication gap in this population had not been so large as expected based on the previously published data [20,25].

Nowadays, concerns about the patients' awareness, choices, and preferences are becoming more important for the complex therapeutic approach, including antithrombotic treatment. Patients want to participate actively in the decision-making about the proposed procedures or treatments and to know all their alternatives [4,5]. The environment in which patients consume medical and health information has changed dramatically during the past decades worldwide [9,10]. The rapid diffusion of Internet technologies within the public sphere has placed an unprecedented amount of health information within reach of general consumers [6]. Nevertheless, according to our data, the prescribing physician continues to be a principal trusted resource for information about the OAC in spite of the variety of new sources of health information. Direct communication between physicians and patients is still an influential factor for the patient's awareness and decisions. The second and third most used sources of information in our study—the printed leaflet (provided together with the box of the medication in Bulgaria) and internet/online forums—could exert positive but also negative influence (particularly the last source) on the patient's attitude and therapeutic choice. We have the impression from our own clinical practice that the reading of the printed leaflet of the drugs (short product characteristics) might discourage the patients. Internet sites are not always reliable for the information they provide, and many could mislead the patients to an inappropriate decision. A study conducted in the USA among Hispanic adult patients with different diseases revealed that common health information sources were doctors (71%), television (68%), family and friends (63%), newspapers and magazines (51%), and radio (40%) [25]. In Europe, the Electrophysiology Wire Survey showed that considerable amount of time and resources were used to inform AF patients about their risk profile and appropriate management. However, a diversity of strategies across the European hospitals was reported [13].

Study limitations: (1) Disproportion of cardiologists, neurologists, and vascular surgeons in our study with the much larger number of the first ones. Patients with AF would attend a cardiologist for examinations and treatment (those without a cerebrovascular or peripheral arterial embolic event would not be referred to neurologist or a vascular surgeon). Patients with DVT were likely to visit a vascular surgeon for evaluation and treatment (a much fewer number in our study) and were less likely to be registered/followed up by a cardiologist or a neurologist unless another condition requiring OAC (AF, prosthetic valve disease, post-stroke, etc.) was present. (2) Our study did not include patients of the inquired physicians to answer the same questions, so we could not compare the answers of both sides. (3) The number of participants was not large enough for our results to be extrapolated nationwide.

5. Conclusions

This questionnaire-based study, conducted among Bulgarian cardiologists, neurologists, and vascular surgeons, shows that patients' attitude and knowledge about OAC depends on their direct communication with the doctor rather than on drug leaflets or internet/online sources. Our patients prefer to discuss thoroughly with the physician the therapeutic options and then to take together the final decision. However, more than one-third of the physicians report their patients do not understand well enough the provided information concerning net clinical benefit of OAC. Moreover, the discontinuation of OAC remains an important issue in our population. These data suggest that physicians' continuous medical education, shared decision-making, and appropriate local strategies for better informing AF/DVT/PE patients are the crucial factors for improvement of OAC management.

Author Contributions: Conceptualization: N.R., T.P., and A.V.; Methodology: N.R., T.P., S.N., and G.G.; Software: S.N. and A.V.; Validation: T.P., G.G., and E.M.; Formal Analysis: N.R., S.N., and E.M.; Investigation: A.V., G.G., and E.M.; Resources: S.N., A.V., and G.G.; Data Curation: N.R., T.P., S.N., and E.M.; Writing-Original Draft Preparation: N.R. and S.N.; Writing-Review & Editing: N.R., T.P., S.N., and E.M.; Visualization: A.V., G.G., and E.M.; Supervision: N.R., T.P., and E.M.; Project Administration: A.V. and G.G.

Acknowledgments: Our study was technically supported by Boehringer Ingelheim RCV GmbH & Co KG Bulgarian Branch. We would like to thank also all clinicians from Bulgaria who volunteered to participate in our study by filling the provided questionnaire.

Appendix A. Questions: Included in the Study Questionnaire

1. What is the average monthly number of patients with the following diagnoses in your practice: atrial fibrillation (AF) or known deep vein thrombosis (DVT) with or without pulmonary embolism (PE)?
2. What is the approximate proportion of your patients with: AF treated with OAC for stroke prevention (%) or known DVT with or without PE on OAC (%)?
3. How often do you see your patients on OAC per month?
4. In your opinion, how satisfied are your patients with the information about the OAC treatment they receive before its initiation?
5. How do you rate your patients' understanding of the provided information about OAC?
6. In your opinion, to what extent would your patients like to be involved in the choice of OAC:
    - They prefer the physician to make the decision
    - They prefer to discuss with the physician, then make the decision by themselves
    - They prefer to discuss with the physician, then make the decision together
7. Did you have to stop the current OAC medication in any of your patients within the past 12 months?
8. In your opinion, how do your patients rate the importance of treatment outcomes and attributes of OAC medication?
9. If you had to discuss with your patients the OAC to be prescribed, which three factors from the ones listed below they would consider the most important in your opinion: drug efficacy; risk of bleeding; other possible adverse reactions; administration frequency of the medication; having to follow a specific diet while on medication; availability of a reversal agent?
10. As a specialist how would you rate the importance of the following complications when choosing an OAC medication: bleeding, fall, surgical emergency, general emergency situations, strokes/DVT/PE?
11. How would your patients rate the importance of the following complications: bleeding, fall, surgical emergency, general emergency situations, stroke/DVT/PE?
12. What sources, in your opinion, do patients use to get information about the OAC they are taking (multiple answers allowed)?

References

1. Ryan, F.; Byrne, S.; O'Shea, S. Managing oral anticoagulation therapy: Improving clinical outcomes. *J. Clin. Pharm. Ther.* **2008**, *33*, 581–590. [CrossRef] [PubMed]
2. Kirley, K.; Qato, D.M.; Kornfield, R.; Stafford, R.S.; Alexander, G.C. National trends in oral anticoagulant use in the United States, 2007 to 2011. *Circ. Cardiovasc. Qual. Outcomes* **2012**, *5*, 615–621. [CrossRef] [PubMed]
3. O'Brien, E.C.; Holmes, D.N.; Ansell, J.E.; Allen, L.A.; Hylek, E.; Kowey, P.R.; Mahaffey, K.W. Physician practices regarding contraindications to oral anticoagulation in atrial fibrillation: Findings from the Outcomes Registry for Better Informed Treatment of Atrial Fibrillation (ORBIT-AF) registry. *Am. Heart J.* **2014**, *167*, 601–609. [CrossRef] [PubMed]
4. Gadisseur, A.P.A.; Kaptein, A.A.; Breukink-Engbers, W.G.M.; Van Der Meer, F.J.M.R.; Rosendaal, F. Patient self-management of oral anticoagulant care vs. management by specialized anticoagulation clinics: Positive effects on quality of life. *J. Thromb. Haemost.* **2004**, *2*, 584–591. [CrossRef] [PubMed]
5. Lane, D.A.; Ponsford, J.; Shelley, A.; Sirpal, A.; Lip, G.Y. Patient knowledge and perceptions of atrial fibrillation and anticoagulant therapy: Effects of an educational intervention programme: The West Birmingham Atrial Fibrillation Project. *Int. J. Cardiol.* **2006**, *110*, 354–358. [CrossRef] [PubMed]
6. Ferrando, F.; Mira, Y. Effective and Safe Management of Oral Anticoagulation Therapy in Patients Who Use the Internet-Accessed Telecontrol Tool SintromacWeb. *Interact. J. Med. Res.* **2015**, *4*, 10. [CrossRef]

7. Runev, N.; Dimitrov, S. Management of stroke prevention in Bulgarian patients with non-valvular atrial fibrillation (BUL-AF Survey). *Int. J. Cardiol.* **2015**, *87*, 683–685. [CrossRef]
8. Naydenov, S.; Runev, N.; Manov, E.; Vasileva, D.; Rangelov, Y.; Naydenova, N. Risk factors, co-morbidities and treatment of in-hospital patients with atrial fibrillation in Bulgaria. *Med. Lith.* **2018**, *54*, 34. [CrossRef]
9. Almeida, G.; de Noblat, L.; Passos, L.; do Nascimento, H.F. Quality of Life analysis of patients in chronic use of oral anticoagulant: An observational study. *Health Qual. Life Outcomes* **2011**, *9*, 91. [CrossRef]
10. Criado-Álvarez, J.J.; González, J.G.; García, S.M.; Barrientos, C.R. Quality of life in patients with oral anticoagulation therapy. *Med. Clin.* **2015**, *144*, 46. [CrossRef]
11. Runev, N.; Manov, E. Atrial fibrillation–epidemiology and prognosis. *Bulg. Cardiol.* **2012**, *18*, 5–10.
12. Runev, N.; Manov, E.; Naydenov, S.; Donova, T. Prevalence of the cardiovascular risk factors in Bulgarian female population. *Eur. J. Prev. Cardiol.* **2015**, *22*, 103.
13. Potpara, T.S.; Pison, L.; Larsen, T.B.; Estner, H.; Madrid, A.; Blomström-Lundqvist, C.; Dagres, N. How are patients with atrial fibrillation approached and informed about their risk profile and available the rapies in Europe? Results of the European Heart Rhythm Association Survey. *Europace* **2015**, *17*, 468–472. [CrossRef] [PubMed]
14. Pancheva, R.; Runev, N.; Manov, E.A. gradient of frequency of rehospitalization of heart failure patients between different types atrial fibrillation and correlation with left atrial diameter. *Eur. J. Heart Fail.* **2018**, *20*, 243.
15. Pancheva, R.; Runev, N.; Manov, E. Predictors of mid-term rehospitalization and mortality rates in Bulgarian patients with heart failure and preserved ejection fraction: A single-center study. *Eur. J. Heart Fail.* **2018**, *20*, 573.
16. Nadar, S.; Begum, N.; Kaur, B.; Sandhu, S.; Lip, G. Patients' understanding of anticoagulant therapy in a multiethnic population. *J. R. Soc. Med.* **2003**, *96*, 175–179. [PubMed]
17. Vasileva, D.; Shabani, R.; Runev, N. Clinical and echocardiographic follow-up of patients with non-valvular atrial fibrillation, treated with Dabigatran–6-months results. *Bulg. Cardiol.* **2017**, *23*, 48–54.
18. Van Geffen, E.C.; Philbert, D.; van Boheemen, C.; van Dijk, L.; Bos, M.B., Bouvy, M.L. Patients' satisfaction with information and experiences with counseling on cardiovascular medication received at the pharmacy. *Patient Educ. Couns.* **2011**, *83*, 303–309. [CrossRef]
19. Hernández Madrid, A.; Potpara, T.S.; Dagres, N.; Chen, J.; Larsen, T.B.; Estner, H.; Cheggour, S. Differences in attitude, education, and knowledge about oral anticoagulation therapy among patients with atrial fibrillation in Europe: Result ofa self-assessment patient survey conducted by the European Heart Rhythm Association. *Europace* **2016**, *18*, 463–467. [CrossRef]
20. Frankel, D.S.; Parker, S.E.; Rosenfeld, L.E.; Gorelick, P.B. HRS/NSA 2014surveyofatrial fibrillation andstroke: Gapsin knowledge and perspective, opportunities for improvement. *Heart Rhythm* **2015**, *12*, 105–113. [CrossRef]
21. Pleis, J.R.; Lethbridge-Cejku, M. Summary Health Statistics for U.S. Adults: National Health Interview Survey. *Natl. Cent. Health Stat. Vital Health Stat. Ser.* **2007**, *10*, 235.
22. Klemes, A.; Solomon, H. The impact of a personalized preventive care model vs. the conventional healthcare model on patient satisfaction. *Open Public Health J.* **2015**, *8*, 1–9. [CrossRef]
23. Pollack, C.V., Jr. Evidence supporting idarucizumab for the reversal of dabigatran. *Am. J. Emerg. Med.* **2016**, *34*, 33–38. [CrossRef] [PubMed]
24. Lane, D.A.; Lip, G. Patient's values and preferences for stroke prevention in atriafibrillation: Balancing stroke and bleeding risk with oral anticoagulation. *Thromb. Haemost.* **2014**, *111*, 381–383.
25. Sanoski, C.A.L. Clinical, economic, and quality of life impact of atrial fibrillation. *J. Manag. Care Pharm.* **2009**, *15*, 4–9. [CrossRef]

20

Subclinical Atrial Fibrillation and Risk of Stroke: Past, Present and Future

Ahmed AlTurki [1,*], Mariam Marafi [2], Vincenzo Russo [3], Riccardo Proietti [4] and Vidal Essebag [1,5]

1 Division of Cardiology, McGill University Health Center, Montreal, QC H3G1A4, Canada; vidal.essebag@mcgill.ca
2 Department of Neurology and Neurosurgery, Montreal Neurological Institute, Montreal, QC H3A2B4, Canada; mariamarafie@gmail.com
3 Depatment of Medical Translational Sciences, University of Campania "Luigi Vanvitelli"—Monaldi Hospital, 80131 Naples, Italy; v.p.russo@libero.it
4 Department of Cardiac, Thoracic, and Vascular Sciences, University of Padua, 35121 Padua, Italy; riccardoproietti6@gmail.com
5 Hôspital Sacré-Coeur de Montréal, Montreal, QC H4J1C5, Canada
* Correspondence: ahmedalturkimd@gmail.com

Abstract: Subclinical atrial fibrillation (SCAF) describes asymptomatic episodes of atrial fibrillation (AF) that are detected by cardiac implantable electronic devices (CIED). The increased utilization of CIEDs renders our understanding of SCAF important to clinical practice. Furthermore, 20% of AF present initially as a stroke event and prolonged cardiac monitoring of stroke patients is likely to uncover a significant prevalence of SCAF. New evidence has shown that implanting cardiac monitors into patients with no history of atrial fibrillation but with risk factors for stroke will yield an incidence of SCAF approaching 30–40% at around three years. Atrial high rate episodes lasting longer than five minutes are likely to represent SCAF. SCAF has been associated with an increased risk of stroke that is particularly significant when episodes of SCAF are greater than 23 h in duration. Longer episodes of SCAF are incrementally more likely to progress to episodes of SCAF >23 h as time progresses. While only around 30–40% of SCAF events are temporally related to stroke events, the presence of SCAF likely represents an important risk marker for stroke. Ongoing trials of anticoagulation in patients with SCAF durations less than 24 h will inform clinical practice and are highly anticipated. Further studies are needed to clarify the association between SCAF and clinical outcomes as well as the factors that modify this association.

Keywords: subclinical atrial fibrillation; atrial high rate episodes; stroke

---

1. Background

Subclinical atrial fibrillation (SCAF) is a term used to describe atrial fibrillation (AF) detected by cardiac devices in an asymptomatic patient [1]. These episodes are presumed to be of relatively short duration. A more accurate term is atrial high rate episodes (AHRE) given the difficulty in establishing that these episodes are indeed SCAF. AF is the one of the common arrhythmias encountered in clinical practice and is a major cause of preventable thromboembolic disease, namely stroke [2]. Early treatment of AF is considered essential to prevent stroke [3]; in up to 20% of AF cases, stroke may be the initial manifestation [4]. Whether SCAF is associated with stroke has been the subject of several studies [1] (references 16–19 should also be cited here).

Cardiac implantable electronic devices (CIED), namely pacemakers, implantable cardioverter defibrillators and implantable monitors are increasingly implanted worldwide. In 2009, 1.3 million CIEDs were implanted with over 400,000 CIEDs implanted in North America alone [5]. Specifically, there has been a significant increase in the implantation of pacemakers for sinus node dysfunction, which is associated with AF, as well as a significant absolute and relative increase in the use of dual-chambered pacemakers that provide an atrial lead which allows monitoring [6]. With an increased prevalence of CIEDs has come an increase in device detected AHRE (SCAF). This presents a conundrum to clinicians with regards to discussing the risk of clinical outcomes, namely stroke, with patients and whether these patients should be receiving oral anticoagulation. Does the duration of these episodes or burden of SCAF increase the risk of stroke? SCAF duration generally refers to the duration of a single episode of SCAF while SCAF burden refers to the daily burden of SCAF average over a certain period of time; the terms are sometimes used interchangeably.

Understanding the significance of SCAF is important with implications for clinical practice. This review assesses the risk of stroke associated with SCAF, the mechanisms underlying the association between SCAF and stroke as well as the effect of SCAF burden on stroke risk; finally ongoing trials that will inform clinical practice will be reviewed.

2. Importance of SCAF

Our initial understanding of the importance of SCAF stems from studies of patients who developed stroke. A significant proportion of strokes appeared to be of embolic origin with no clear cause after guideline-directed investigation for embolic causes [7]. This usually includes cardiac monitors for 24–48 h after the admission to screen for AF [8]. Despite extensive investigations, often no cause is found, and these patients are described to have an embolic stroke of undetermined source (ESUS) or cryptogenic stroke [7,9,10]. The Cryptogenic Stroke and Underlying Atrial Fibrillation (CRYSTAL AF) and the 30-Day Cardiac Event Monitor Belt for Recording Atrial Fibrillation after a Cerebral Ischemic Event (EMBRACE) trials have shown that with prolonged monitoring, including those via implantable cardiac devices, a significant proportion of patients with cryptogenic strokes have underlying asymptomatic AF episodes [11,12]. The importance of the detection of AF lies in its impact on subsequent management of stroke secondary prevention: Standard anti-platelet therapy if not related to AF and anticoagulation if due to AF [13]. Evidence from the EMBRACE and the CRYSTAL-AF emphasize the importance of undetected AF in terms of stroke risk [11,12]. While the majority (60%) of strokes are due to documented cerebrovascular disease, 15% are due to documented AF and 25% are due to ESUS [14]. Understanding the relationship between SCAF and stroke is thus imperative.

In the EMBRACE trial, patients were enrolled if they were 55 years or older, had experienced an ESUS event in the preceding six months which was confirmed by a stroke neurologist, and did not have AF and or another cause of stroke after extensive testing [12]. Patients were randomized in this open-label trial to undergo ambulatory electrocardiogram monitoring with a 30-day event-triggered loop recorder or one additional round of 24-h Holter monitoring [12]. Results of this trial showed AF lasting 30 s or longer was detected in 16.1% with the a 30-day event-triggered loop recorder compared to 3.2% in the control group (absolute difference, 12.9 percentage points; 95% confidence interval (CI), 8.0 to 17.6; $p < 0.001$; number needed to screen, eight) [12]. In the CRYSTAL-AF trial, investigators similarly enrolled patients who were 40 years and older who had experienced an ESUS event in the preceding three months that was supported by both symptoms and brain imaging and did not have a cause of ESUS after extensive testing [11]. Patients were randomized to receive either an implantable loop recorder (REVEAL XT) or conventional follow-up. At 12 months of follow-up, AF had been detected in 12.4% who received an implantable monitor compared to 2.0% of patients who received conventional therapy (hazard ratio (HR) 7.3; 95% CI, 2.6 to 20.8; $p < 0.001$) [11].

Two trials, New Approach Rivaroxaban Inhibition of Factor Xa in a Global Trial versus ASA to Prevent Embolism in Embolic Stroke of Undetermined Source (NAVIGATE-ESUS) and Randomized, Double-Blind, Evaluation in Secondary Stroke Prevention Comparing the Efficacy and Safety of the Oral Thrombin Inhibitor Dabigatran Etexilate versus Acetylsalicylic Acid in Patients with Embolic Stroke of Undetermined Source (RESPECT-ESUS), have evaluated a strategy of empiric anticoagulation for all patients with cryptogenic stroke [9,10]. These trials failed to demonstrate the superiority of oral anticoagulation over aspirin in the reduction of recurrent strokes in patients with ESUS [9,10]. This further highlights the importance of the detection of SCAF as well as understanding which patients with SCAF should receive treatment.

3. Stroke Risk

Several studies have assessed patients who had an implantable device for any indication and followed them for the development of AHRE [14–19]. These studies are summarized in Table 1. An implanted atrial lead allows for continuous detection and characterization of AHRE over a prolonged period of time [1]. Pollak and colleagues showed that a cut-off of five minutes for AHRE significantly reduces the risk that oversensing episodes are classified as SCAF [20].

Table 1. The incidence of subclinical atrial fibrillation (SCAF) and associated stroke in patients with cardiac implantable electronic devices (CIEDs).

Study (First Author, Year)	Study Population	Design	Mode of SCAF Detection	SCAF Criteria + Burden	Clinical Outcome	Annual Stroke and Systemic Embolism Event Rate (%)	Comparative Outcomes (HR, 95% CI)	F/u	Incidence of SCAF (%)
ASSERT (Healey et al., 2013) [1]	2580 patients Inclusion criteria: 1. ≥65 years 2. HTN requiring medical therapy 3. Initial implantation of a St. Jude Medical dual-chamber pacemaker (for sinus-node or atrioventricular-node disease) or defibrillator (for any indication) in the preceding 8 weeks. Exclusions: History of atrial fibrillation or flutter or an indication for oral anticoagulation	Prospective cohort study	Dual chamber pacemaker or defibrillator	>190 bpm + ≥6 min	Stroke or systemic embolism	SCAF = 1.69 No SCAF = 0.69	5.56, 1.28–4.85	2.5 years	10.1
ASSERT II (Healey et al., 2017) [21]	256 patients Inclusion criteria: 1. ≥65 years AND 2. CHA2DS2-VASc score > 2, OR 3. obstructive sleep apnea, OR 4. BMI > 30, AND 5. Left atrial enlargement 6. OR 7. elevated serum N-terminal pro–brain-type natriuretic peptide level ≥ 290 pg/mL	Prospective cohort study	CCNFIRM AF subcutaneous cardiac monitor	+ ≥6 min	NA	6 events occurred (4 stroke, 1 TIA and 1 systemic embolism) but none in patients who had SCAF detected	NA	16 months	34.4

Table 1. *Cont.*

Study (First Author, Year)	Study Population	Design	Mode of SCAF Detection	SCAF Criteria + Burden	Clinical Outcome	Annual Stroke and Systemic Embolism Event Rate (%)	Comparative Outcomes (HR, 95% CI)	F/u	Incidence of SCAF (%)
AT 500 registry (Capucci et al., 2005) [18]	225 patients Inclusion criteria: 1. Bradycardia 2. Guideline indication for dual-chamber pacing 3. History of documented symptomatic atrial tachyarrhythmias	Prospective cohort study	Dual chamber pacemaker	NA + 24 h	Stroke or systemic embolism	NA	3.10, 1.10–10.50	22 months	NA
MOST (Glotzer et al., 2003) [16]	312 patients Inclusion criteria: 1. ≥21 years 2. Dual-chamber pacemaker for sinus node dysfunction 3. In sinus rhythm at onset of study	Prospective cohort study	Dual chamber pacemaker	>220 bpm + ≥5 min	Stroke and all-cause mortality	SCAF = 1.82 No SCAF = 0.48	2.79, 1.51–5.15	33 months	51.3
HOME CARE and EVEREST (Shanmugam et al., 2011) [19]	560 patients All patients had heart failure and a biventricular pacemaker capable of continuous heart rhythm monitoring though home monitoring. Patients in sinus rhythm (including patients with a prior history of AF) with >70% home monitored transmissions during follow up (minimum >3 months follow-up)	Prospective cohort study	Biventricular pacemaker or defibrillator	>180 bpm + ≥3.8 h	Stroke or systemic embolism	NA	9.40, 1.80–47.00	12 months	40

Table 1. *Cont.*

Study (First Author, Year)	Study Population	Design	Mode of SCAF Detection	SCAF Criteria + Burden	Clinical Outcome	Annual Stroke and Systemic Embolism Event Rate (%)	Comparative Outcomes (HR, 95% CI)	F/u	Incidence of SCAF (%)
SOS-AF (Boriani et al., 2014) [17]	10,016 patients Inclusion: CIED able to monitor for atrial high rate episodes At least 3 months of follow-up Device diagnostic data available Did not have permanent AF	Prospective cohort study	CIED	>175 bpm + ≥5 min	Stroke	SCAF = 0.49 No SCAF = 0.31	1.76, 1.02–3.02	24 months	43
TRENDS (Glotzer et al., 2009) [15]	2486 patients Inclusion criteria: 1. Guideline indication for an implantable cardiac rhythm device capable of long-term monitoring 2. At least 1 risk factor for stroke Exclusion criteria: 1. Replacement devices 2. : Long-standing persistent AF 3. Known re-entrant supraventricular tachycardias, 4. Terminal illness limiting survival 5. Unable or unwilling to consent 6. Enrolled in a conflicting drug or device study.	Prospective cohort study	CIED	>175 bpm + ≥5.6 h	Stroke or systemic embolism	SCAF = 2.4 No SCAF = 1.1	2.20, 0.96–5.05	1.4 years	55.9

SCAF = Subclinical atrial fibrillation; HR = hazard ratio; CI = confidence interval; FU = follow up; CIED = cardiac implantable electronic device; TIA = transient ischemic attack; NA = not available; HTN = hypertension; BMI= body mass index; CHA2DS2-VASc = congestive heart failure, hypertension age, diabetes mellitus, stroke, vascular disease, age and sex.

In an ancillary study of the Mode Selection Trial (MOST) trial which randomized 2010 patients with sinus node dysfunction to dual chamber versus single chamber pacing, Glotzer et al. enrolled 312 patients and followed them for 27 months (median) with the atrial detection rate programmed to 220 beats per minute for at least 10 beats [16]. Analysis was limited to episodes of at least five minutes in keeping with the data by Pollack et al. [20]. Of the patients enrolled, 51% experienced at least one episode of AHRE (≥five minutes). In 160 patients with an AHRE, the primary endpoint of death or nonfatal stroke occurred in 33 patients (20.6%) compared to 10.5% in those without AHRE. AHRE was an independent predictor of death or stroke [16]. The Asymptomatic Atrial Fibrillation and Stroke Evaluation in Pacemaker Patients and the Atrial Fibrillation Reduction Atrial Pacing Trial (ASSERT) trial enrolled 2580 patients who were ≥65 years old, had hypertension but no history of AF who had received a CIED (from St Jude Medical) for sinus node or atrioventricular node dysfunction in the eight weeks prior to enrollment [1]. Patients were excluded if they had any history of AF or atrial flutter or if they required oral anticoagulation for any indication. These patients were then monitored for three months to assign patients into two groups, those with AHRE (defined as an atrial rate of 190 beats or more lasting more than six minutes) and those without AHRE. The patients were subsequently followed every six months for a mean of 30 months for the primary outcome which consisted of systemic embolism or stroke [1]. At the three-month monitoring period, SCAF had occurred in 10.1% of patients. SCAF was associated with a five-fold increased risk of clinical AF (HR 5.56; 95% CI 3.78 to 8.17; $p < 0.001$) and a 2.5-fold increased risk of stroke or systemic embolism (HR 2.49; 95% CI, 1.28 to 4.85; $p = 0.007$). After adjustment for stroke predictors, SCAF remained predictive of the stroke or systemic embolism [1]. Though the stroke risk is not as high as that seen with clinical AF, which is four to five times the general population, it is still significant at two to two-and-a-half times the general population [22]. The major limitation of the ASSERT trial is that SCAF was defined using a limited sampling period of three months post device implantation. SCAF, in that time-period may have been transient due to lead implantation (Mittal et al. 2008). These trials also do not differentiate the type of strokes due to limitations with data. The data from MOST and ASSERT clearly demonstrate that patients with SCAF have an associated risk of stroke but a risk lower than clinical AF. Further studies and analyses are required to better improve our understanding of SCAF

An important observation of the above-mentioned studies is that SCAF was detected in patients with implantable pacemaker and defibrillators who were therefore at higher risk of developing AF. Whether this risk translates into increased risk in the general population were they to be monitored remained controversial. Several studies have attempted to address this issue by having cardiac monitors implanted for the purpose of monitoring for SCAF. These studies are also included in Table 1. In an international prospective, single-arm, multicenter study (REVEAL-AF), conducted from November 2012 to January 2017, 386 patients with at least three risk factors for stroke were enrolled after initial screening [23]. Participants received an implanted cardiac monitor for a mean of 22.5 months (Reveal XT or Reveal LINQ; Medtronic). The primary end point was adjudicated AF lasting six or more minutes and was assessed at 18 months. In addition, the median time from device insertion to SCAF detection was also assessed as was the subsequent prescription rate for anticoagulation. The incidence rate of significant SCAF ≥ six minutes progressively increased with longer monitoring: 6% at 30 days, 20% at six months, 27% at one year, 34% at two years and finally 40% at 30 months. The median time from insertion to detection of SCAF was three months and 72 patients (56% of those who developed SCAF at the 18-month primary end-point of the trial) received oral anticoagulation [23]. Similarly, ASSERT-II was a prospective single-arm multi-center study that enrolled 256 patients from cardiology and neurology clinics who had no history of AF and at least two risk factors for stroke [21]. In addition, patients were required to have an element of cardiomyopathy manifest as either an enlarged left atrium or elevated brain natriuretic peptides. Significant SCAF was defined as episodes lasting longer than five minutes and follow-up was for 17 months. The incidence of SCAF was 34% which was predicted by age, hypertension and an enlarged left atrium [21]. The major knowledge gap in this area is patient selection given the lack of clinical outcomes and cost-effectiveness analyses.

4. SCAF Burden

Whilst SCAF was clearly associated with an increased risk of stroke, uncertainty remained as to whether longer episodes were more likely to be associated with stroke. In a scientific statement, the American Heart Association acknowledges the large knowledge gaps pertaining to AF burden. In particular, the statement notes the burden at which clinical outcomes increase remains unknown [24]. TRENDS (A Prospective Study of the Clinical Significance of Atrial Arrhythmias Detected by Implanted Device Diagnostics) was a prospective observational study in patients with a CIED and at least one risk factor for stroke [15]. Patients were excluded if they had long-standing persistent AF, re-entrant supraventricular arrhythmias or a terminal illness. Interestingly, patients with paroxysmal AF were included in this study. Follow-up visits occurred every three months, but the study was terminated early due to a low event rate. AHRE detection settings were set at an atrial rate of greater than 175 beats per minute lasting greater than 20 s. The authors concede that these settings would not help differentiate AF from other atrial tachyarrhythmias [15]. In addition, with such a short detection duration, the device was liable to record over-sensed events as AHRE. Patients were classified into three groups based on the longest duration of AHRE during 30-day window subsets: Zero burden, low burden (≤5.5 h) and high burden (>5.5 h). During a mean follow-up of 1.4 years, the annualized thromboembolic (stroke and transient ischemic (TIA)) risk was 1.1% in the zero-burden group, 1.1% in the low burden group, and 2.4% in the high burden group. In comparison to those with zero-burden, the adjusted HR in the low and high burden subsets were 0.98 (95% CI 0.34 to 2.82, $p = 0.97$) and 2.20 (95% CI 0.96 to 5.05, $p = 0.06$), respectively [15]. The inclusion of patients with history of paroxysmal AF was a major limitation of this study. In a systematic review and meta-analysis, Mahajan et al. pooled data from seven studies. The duration cut-off for AHRE varied among the included studies. In patients with subclinical AF exceeding the defined cut-off SCAF duration of the study, the annual stroke rate was 1.89/100 person-year with a 2.4-fold (95% CI 1.8–3.3, $p < 0.001$) increased risk of stroke compared to patients with subclinical AF who did not reach the cut-off duration; the absolute risk was 0.93/100 person-years [25].

Attempts were made to assess whether increased AF burden was associated with an increased risk of stroke. Proietti and colleagues performed a systematic review and meta-analysis to assess whether SCAF burden is associated with stroke risk [26]. This analysis was limited by a small number of studies that reported such data and the varying cut-off points used in the studies. The authors concluded that a direct correlation between burden of asymptomatic AF and HR for stroke cannot be confirmed [26]. Van Gelder and colleagues performed an important analysis of the ASSERT study which showed that SCAF for a duration >24 h is associated with an increased risk of ischemic stroke or systemic embolism [27]. Patients were divided into groups depending on the duration of the single longest duration of SCAF: 19% > six minutes to 6 h, 7% > six hours to 24 h and 10.7% > 24 h; patients with SCAF for <6 min were excluded from this analysis; patients were followed for 2.5 years. In patients in whom the longest episode of SCAF exceeded 24 h, there was an associated significant increased risk of stroke (adjusted HR 3.24, 95% CI 1.51–6.95, $p = 0.003$). In patients with SCAF between six minutes and 24 h, the risk of stroke was not significantly different from patients without SCAF [27]. Patients who had SCAF for ≥24 h had an annual stroke risk of approximately 5% which is similar to the risk observed in patients with clinical AF. The significant increase in stroke risk with episodes > 24 h was also noted in the AT500 registry [18]. These studies have informed the current practice of prescribing oral anticoagulation in patients with SCAF episodes > 24 h but questions remained regarding patients with long episodes of SCAF not reaching 24 h and those who experience progression to longer SCAF episodes. Going forward, another metric, such as AF density may become clinically relevant. AF density incorporates the temporal dispersion of AF burden (Charitos et al.); further studies are needed to compare the effects of AF burden and AF density.

5. Progression

Whether progression to longer episodes of SCAF is associated with an increased risk of stroke is unclear. Initial data came from anticoagulation studies that compared the risk of stroke in patients with paroxysmal compared to more persistent forms of AF. In the Apixaban for Reduction in Stroke and Other Thromboembolic Events in Atrial Fibrillation (ARISTOTLE) trial, in which patients with AF were randomized to apixaban versus warfarin, the incidence of stroke or systemic embolism was significantly higher in patients with persistent or permanent AF compared to patients with paroxysmal AF (1.52 vs. 0.98%; $p = 0.003$, adjusted $p = 0.015$) [28]. In the Rivaroxaban Once Daily Oral Direct Factor Xa Inhibition Compared with Vitamin K Antagonism for Prevention of Stroke and Embolism Trial in Atrial Fibrillation (ROCKET-AF) trial, patients with AF were randomized to receive either rivaroxaban or warfarin.

There was a significantly higher risk or stroke (2.18 vs. 1.73 events per 100-patient-years, $p = 0.048$) and death (4.78 vs. 3.52 events per 100-patient years, $p = 0.006$) in patients with persistent AF compared to paroxysmal AF [29]. Data from clinical AF suggests that progression to a greater AF burden increases stroke risk. De Vos showed that approximately 15% of patients with paroxysmal AF progress to persistent AF at one year of follow-up [30]; this progression is predictable using clinical risk scores such as the Hypertension, Age, Transient ischaemic attack or stroke, Chronic obstructive pulmonary disease, and Heart failure (HATCH) score [30,31] and may be preventable with catheter ablation [32]. Patients who progress are more likely to become symptomatic or experience a stroke or TIA [30].

Similar findings were found in patients with SCAF. Boriani et al. pooled patient level data from three prospective studies: TRENDS, Stroke preventiOn Strategies based on Atrial Fibrillation information from implanted devices (SOS) and Phase IV Long Term Observational Study of Patients Implanted With Medtronic CRDM Implantable Cardiac Devices (PANORAMA) [33]. Among the study population of 6580 patients, de novo AF with a SCAF burden of ≥5 min, was detected in 2244 patients (34%) during a follow-up period of 2.4 ± 1.7 years. Among these patients, 1091 (49.8%) transitioned to a higher SCAF-burden threshold during follow-up. Approximately 24% of patients transitioned from a lower threshold to a daily SCAF burden of ≥23 h during follow-up. Factors associated with transition to a greater SCAF burden on multivariate analysis included male gender and a CHADS2 (Congestive heart failure, Hypertension, Age>75, Diabetes mellitus and Stroke or transient ischemic attack) score of two or greater (33)]. Figure 1 shows the risk associated with a SCAF burden ≥ 23 h in various studies compared to no SCAF. Wong et al. also performed a sub study of ASSERT to assess the impact of SCAF burden progression. Patients in whom the longest SCAF episode was >6 min but <24 h during the first year (415 patients) were included [34]. The authors assessed the association between progression to SCAF >24 h or the development of clinical AF and heart failure hospitalizations. During a mean follow-up of two years, 15.7% of patients progressed. The rate of heart failure hospitalization among patients with SCAF progression was 8.9% per year compared with 2.5% per year for those without progression. After multivariable adjustment, SCAF progression was independently associated with HF hospitalization (HR 4.58; 95%; CI: 1.64 to 12.80; $p = 0.004$). These results remained significant even if patients with a history of heart failure were excluded or when the analysis was limited to only progression to SCAF >24 h and not clinical AF [34]. Therefore, it seems that a significant SCAF burden of greater >24 h is associated not only with an increased risk of stroke but also an increased risk of heart failure hospitalizations [22]. This is consistent with the relationship seen between clinical AF and heart failure in which a vicious cycle can develop [35].

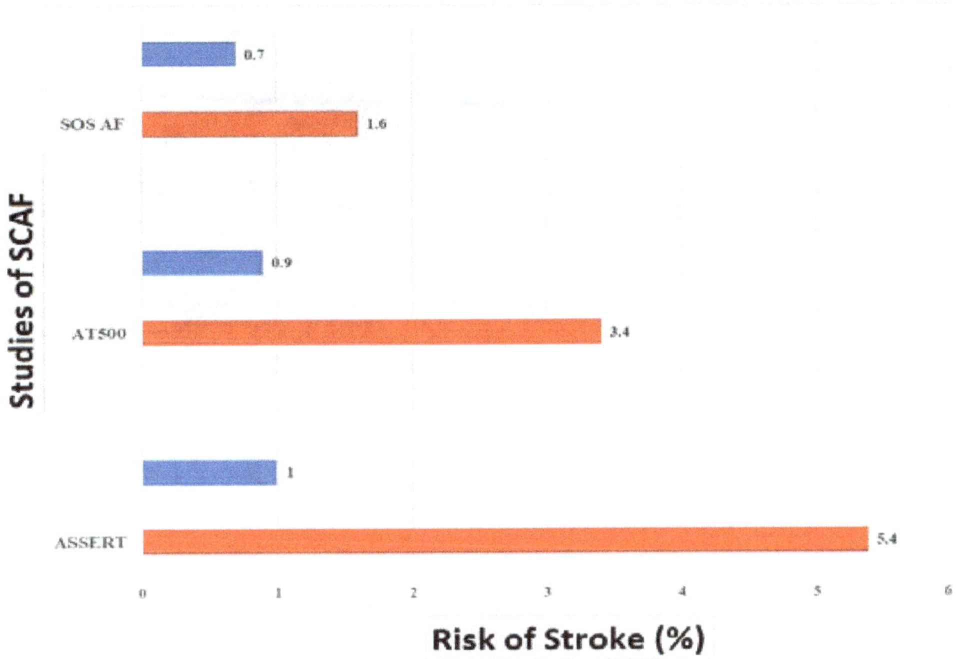

Figure 1. The risk of stroke associated with a SCAF burden ≥23 h in different studies compared to no SCAF. Risk of stroke in patients with SCAF ≥23 h (red) compared to no SCAF (blue). SCAF = subclinical atrial fibrillation.

6. Mechanism of Increased Stroke in SCAF

A direct and causal relationship between SCAF and stroke is not entirely clear. In its scientific statement the American Heart Association recognizes the presence of an important knowledge gap with regard to whether a temporal relationship exists between AF burden and stroke risk [24]. The association between AF and stroke is complex. There is a strong causal association between AF and embolic stroke but also an association with ischemic stroke [36]. In addition to causing atrial thromboembolism through stasis and clot formation, other factors such endothelial dysfunction, left atrial fibrosis myocyte dysfunction, chamber dilatation and left atrial appendage mechanical dysfunction may also have a role in stroke risk [37].

Brambatti and colleagues performed a sub-analysis of the ASSERT trial to assess the temporal association between SCAF and stroke and systemic embolism; the analysis included SCAF >6 min [38]. Of all the patients who experienced a stroke or systemic embolism, 51% had SCAF in keeping with previous data that shows that 50–60% of strokes are due to atherosclerosis and not thromboembolism. However, of the patients experiencing SCAF, only 16% had SCAF in the 30 days preceding the stroke or systemic embolism event [38]. A sub-analysis of the TRENDS study had similar findings; only 11 (27.5%) of the 40 patients developing clinical thromboembolism exhibited SCAF within 30 days before the event [39]. Figure 2 depicts the temporal relationship between SCAF and stroke in three studies [40].

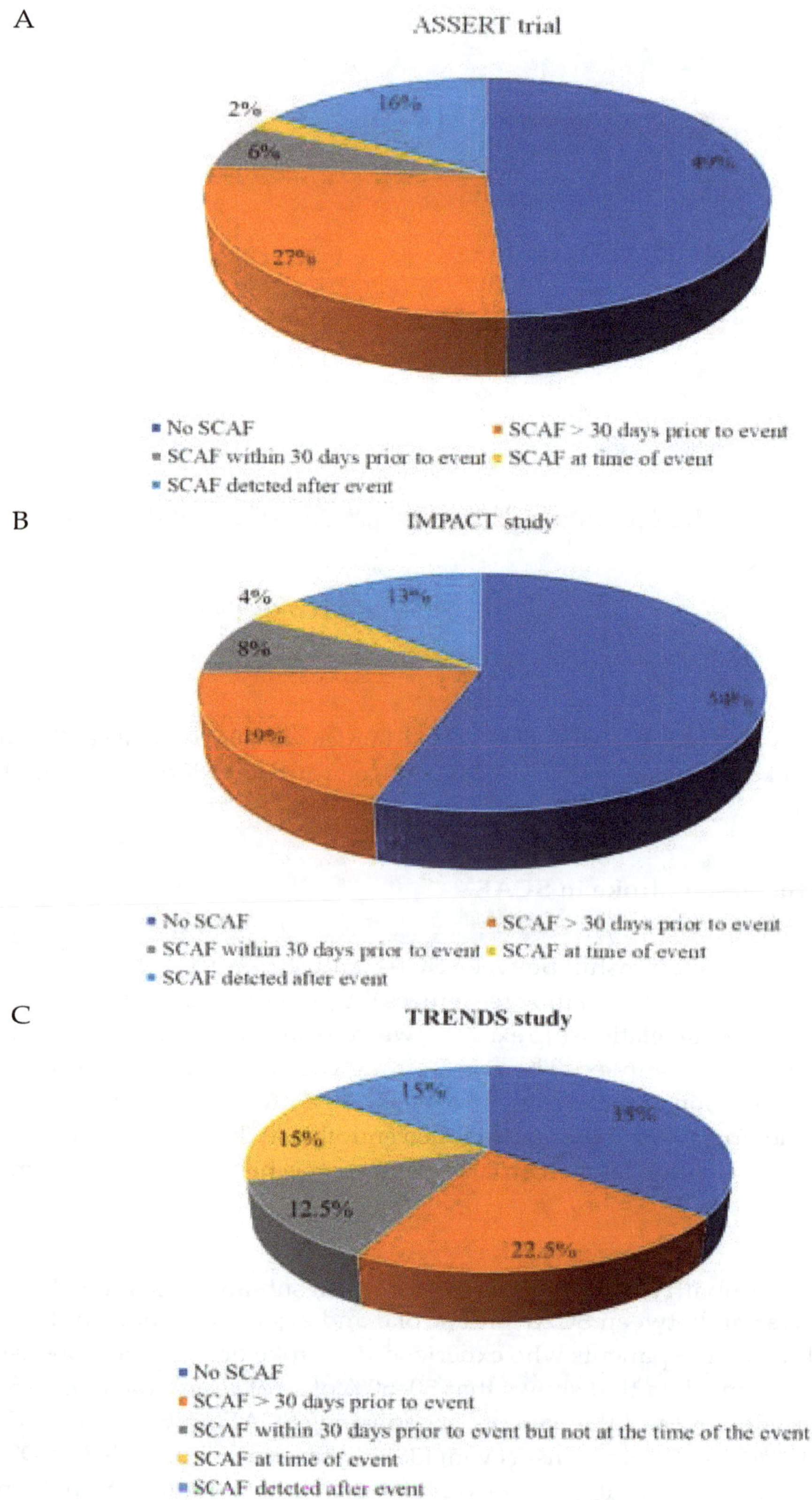

Figure 2. SCAF and stroke: A temporal relationship based on data from (**A**) ASSERT, (**B**) IMPACT and (**C**) TRENDS. All stroke or systemic embolism events are correlated with SCAF.

There are several important points to note from this data in the context of our current understanding of AF. For the majority of stroke or systemic embolism events, there was no temporal relationship with SCAF. When a temporal relationship existed, the duration of SCAF was almost always much shorter in duration than the 48 h commonly believed to be the minimum duration required for thrombus to form in the left atrial appendage; this is the time period considered safe for cardioversion [41]. Furthermore, those with SCAF who experienced stroke did not require progression to longer episodes in order to develop stroke or systemic embolism. Therefore, SCAF is likely an important risk marker for stroke and systemic embolism and if there is a direct causal relationship this is not as simple as a direct predictable relationship.

7. Treatment

The treatment of SCAF presents several challenges due to the issues raised above. There are several factors to keep in mind when considering the treatment of SCAF. In clinical AF, oral anticoagulation is recommended regardless of AF subtype and depending on the presence of clinical factors (age, hypertension, diabetes mellitus, heart failure and stroke) which have consistently been shown to increase stroke risk [42]. Given that oral anticoagulation has been shown to significantly decrease stroke risk in clinical AF, this risk reduction should theoretically translate to SCAF. However, in SCAF the increased risk is of a lower magnitude (2–2.5 times) compared to clinical AF (5 times) and this may reduce the net clinical benefit observed with anticoagulation in SCAF. Patients with SCAF >24 h have an absolute risk profile that is similar to that observed in clinical AF and are the subgroup of SCAF most likely to derive benefit from oral anticoagulation. This is consistent with current guidelines [42]. An algorithm for the management of SCAF is proposed in Figure 3.

The equipoise in whether patients with SCAF should receive oral anticoagulation can be observed in clinical practice. Healey et al. performed a retrospective analysis of all patients at a single academic hospital who had pacemakers capable of documenting AF [43]. In 445 patients studied, SCAF was found in 55% of patients who were more likely to be older, have history of clinical AF and a large left atrium. Anticoagulants were used more frequently among patients who also had clinical AF (58.9%) compared with those without (23.7%, $p < 0.001$) [43].

One strategy that was attempted is intermittent anticoagulation during episodes of SCAF with the premise that stroke risk is highest at that time-point while avoiding the risk of bleeding at other times. In the Multicenter Randomized Trial of Anticoagulation Guided by Remote Rhythm Monitoring in Patients with Implanted Cardioverter-Defibrillator and Resynchronization Devices (IMPACT) trial, 2718 patients with CIEDs were randomized to start and stop anticoagulation based on remote rhythm monitoring compared to usual office-based follow-up with anticoagulation determined by standard clinical criteria [44]. The primary endpoint was a composite of stroke, systemic embolism, and major bleeding. The trial was stopped early after a two-year median follow-up due to futility. Primary events (2.4 vs. 2.3 per 100 patient-years) were similar between the two groups (HR 1.06; 95% CI 0.75–1.51; $p = 0.732$) [44]. There are multiple issues that limit inferences from this trial. Firstly, it was performed in the era of warfarin which limits the ability to provide rapid intermittent anticoagulation and which increases the risk of bleeding. In addition, because major bleeding was used in the primary endpoint composite, this may have led to the neutral result (observed and early termination. In addition, the algorithm for home monitoring was complex with poor adherence. In the end, anticoagulation use was similar in both arms [44].

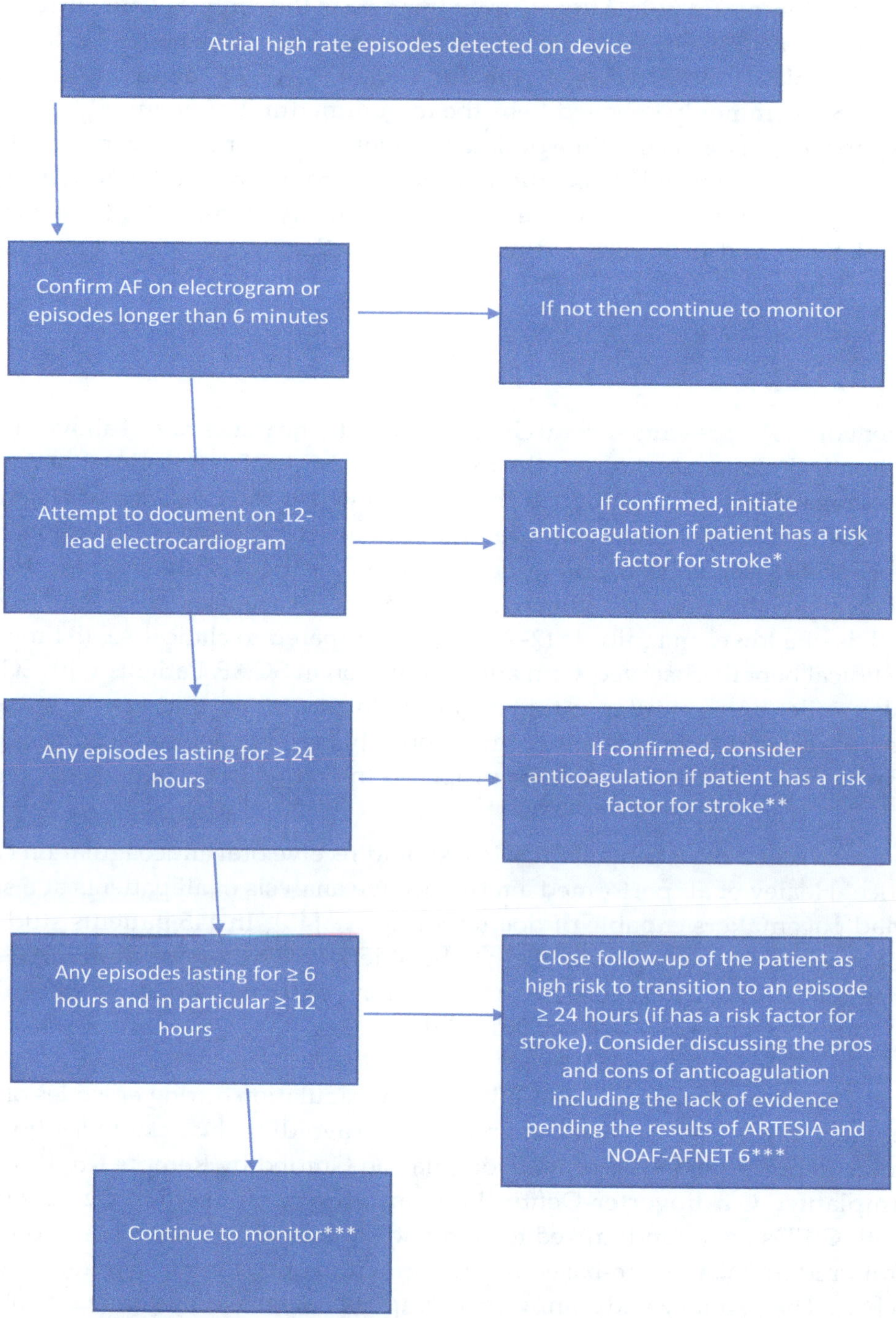

Figure 3. Suggested clinical algorithm for the management of SCAF. * Based on current atrial fibrillation guidelines [2,42]; ** based on current guidelines to consider anticoagulation when a device detected episode is for 24 h or longer [42]; *** data suggests that these patients are at high risk to transition to episodes lasting 24 h or longer [33]. *** Management for patients with an episode > 6 min is currently unclear and such patients may be eligible for enrolment in the ARTESIA and NOAH-AFNET 6 trials depending on the presence of other risk factors for stroke.

8. Future Directions

Current guidelines suggest that patients with AHRE (SCAF) greater than 24 h as well as at least one risk factor for stroke should receive oral anticoagulation [42]. In addition, the guidelines also suggest that patients with shorter durations of AHRE who are at high risk such as those with cryptogenic stroke should be considered for oral anticoagulation [42]. The gap in knowledge exists for patients who have episodes between 6 min and 24 h, particularly in patients with relatively longer episodes. Given the clinical equipoise in this population, two trials are currently underway to try and provide clarity: The Apixaban for the Reduction of Thrombo-Embolism in Patients With Device-Detected Sub-Clinical Atrial Fibrillation (ARTESIA) trial and the Non-vitamin K Antagonist Oral Anticoagulants in Patients With Atrial High Rate Episodes (NOAH-AFNET 6) trial [45,46].

ARTESIA is a prospective, multicenter, double-blind, randomized controlled trial, enrolling patients with SCAF detected by a CIED who have additional risk factors for stroke [46]. To be eligible, participants must have had at least one episode of SCAF ≥6 min in duration on device interrogation, be at least 55 years of age or older and have risk factors for stroke (the number of risk factors depends on the age with those 75 years of age or older not requiring any further risk factors) [46]. The trial will exclude patients with documented AF on a 12-lead electrocardiogram or those who have an indication for oral anticoagulant therapy. Participants will be randomized to apixaban or aspirin 81 mg daily and will receive placebo pills accordingly (aspirin and two placebo pills instead of apixaban or apixaban and placebo aspirin) [46]. The primary outcome is the composite of stroke, TIA (with magnetic resonance imaging evidence of a cerebral infarction on diffusion-weighting) and systemic embolism. The trial is aiming to recruit around 4000 patients from 230 international clinical sites. ARTESIA is expected to have 36 months of follow-up until 248 adjudicated primary outcome events have occurred [46].

NOAH-AFNET 6 is an investigator-driven, prospective, parallel-group, randomized, event-driven, double-blind, multicenter trial [45]. The trial will recruit patients with SCAF detected by a CIED with at least one risk factor for stroke. To be eligible, participants must have AHRE, be aged ≥ 65 years with at least one other stroke risk factor. Excluded will be patients with documented AF or an indication for oral anticoagulation. These broad inclusion/exclusion criteria were put in place to mimic clinical practice. NOAH-AFNET 6 will randomize 3400 patients to edoxaban or no anticoagulation (aspirin depending on clinical indications) in a superiority trial. The primary efficacy outcome is stroke or cardiovascular death and the primary safety outcome will be major bleeding. All patients will be followed until the 222 target primary outcomes are reached. Patients will be censored when they develop AF and offered open-label anticoagulation [45].

Further studies are needed to improve our understanding of SCAF, its clinical impact and the role of different therapies. A prospective study of well-matched patients with SCAF compared to clinical AF would provide insight into the true incidence of thromboembolic events in both groups. In addition, a greater understanding of the temporal relationship between SCAF and thromboembolic events is needed which would need a larger study. Does atrial AF burden or density significantly increase risk; and consequently, does the reduction of SCAF burden mitigate this risk? Studies in clinical AF suggest that this is unlikely to be the case. Finally, does anticoagulation therapy in patients with high SCAF burden/density, those who have significant progression of SCAF or patients with evidence of an underlying cardiomyopathy (enlarged left atrium or elevated natriuretic peptides) significantly reduce the risk of thromboembolic events?

There are several noteworthy limitations and unanswered questions regarding SCAF with current data. Not all stroke events in SCAF studies are embolic strokes and as shown above with the timing of stroke relative to the SCAF episode, SCAF may be a risk marker for stroke. Another important element to consider when discussing AF and SCAF burden is the large discrepancy between clinical and device detected categorization of the pattern of AF. Charitos and colleagues showed that while the majority of patients with AF are clinically classified as paroxysmal AF, this correlates poorly with the temporal persistence of AF based on continuous device monitoring [47]. The impact of this discrepancy on clinical practice remains unclear. Finally, the highly anticipated results of the two anticoagulation in SCAF trials should be released in 2022 with the large potential to change clinical practice.

9. Conclusions

Cardiac implantable electronic devices have led to the detection of SCAF which has clearly been shown to be associated with an increased risk of stroke. Based on current data, patients with episodes of

SCAF lasting for 24 h or greater and at least one risk factor for stroke should receive oral anticoagulation. Longer episodes of SCAF and progression to longer episodes also confer an increased risk of stroke. Trials are now underway to assess the efficacy and safety or oral anticoagulation in patients with SCAF lasting less than 24 h.

Author Contributions: A.A., M.M., R.P., V.R. and V.E. were involved in the conception of this manuscript. A.A. and M.M. drafted the manuscript. R.P., V.R. and V.E. helped draft and critically revised the manuscript.

References

1. Healey, J.S.; Connolly, S.J.; Gold, M.R.; Israel, C.W.; Van Gelder, I.C.; Capucci, A.; Lau, C.P.; Fain, E.; Yang, S.; Bailleul, C.; et al. Subclinical Atrial Fibrillation and the Risk of Stroke. *N. Engl. J. Med.* **2012**, *366*, 120–129. [CrossRef] [PubMed]
2. Kirchhof, P.; Benussi, S.; Kotecha, D.; Ahlsson, A.; Atar, D.; Casadei, B.; Castella, M.; Diener, H.-C.; Heidbuchel, H.; Hendriks, J.; et al. 2016 ESC Guidelines for the management of atrial fibrillation developed in collaboration with EACTS. *Eur. Heart J.* **2016**, *37*, 2893–2962. [CrossRef] [PubMed]
3. Nattel, S.; Guasch, E.; Savelieva, I.; Cosio, F.G.; Valverde, I.; Halperin, J.L.; Conroy, J.M.; Al-Khatib, S.M.; Hess, P.L.; Kirchhof, P.; et al. Early management of atrial fibrillation to prevent cardiovascular complications. *Eur. Heart J.* **2014**, *35*, 1448–1456. [CrossRef] [PubMed]
4. Lubitz, S.A.; Yin, X.; McManus, D.D.; Weng, L.-C.; Aparicio, H.J.; Walkey, A.J.; Romero, J.R.; Kase, C.S.; Ellinor, P.T.; Wolf, P.A.; et al. Stroke as the Initial Manifestation of Atrial Fibrillation. *Stroke* **2017**, *48*, 490–492. [CrossRef]
5. Mond, H.G.; Proclemer, A. The 11th world survey of cardiac pacing and implantable cardioverter-defibrillators: Calendar year 2009—A World Society of Arrhythmia's project. *Pacing Clin. Electrophysiol.* **2011**, *34*, 1013–1027. [CrossRef] [PubMed]
6. Birnie, D.; Williams, K.; Guo, A.; Mielniczuk, L.; Davis, D.; Lemery, R.; Green, M.; Gollob, M.; Tang, A. Reasons for Escalating Pacemaker Implants. *Am. J. Cardiol.* **2006**, *98*, 93–97. [CrossRef] [PubMed]
7. Saver, J.L. Cryptogenic Stroke. *N. Engl. J. Med.* **2016**, *374*, 2065–2074. [CrossRef] [PubMed]
8. Kishore, A.; Vail, A.; Majid, A.; Dawson, J.; Lees, K.R.; Tyrrell, P.J.; Smith, C.J. Detection of Atrial Fibrillation After Ischemic Stroke or Transient Ischemic Attack. *Stroke* **2014**, *45*, 520–526. [CrossRef]
9. Diener, H.-C.; Sacco, R.L.; Easton, J.D.; Granger, C.B.; Bernstein, R.A.; Uchiyama, S.; Kreuzer, J.; Cronin, L.; Cotton, D.; Grauer, C.; et al. Dabigatran for Prevention of Stroke after Embolic Stroke of Undetermined Source. *N. Engl. J. Med.* **2019**, *380*, 1906–1917. [CrossRef]
10. Hart, R.G.; Sharma, M.; Mundl, H.; Kasner, S.E.; Bangdiwala, S.I.; Berkowitz, S.D.; Swaminathan, B.; Lavados, P.; Wang, Y.; Wang, Y.; et al. Rivaroxaban for Stroke Prevention after Embolic Stroke of Undetermined Source. *N. Engl. J. Med.* **2018**, *378*, 2191–2201. [CrossRef]
11. Sanna, T.; Diener, H.-C.; Passman, R.S.; Di Lazzaro, V.; Bernstein, R.A.; Morillo, C.A.; Rymer, M.M.; Thijs, V.; Rogers, T.; Beckers, F.; et al. Cryptogenic Stroke and Underlying Atrial Fibrillation. *N. Engl. J. Med.* **2014**, *370*, 2478–2486. [CrossRef] [PubMed]
12. Gladstone, D.J.; Spring, M.; Dorian, P.; Panzov, V.; Thorpe, K.E.; Hall, J.; Vaid, H.; O'Donnell, M.; Laupacis, A.; Côté, R.; et al. Atrial Fibrillation in Patients with Cryptogenic Stroke. *N. Engl. J. Med.* **2014**, *370*, 2467–2477. [CrossRef] [PubMed]
13. Wein, T.; Lindsay, M.P.; Cote, R.; Foley, N.; Berlingieri, J.; Bhogal, S.; Bourgoin, A.; Buck, B.H.; Cox, J.; Davidson, D.; et al. Canadian stroke best practice recommendations: Secondary prevention of stroke, sixth edition practice guidelines, update 2017. *Int. J. Stroke* **2018**, *13*, 420–443. [CrossRef] [PubMed]
14. Hart, R.G.; Diener, H.C.; Coutts, S.B.; Easton, J.D.; Granger, C.B.; O'Donnell, M.J.; Sacco, R.L.; Connolly, S.J.; Cryptogenic Stroke, E.I.W.G. Embolic strokes of undetermined source: The case for a new clinical construct. *Lancet Neurol.* **2014**, *13*, 429–438. [CrossRef]
15. Glotzer, T.V.; Daoud, E.G.; Wyse, D.G.; Singer, D.E.; Ezekowitz, M.D.; Hilker, C.; Miller, C.; Qi, D.; Ziegler, P.D. The Relationship Between Daily Atrial Tachyarrhythmia Burden from Implantable Device Diagnostics and Stroke Risk. *Circ. Arrhythmia Electrophysiol.* **2009**, *2*, 474–480. [CrossRef]

16. Glotzer, T.V.; Hellkamp, A.S.; Zimmerman, J.; Sweeney, M.O.; Yee, R.; Marinchak, R.; Cook, J.; Paraschos, A.; Love, J.; Radoslovich, G.; et al. Atrial High Rate Episodes Detected by Pacemaker Diagnostics Predict Death and Stroke. *Circulation* **2003**, *107*, 1614–1619. [CrossRef]
17. Boriani, G.; Glotzer, T.V.; Santini, M.; West, T.M.; De Melis, M.; Sepsi, M.; Gasparini, M.; Lewalter, T.; Camm, J.A.; Singer, D.E. Device-detected atrial fibrillation and risk for stroke: An analysis of >10 000 patients from the SOS AF project (Stroke prevention Strategies based on Atrial Fibrillation information from implanted devices). *Eur. Heart J.* **2013**, *35*, 508–516. [CrossRef]
18. Capucci, A.; Santini, M.; Padeletti, L.; Gulizia, M.; Botto, G.; Boriani, G.; Ricci, R.; Favale, S.; Zolezzi, F.; Di Belardino, N.; et al. Monitored Atrial Fibrillation Duration Predicts Arterial Embolic Events in Patients Suffering from Bradycardia and Atrial Fibrillation Implanted with Antitachycardia Pacemakers. *J. Am. Coll. Cardiol.* **2005**, *46*, 1913–1920. [CrossRef]
19. Shanmugam, N.; Boerdlein, A.; Proff, J.; Ong, P.; Valencia, O.; Maier, S.K.G.; Bauer, W.R.; Paul, V.; Sack, S. Detection of atrial high-rate events by continuous Home Monitoring: Clinical significance in the heart failure–cardiac resynchronization therapy population. *Europace* **2011**, *14*, 230–237. [CrossRef]
20. Pollak, W.M.; Simmons, J.D.; Interian, A., Jr.; Atapattu, S.A.; Castellanos, A.; Myerburg, R.J.; Mitrani, R.D. Clinical utility of intraatrial pacemaker stored electrograms to diagnose atrial fibrillation and flutter. *Pacing Clin. Electrophysiol.* **2001**, *24*, 424–429. [CrossRef]
21. Healey, J.S.; Alings, M.; Ha, A.; Leong-Sit, P.; Birnie, D.H.; Graaf JJd Freericks, M.; Verma, A.; Wang, J.; Leong, D.; Dokainish, H.; et al. Subclinical Atrial Fibrillation in Older Patients. *Circulation* **2017**, *136*, 1276–1283. [CrossRef] [PubMed]
22. Healey, J.S.; Wong, J.A. Subclinical atrial fibrillation: The significance of progression to longer episodes. *Heart Rhythm* **2018**, *15*, 384–385. [CrossRef] [PubMed]
23. Reiffel, J.A.; Verma, A.; Kowey, P.R.; Halperin, J.L.; Gersh, B.J.; Wachter, R.; Pouliot, E.; Ziegler, P.D. Incidence of Previously Undiagnosed Atrial Fibrillation Using Insertable Cardiac Monitors in a High-Risk Population: The Reveal AF Study. *JAMA Cardiol.* **2017**, *2*, 1120–1127. [CrossRef] [PubMed]
24. Chen, L.Y.; Chung, M.K.; Allen, L.A.; Ezekowitz, M.; Furie, K.L.; McCabe, P.; Noseworthy, P.A.; Perez, M.V.; Turakhia, M.P. Atrial Fibrillation Burden: Moving Beyond Atrial Fibrillation as a Binary Entity: A Scientific Statement from the American Heart Association. *Circulation* **2018**, *137*, e623–e644. [CrossRef] [PubMed]
25. Mahajan, R.; Perera, T.; Elliott, A.D.; Twomey, D.J.; Kumar, S.; Munwar, D.A.; Khokhar, K.B.; Thiyagarajah, A.; Middeldorp, M.E.; Nalliah, C.J.; et al. Subclinical device-detected atrial fibrillation and stroke risk: A systematic review and meta-analysis. *Eur. Heart J.* **2018**, *39*, 1407–1415. [CrossRef] [PubMed]
26. Proietti, R.; Labos, C.; AlTurki, A.; Essebag, V.; Glotzer, T.V.; Verma, A. Asymptomatic atrial fibrillation burden and thromboembolic events: Piecing evidence together. *Expert Rev. Cardiovasc. Ther.* **2016**, *14*, 761–769. [CrossRef] [PubMed]
27. Van Gelder, I.C.; Healey, J.S.; Crijns, H.J.G.M.; Wang, J.; Hohnloser, S.H.; Gold, M.R.; Capucci, A.; Lau, C.-P.; Morillo, C.A.; Hobbelt, A.H.; et al. Duration of device-detected subclinical atrial fibrillation and occurrence of stroke in ASSERT. *Eur. Heart J.* **2017**, *38*, 1339–1344. [CrossRef]
28. Al-Khatib, S.M.; Thomas, L.; Wallentin, L.; Lopes, R.D.; Gersh, B.; Garcia, D.; Ezekowitz, J.; Alings, M.; Yang, H.; Alexander, J.H.; et al. Outcomes of apixaban vs. warfarin by type and duration of atrial fibrillation: Results from the ARISTOTLE trial. *Eur. Heart J.* **2013**, *34*, 2464–2471. [CrossRef]
29. Steinberg, B.A.; Hellkamp, A.S.; Lokhnygina, Y.; Patel, M.R.; Breithardt, G.; Hankey, G.J.; Becker, R.C.; Singer, D.E.; Halperin, J.L.; Hacke, W.; et al. Investigator. Higher risk of death and stroke in patients with persistent vs. paroxysmal atrial fibrillation: Results from the ROCKET-AF Trial. *Eur. Heart J.* **2015**, *36*, 288–296. [CrossRef]
30. De Vos, C.B.; Pisters, R.; Nieuwlaat, R.; Prins, M.H.; Tieleman, R.G.; Coelen, R.J.; van den Heijkant, A.C.; Allessie, M.A.; Crijns, H.J. Progression from paroxysmal to persistent atrial fibrillation clinical correlates and prognosis. *J. Am. Coll. Cardiol.* **2010**, *55*, 725–731. [CrossRef]
31. Barrett, T.W.; Self, W.H.; Wasserman, B.S.; McNaughton, C.D.; Darbar, D. Evaluating the HATCH score for predicting progression to sustained atrial fibrillation in ED patients with new atrial fibrillation. *Am. J. Emerg. Med.* **2013**, *31*, 792–797. [CrossRef] [PubMed]
32. Proietti, R.; Hadjis, A.; AlTurki, A.; Thanassoulis, G.; Roux, J.F.; Verma, A.; Healey, J.S.; Bernier, M.L.; Birnie, D.; Nattel, S.; et al. A Systematic Review on the Progression of Paroxysmal to Persistent Atrial Fibrillation: Shedding New Light on the Effects of Catheter Ablation. *JACC Clin. Electrophysiol.* **2015**, *1*, 105–115. [CrossRef]

33. Boriani, G.; Glotzer, T.V.; Ziegler, P.D.; De Melis, M.; di Mangoni, S.S.L.; Sepsi, M.; Landolina, M.; Lunati, M.; Lewalter, T.; Camm, A.J. Detection of new atrial fibrillation in patients with cardiac implanted electronic devices and factors associated with transition to higher device-detected atrial fibrillation burden. *Heart Rhythm* **2018**, *15*, 376–383. [CrossRef] [PubMed]
34. Wong, J.A.; Conen, D.; Van Gelder, I.C.; McIntyre, W.F.; Crijns, H.J.; Wang, J.; Gold, M.R.; Hohnloser, S.H.; Lau, C.P.; Capucci, A.; et al. Progression of Device-Detected Subclinical Atrial Fibrillation and the Risk of Heart Failure. *J. Am. Coll. Cardiol.* **2018**, *71*, 2603–2611. [CrossRef] [PubMed]
35. Glotzer, T.V. The Cacophony of Silent Atrial Fibrillation. *J. Am. Coll. Cardiol.* **2018**, *71*, 2612–2615. [CrossRef] [PubMed]
36. D'Souza, A.; Butcher, K.S.; Buck, B.H. The Multiple Causes of Stroke in Atrial Fibrillation: Thinking Broadly. *Can. J. Cardiol.* **2018**, *34*, 1503–1511. [CrossRef] [PubMed]
37. Kamel, H.; Okin, P.M.; Elkind, M.S.V.; Iadecola, C. Atrial Fibrillation and Mechanisms of Stroke: Time for a New Model. *Stroke* **2016**, *47*, 895–900. [CrossRef]
38. Brambatti, M.; Connolly, S.J.; Gold, M.R.; Morillo, C.A.; Capucci, A.; Muto, C.; Lau, C.P.; Gelder, I.C.V.; Hohnloser, S.H.; Carlson, M.; et al. Temporal Relationship Between Subclinical Atrial Fibrillation and Embolic Events. *Circulation* **2014**, *129*, 2094–2099. [CrossRef]
39. Daoud, E.G.; Glotzer, T.V.; Wyse, D.G.; Ezekowitz, M.D.; Hilker, C.; Koehler, J.; Ziegler, P.D. Temporal relationship of atrial tachyarrhythmias, cerebrovascular events, and systemic emboli based on stored device data: A subgroup analysis of TRENDS. *Heart Rhythm* **2011**, *8*, 1416–1423. [CrossRef]
40. Hirsh, B.J.; Copeland-Halperin, R.S.; Halperin, J.L. Fibrotic Atrial Cardiomyopathy Atrial, Fibrillation, and Thromboembolism: Mechanistic Links and Clinical Inferences. *J. Am. Coll. Cardiol.* **2015**, *65*, 2239–2251. [CrossRef]
41. Klein, A.L.; Grimm, R.A.; Murray, R.D.; Apperson-Hansen, C.; Asinger, R.W.; Black, I.W.; Davidoff, R.; Erbel, R.; Halperin, J.L.; Orsinelli, D.A.; et al. Use of Transesophageal Echocardiography to Guide Cardioversion in Patients with Atrial Fibrillation. *N. Engl. J. Med.* **2001**, *344*, 1411–1420. [CrossRef] [PubMed]
42. Macle, L.; Cairns, J.A.; Andrade, J.G.; Mitchell, L.B.; Nattel, S.; Verma, A.; Verma, A.; Macle, L.; Andrade, J.; Atzema, C.; et al. The 2014 Atrial Fibrillation Guidelines Companion: A Practical Approach to the Use of the Canadian Cardiovascular Society Guidelines. *Can. J. Cardiol.* **2015**, *31*, 1207–1218. [CrossRef] [PubMed]
43. Healey, J.S.; Martin, J.L.; Duncan, A.; Connolly, S.J.; Ha, A.H.; Morillo, C.A.; Nair, G.M.; Eikelboom, J.; Divakaramenon, S.; Dokainish, H. Pacemaker-Detected Atrial Fibrillation in Patients with Pacemakers: Prevalence, Predictors, and Current Use of Oral Anticoagulation. *Can. J. Cardiol.* **2013**, *29*, 224–228. [CrossRef] [PubMed]
44. Martin, D.T.; Bersohn, M.M.; Waldo, A.L.; Wathen, M.S.; Choucair, W.K.; Lip, G.Y.H.; Ip, J.; Holcomb, R.; Akar, J.G.; Halperin, J.L.; et al. Randomized trial of atrial arrhythmia monitoring to guide anticoagulation in patients with implanted defibrillator and cardiac resynchronization devices. *Eur. Heart J.* **2015**, *36*, 1660–1668. [CrossRef] [PubMed]
45. Kirchhof, P.; Blank, B.F.; Calvert, M.; Camm, A.J.; Chlouverakis, G.; Diener, H.-C.; Goette, A.; Huening, A.; Lip, G.Y.H.; Simantirakis, E.; et al. Probing oral anticoagulation in patients with atrial high rate episodes: Rationale and design of the Non-Vitamin K antagonist Oral anticoagulants in patients with Atrial High rate episodes (NOAH–AFNET 6) trial. *Am. Heart J.* **2017**, *190*, 12–18. [CrossRef] [PubMed]
46. Vinereanu, D.; Lopes, R.D.; Bahit, M.C.; Xavier, D.; Jiang, J.; Al-Khalidi, H.R.; He, W.; Xian, Y.; Ciobanu, A.O.; Kamath, D.Y. A multifaceted intervention to improve treatment with oral anticoagulants in atrial fibrillation (IMPACT-AF): an international, cluster-randomised trial. *The Lancet* **2017**, *390*, 1737–1746.8. [CrossRef]
47. Charitos, E.I.; Pürerfellner, H.; Glotzer, T.V.; Ziegler, P.D. Clinical Classifications of Atrial Fibrillation Poorly Reflect Its Temporal Persistence: Insights from 1195 Patients Continuously Monitored with Implantable Devices. *J. Am. Coll. Cardiol.* **2014**, *63*, 2840–2848. [CrossRef] [PubMed]

Permissions

All chapters in this book were first published by MDPI; hereby published with permission under the Creative Commons Attribution License or equivalent. Every chapter published in this book has been scrutinized by our experts. Their significance has been extensively debated. The topics covered herein carry significant findings which will fuel the growth of the discipline. They may even be implemented as practical applications or may be referred to as a beginning point for another development.

The contributors of this book come from diverse backgrounds, making this book a truly international effort. This book will bring forth new frontiers with its revolutionizing research information and detailed analysis of the nascent developments around the world.

We would like to thank all the contributing authors for lending their expertise to make the book truly unique. They have played a crucial role in the development of this book. Without their invaluable contributions this book wouldn't have been possible. They have made vital efforts to compile up to date information on the varied aspects of this subject to make this book a valuable addition to the collection of many professionals and students.

This book was conceptualized with the vision of imparting up-to-date information and advanced data in this field. To ensure the same, a matchless editorial board was set up. Every individual on the board went through rigorous rounds of assessment to prove their worth. After which they invested a large part of their time researching and compiling the most relevant data for our readers.

The editorial board has been involved in producing this book since its inception. They have spent rigorous hours researching and exploring the diverse topics which have resulted in the successful publishing of this book. They have passed on their knowledge of decades through this book. To expedite this challenging task, the publisher supported the team at every step. A small team of assistant editors was also appointed to further simplify the editing procedure and attain best results for the readers.

Apart from the editorial board, the designing team has also invested a significant amount of their time in understanding the subject and creating the most relevant covers. They scrutinized every image to scout for the most suitable representation of the subject and create an appropriate cover for the book.

The publishing team has been an ardent support to the editorial, designing and production team. Their endless efforts to recruit the best for this project, has resulted in the accomplishment of this book. They are a veteran in the field of academics and their pool of knowledge is as vast as their experience in printing. Their expertise and guidance has proved useful at every step. Their uncompromising quality standards have made this book an exceptional effort. Their encouragement from time to time has been an inspiration for everyone.

The publisher and the editorial board hope that this book will prove to be a valuable piece of knowledge for researchers, students, practitioners and scholars across the globe.

List of Contributors

Minho Han, Young Dae Kim, Jin Kyo Choi, Ji Hoe Heo and Hyo Suk Nam
Department of Neurology, Yonsei University College of Medicine, Seoul 03722, Korea

Joonsang Yoo
Department of Neurology, Keimyung University School of Medicine, Daegu 42601, Korea

Hyungjong Park
Department of Neurology, Yonsei University College of Medicine, Seoul 03722, Korea
Department of Neurology, Keimyung University School of Medicine, Daegu 42601, Korea

Hye Sun Lee
Biostatistics Collaboration Unit, Yonsei University College of Medicine, university, Seoul 03722, Korea

Jan C. Purrucker, Kyra Hölscher and Peter A. Ringleb
Department of Neurology, Heidelberg University Hospital, 69120 Heidelberg, Germany

Jennifer Kollmer
Department of Neuroradiology, Heidelberg University Hospital, 69120 Heidelberg, Germany

Doralisa Morrone
Division of Cardiology, Department of Surgical, Medical and Molecular Pathology and Critical Care Medicine, University of Pisa, 50124 Pisa, Italy

Sonja Kroep and Ling-Hsiang Chuang
Pharmerit—An OPEN Health Company, 3068 AV Rotterdam, The Netherlands

Fabrizio Ricci
Institute of Cardiology and Center of Excellence on Aging, G. d'Annunzio University, 66100 Chieti-Pescara Fondazione VillaSerena per la Ricerca, Città Sant'Angelo, 65013 Pescara, Italy

Raffaele De Caterina
Division of Cardiology, Department of Surgical, Medical and Molecular Pathology and Critical Care Medicine, University of Pisa, 50124 Pisa, Italy
Fondazione VillaSerena per la Ricerca, Città Sant'Angelo, 65013 Pescara, Italy

Christian Arndt
Department of Anaesthesiology, University Hospital Marburg, 35033 Marburg, Germany

Giulia Renda
Institute of Cardiology and Center of Excellence on Aging, G. d'Annunzio University, 66100 Chieti-Pescara, Italy

Giuseppe Patti
Department of Thoracic and Cardiovascular Diseases, University of Eastern Piedmont, 28100 Novara, Italy

Paulus Kirchhof
University of Birmingham Institute of Cardiovascular Sciences, University of Birmingham, UHB and SWBH NHS Trusts, Birmingham B15 2TT, UK
Heart and Vascular Center, Hamburg University, 20251 Hamburg, Germany

Ben van Hout
Pharmerit—An OPEN Health Company, 3068 AV Rotterdam, The Netherlands
School of Health and Related Research (ScHARR), The University of Sheffeld, Sheffeld S10 2TN, UK

Daniela Vasileva and Yavor Rangelov
Department of Internal Diseases "Prof. St. Kirkovich", Medical University of Sofia, Sofia 1431, Bulgaria

Nadya Naydenova
Clinic of Cardiology, UMHAT "St. Ekaterina", Medical University of Sofia, Sofia 1431, Bulgaria

Gediminas Urbonas, Leonas Valius, Kęstutis Petniūnas and Inesa Petniūnienė
Department of Family medicine, Medical Academy, Lithuanian University of Health Sciences, LT-50161 Kaunas, Lithuania

Gintarė Šakalytė
Department of Cardiology, Medical Academy, Lithuanian University of Health Sciences, LT-50161 Kaunas, Lithuania

Giuseppe Coppola, Girolamo Manno, Antonino Mignano, Mirko Luparelli, Antonino Zarcone, Giuseppina Novo and Egle Corrado
Division of Cardiology, University Hospital "P. Giaccone", University of Palermo, Via del Vespro 129, p.c. 90127 Palermo, Italy

Antonino Salvatore Rubino
Department of Translational Medical Sciences, University of Campania "Luigi Vanvitelli", 80131 Naples, Italy

Iwona Gorący, Mariusz Kaczmarczyk, Andrzej Ciechanowicz, Klaudyna Lewandowska and Paweł Jakubiszyn
Department of Clinical and Molecular Biochemistry, Pomeranian Medical University, 70-111 Szczecin, Poland

Oksana Bodnar
Department of General and Dental Radiology, Pomeranian Medical University, 70-111 Szczecin, Poland

Bartosz Kopijek and Andrzej Brodkiewicz
Department of Pediatrics, Child Nephrology, Dialysotherapy and Management of Acute Poisoning, Pomeranian Medical University, 71-899 Szczecin, Poland

Lech Cyryłowski
Department of Intervention Radiology, Pomeranian Medical University, 70-111 Szczecin, Poland

Enrico Melillo, Giuseppe Palmiero, Vittorio Monda and Luigi Ascione
Department of Cardiology, AO dei Colli, Monaldi Hospital, 80131 Naples, Italy

Adele Ferro
Institute of Biostructure and Bioimaging, National Council Research, 80131 Naples, Italy

Paola Elvira Mocavero
Anesthesiology and Intensive Care Unit, AO dei Colli, Monaldi Hospital, 80131 Naples, Italy

Ahmed AlTurki and Jakub B. Maj
Division of Cardiology, McGill University Health Center, Montreal, QC H3G1A4, Canada

Mariam Marafi
Department of Neurology and Neurosurgery, Montreal Neurological Institute, Montreal, QC H3A2B4, Canada

Filippo Donato, Giovanni Vescovo and Riccardo Proietti
Department of Cardiac, Thoracic, and Vascular Sciences, University of Padua, 35121 Padua, Italy

Vincenzo Russo
Department of Medical Translational Sciences, University of Campania "Luigi Vanvitelli"-Monaldi Hospital, 80131 Naples, Italy

Fabio Angeli and Giuseppe Ambrosio
Division of Cardiology and Cardiovascular Pathophysiology, Hospital S. Maria della Misericordia, 06156 Perugia, Italy

Gianpaolo Reboldi and Monica Trapasso
Department of Medicine, University of Perugia, 06156 Perugia, Italy

Adolfo Aita and Paolo Verdecchia
Fondazione Umbra Cuore e Ipertensione-ONLUS and Division of Cardiology, Hospital S. Maria Della Misericordia, 06156 Perugia, Italy

Alfredo Caturano, Raffaele Galiero and Pia Clara Pafundi
Department of Advanced Medical and Surgical Sciences, University of Campania "Luigi Vanvitelli", Piazza Luigi Miraglia 2, IT-80138 Naples, Italy

Francesca Pescini
Stroke Unit, Careggi University Hospital, 50134 Florence, Italy

Giovanni Pracucci, Carmen Barbato, Francesco Galmozzi, Anna Melone and Damiano Mistri
NEUROFARBA Department, Neuroscience Section, University of Florence, 50134 Florence, Italy

Cristina Sarti
Stroke Unit, Careggi University Hospital, 50134 Florence, Italy
NEUROFARBA Department, Neuroscience Section, University of Florence, 50134 Florence, Italy

Anna Poggesi, Valentina Rinnoci and Emilia Salvadori
Stroke Unit, Careggi University Hospital, 50134 Florence, Italy
NEUROFARBA Department, Neuroscience Section, University of Florence, 50134 Florence, Italy
IRCCS Don Carlo Gnocchi, 50143 Florence, Italy

Eleonora Camilleri, Silvia Galora, Betti Giusti, Anna Maria Gori and Rossella Marcucci
Department of Experimental and Clinical Medicine, University of Florence, 50134 Florence, Italy

Francesca Cesari
Central Laboratory, Careggi University Hospital, 50134 Florence, Italy

Stefano Chiti
Department Health Professions, U.O.c Research and Development, 50134 Careggi University Hospital, 50134 Florence, Italy

Stefano Diciotti and Chiara Marzi
Department of Electrical, Electronic, and Information Engineering "Guglielmo Marconi", University of Bologna, 40136 Bologna, Italy

Enrico Fainardi
Neuroradiology Unit, Department of Experimental and Clinical Biomedical Sciences, University of Florence, Careggi University Hospital, 50134 Florence, Italy

Davide Castagno, Mara Morello and Simone Frea
Division of Cardiology, "Città della Salute e della Scienza di Torino" Hospital, Department of Medical Sciences, University of Turin, 10124 Torino, Italy

Chiara Rovera
Cardiology Unit, "Ospedale Civico", Chivasso, 10034 Torino, Italy

Giovanni Marchetto and Mauro Rinaldi
Division of Cardiac Surgery, "Città della Salute e della Scienza di Torino" Hospital, University of Turin, 10124 Torino, Italy

Elena-Daniela Grigorescu
Diabetes, Nutrition and Metabolic Diseases, "Grigore T. Popa" University of Medicine and Pharmacy, 700115 Iaşi, Romania

Cristina-Mihaela Lăcătuşu, Alina Onofriescu and Bogdan-Mircea Mihai
Diabetes, Nutrition and Metabolic Diseases, "Grigore T. Popa" University of Medicine and Pharmacy, 700115 Iaşi, Romania
"Sf. Spiridon" Emergency Hospital, 700111 Iaşi, Romania

Cristian Stătescu and Radu Andy Sascău
Internal Medicine, "Grigore T. Popa" University of Medicine and Pharmacy, 700115 Iaşi, Romania
"George I.M. Georgescu" Cardiovascular Diseases Institute, Cardiology Department, 700503 Iaşi, Romania

Benjamin Voellger, Rosita Rupa, Barbara Carl and Christopher Nimsky
Department of Neurosurgery, University Hospital Marburg, 35033 Marburg, Germany

Andrea Ballatore, Andrea Saglietto, Paolo Desalvo, Pier Paolo Bocchino and Gaetano Maria De Ferrari
Division of Cardiology, "Città della Salute e della Scienza di Torino" Hospital, Department of Medical Sciences, University of Turin, 10126 Turin, Italy

Fiorenzo Gaita
Cardiology Department, Clinica Pinna Pintor, 10129 Torino, Italy

Matteo Anselmino
Division of Cardiology, "Città della Salute e della Scienza di Torino" Hospital, Department of Medical Sciences, University of Turin, 10126 Turin, Italy
Division of Cardiology, "Città della Salute e della Scienza di Torino" Hospital, Department of Medical Sciences, University of Turin, 10124 Torino, Italy

Mario Matta
Division of Cardiology, Electrophysiology Lab, Sant'Andrea Hospital, 13100 Vercelli, Italy

Francesco De Sensi, Gennaro Miracapillo, Luigi Addonisio, Marco Breschi, Alberto Cresti, Pasquale Baratta and Ugo Limbruno
Cardiology Department, Misericordia Hospital, 58100 Grosseto, Italy

Francesco Paneni
Center for Molecular Cardiology, University Hospital, 8057 Zürich, Switzerland

Nikolay Runev, Stefan Naydenov and Emil Manov
Department of Internal Diseases, Medical University of Sofia, 1431 Sofia, Bulgaria
Department of Internal Diseases "Prof. St. Kirkovich", Medical University of Sofia, Sofia 1431, Bulgaria

Tatjana Potpara
Faculty of Medicine, University of Belgrade, 11000 Belgrade, Serbia

Anita Vladimirova and Gergana Georgieva
Boehringer Ingelheim RCV GmbH & Co KG Bulgarian Branch, 1505 Sofia, Bulgaria

Vidal Essebag
Division of Cardiology, McGill University Health Center, Montreal, QC H3G1A4, Canada
Hôspital Sacré-Coeur de Montréal, Montreal, QC H4J1C5, Canada

Index

www.ingramcontent.com/pod-product-compliance
Lightning Source LLC
LaVergne TN
LVHW060544210926
848485LV00005B/1256